A MOTHER'S MANUAL FOR
THE WOMEN OF FERRARA

The Other Voice in Early Modern Europe:
The Toronto Series, 89

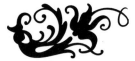

MICHELE SAVONAROLA

A Mother's Manual for the Women of Ferrara:
A Fifteenth-Century Guide to Pregnancy and Pediatrics

~

Edited, with introduction and notes, by
GABRIELLA ZUCCOLIN

Translated by
MARTIN MARAFIOTI

Iter Press
NEW YORK | TORONTO

2022

978-1-64959-030-5 (paper)
978-1-64959-031-2 (pdf)
978-1-64959-032-9 (epub)

Library of Congress Cataloging-in-Publication Data

Names: Savonarola, Michele, 1385?-1466?, author. | Zuccolin, Gabriella, editor.
Title: A mother's manual for the women of Ferrara : a fifteenth-century guide to pregnancy and
    pediatrics / Michele Savonarola ; edited, with introduction and notes, by Gabriella Zuccolin ;
    translated by Martin Marafioti.
Description: New York : Iter Press, 2022. | Series: The other voice in early modern Europe. The Toronto
    series ; 89 | Includes bibliographical references and index. | Summary: "English translation of
    the fifteenth-century obstetrical and pediatric treatise written in the Italian vernacular for the
    women of Ferrara by the learned court physician Michele Savonarola, grandfather of Girolamo
    Savonarola, religious reformer and Florentine leader"-- Provided by publisher.
Identifiers: LCCN 2022004057 (print) | LCCN 2022004058 (ebook) | ISBN 9781649590305
    (paperback) | ISBN 9781649590312 (pdf) | ISBN 9781649590329 (epub)
Subjects: LCSH: Savonarola, Michele, 1385?-1466? | Obstetrics--Italy--Ferrara--History--15th
    century. | Pediatrics--Italy--Ferrara--History--15th century. | Pregnancy--Italy--Ferrara--History-
    -15th century.
Classification: LCC RG67.I8 S28 2022 (print) | LCC RG67.I8 (ebook) | DDC 618.2009454/51--dc23/
    eng/20220224
LC record available at https://lccn.loc.gov/2022004057
LC ebook record available at https://lccn.loc.gov/2022004058

Cover Illustration

Genève, Bibliothèque de Genève, Ms. fr. 76 – Quintus Curtius Rufus, *Faits et gestes d'Alexandre* / f. 18r
(dated around 1475).

Cover Design

Maureen Morin, Library Communications, University of Toronto Libraries.

To our mothers and Lorenzo

Contents

Acknowledgments

I owe a huge debt of thanks to everyone who offered their support in the realization of this volume. Many thanks to the thoughtful and extraordinary editors of The Other Voice in Early Modern Europe – The Toronto Series, Margaret L. King and the late Albert Rabil Jr., for encouraging this project, and for accepting the volume in the series. I am especially grateful to Martin Marafioti, for involving me in the incredible adventure of the English edition of Savonarola's *Mother's Manual.* Martin deserves special thanks also for the chivalrous patience with which he waited for me to complete my part of the work, whose gestation took much more than nine months. Special thanks to Monica H. Green, whose magisterial studies on women's medicine provided crucial help in tackling the Introduction to the volume.

There are countless others who deserve thanks, among whom are the volume's peer reviewers, for their helpful feedback, and the staff at Iter Press. Special thanks to Chiara Crisciani, for introducing me to Savonarola's works many years ago, when I was still a student at the University of Pavia. I am grateful to Helen King, Lauren Kassell, and Mary Fissell, for their help and encouragement in seeing this book to the end during my Cambridge years, when everything still seemed very foggy and far away. A Wellcome fellowship at the University of Cambridge allowed me both to begin this project and to broaden my engagement with women's medicine in the Middle Ages, as did a fellowship at Villa I Tatti, the Harvard University Center for Italian Renaissance Studies in Florence. Funds provided by the University of Pavia supported the last phases of the work. I would also like to thank Carla Casagrande for her continuous encouragement. Thanks to Outi Merisalo and Iolanda Ventura, for their support in resolving some source-related doubts, and to Francesca Dantini, the wonderfully kind librarian of the Biblioteca Panizzi in Reggio Emilia, for her continued availability.

Many thanks to my family and children too, especially to Pasquale, for their support, good humor as well as the countless gorgeous meals as I wrote and checked over the footnotes of this work.

GZ

My deepest thanks to the Editors of the "Other Voice in Early Modern Europe" series, Margaret L. King and the late Albert Rabil Jr. for their enthusiasm and stewardship of this project. I am grateful to the National Endowment for the Humanities for their generous support in the form of a Scholarly Editions and Translations Grant. Thank you to the Dyson College of Arts and Sciences at Pace University for support in the form of Summer Research Grants and a sabbatical leave. I am especially grateful to Dean Nira Herrmann, and my department chairs Antonia Garcia-Rodriguez, Iride Lamartina-Lens, and Susan Berardini for their faith in me and in this project.

My sincere gratitude to the kind and helpful staffs at libraries, special collections, and archives I have consulted for this project especially the Special Collections Archives and Manuscripts Collection at the Wellcome Library; the Library of the Warburg Institute; the Institute of the History of Medicine at the Welch Medical Library of the Johns Hopkins University.

I am indebted to to one of the pioneers in the field of the history of women's medicine, Monica H. Green for her encouragement, guidance, and collaboration. Thank you, Monica for your assistance with Savonarola's Latin and the "medicalese" in the text.

To Guido Giglioni and Roberto Poma: *grazie infinite* for helping me to unpack the medical and philosophical contexts in Savonarola's words. For their guidance, multiple readings, and valuable feedback on this translation, I thank Roberta Ricci and Heather Dubnick. How do I show my appreciation to Valeria Finucci? Valeria, without your support and guidance, this project would not have been possible. Thank you, dear mentor and friend.

My heartfelt gratitude to my colleague and collaborator in this project, Gabriella Zuccolin. Your inexhaustive generosity of time and your erudition made the publication of this translation possible.

For their unwavering support and patience, I thank my husband Philip Clemmey and our nephew Gedeon Weinberg.

MM

Illustrations

Introduction

The Other Voice

Around 1460, the Italian physician Michele Savonarola—paternal grandfather of the religious reformer Girolamo Savonarola, and paragon of the learned court physician encountered in this era of European history—composed a vernacular work on pregnancy, obstetrics, and pediatrics, addressed to the women and midwives of Ferrara. The work bore the Latin title *De regimine praegnantium et noviter natorum usque ad septennium*—literally, *Regimen for Pregnant Women and Newborns up to the Seventh Year*—and is translated here as *A Mother's Manual for the Women of Ferrara*.[1] He writes in a male voice, but has made two unconventional choices: to write in the vernacular, not the Latin of learned professionals, and to address the treatise explicitly to the women actively concerned with childbirth: the mothers and midwives of Ferrara.

Having taken this bold step, Savonarola set about seeking ways of protecting his choice from criticism. It is the first time since late antiquity that a treatise on obstetrics and generation is addressed to midwives. It is the first time, within the Latin West, that such a monographic work, despite its Latin title, is written directly in the vernacular.[2] The brief introduction in which the author

---

1. The work was first edited in 1952 as *Il trattato ginecologico-pediatrico in volgare "Ad mulieres ferrarienses de regimine pregnantium" di Michele Savonarola*, ed. Luigi Belloni (Milan: Stucchi, 1952). See the Bibliography, *Works by Michele Savonarola*, #13, for manuscripts and relevant studies. The translated text will be cited henceforth as *MM*. Where the original Italian work is discussed, it will be cited as *DRP*.

2. Vernacular translations of originally Latin works on women's medicine already circulated throughout medieval Europe, especially those connected with the Trotula texts at Salerno, masterfully studied by Monica H. Green especially in her edition and translation *The Trotula: A Medieval Compendium of Women's Medicine* (Philadelphia: University of Pennsylvania Press, 2001). The few vernacular *regimina* (the plural, in Latin, of "regimen") that included gynecological and pediatric topics written prior to the fifteenth century are too schematic and general to set a precedent when compared to Savonarola's *MM*. Examples are the brief instructions in the three chapters devoted to the delivery and care of newborn babies in the *Régime du corps* by Aldobrandino of Siena (written for Beatrice of Savoy in 1256, and translated from French into Florentine dialect in 1310), or the equally generic guidelines provided by Francesco da Barberino in the fourteenth-century *Reggimento e costumi di donna*; for these, see respectively Aldobrandino da Siena, *Le régime du corps de Maître Aldebrandin de Sienne: Texte français du 13e siecle*, ed. Louis Landouzy and Roger Pépin (Paris: Honoré Champion, 1911), and Francesco da Barberino, *Un galateo femminile italiano del Trecento: Il "Reggimento e costumi di donna,"* ed. Giovanni Battista Festa (Bari: Laterza, 1910). Regarding the Trotula ensemble of texts and their vernacular translations, in addition to Green's edition of *The Trotula*, see especially the bibliography in Green, *Making Women's Medicine Masculine: The Rise of Male Authority in Pre-Modern Gynaecology* (Oxford:

comments on his wish to dedicate his work to women and his choice of writing in the vernacular is a small rhetorical masterpiece, brimming with justifications and appeals to the reader, delivered in a markedly pedagogical-moral tone. What has moved Savonarola to choose the vernacular is his feeling of gratitude towards his "Ferrarese daughters," his desire to be a good father to them, and, as a good Christian, his respect for the sanctity of human life. His concern to correct what he sees as the ignorance of midwives is also central to his purpose, although Savonarola does not berate them for this failing as much as will the authors of later midwifery handbooks.[3] Rather, his fatherly desire to save future mothers and their unborn children from the awful destiny of death underlies his brave linguistic choice. By writing in the vernacular, Savonarola waives any rights to the fame, honor, and glory that a Latin version of this work might have procured him, in order to ensure that "through my book you will become both physical and spiritual healers for your children."[4]

Oxford University Press, 2008). See also Elizabeth Dearnley, "'Women of oure tunge cunne bettir reede and vnderstonde this langage': Women and Vernacular Translation in Later Medieval England," in *Multilingualism in Medieval Britain, c. 1066–1520: Sources and Analysis*, ed. by Judith A. Jefferson and Ad Putter (Turnhout: Brepols, 2013), 259–72; and Orlanda S. H. Lie, "What Every Midwife Needs to Know: The Trotula," in *Women's Writing from the Low Countries, 1200–1875: A Bilingual Anthology*, ed. Lia van Gemert et al. (Amsterdam: Amsterdam University Press, 2010), 138–43. For a comparison with the French context, albeit during a later period, see Valerie Worth-Stylianou, *Pregnancy and Birth in Early Modern France: Treatises by Caring Physicians and Surgeons, 1581–1625: François Rousset, Jean Liebault, Jacques Guillemeau, Jacques Duval, and Louis de Serres* (Toronto: Iter Press and Centre for Reformation and Renaissance Studies, 2013); and Worth-Stylianou, *Les traités d'obstétrique en langue française au seuil de la modernité: Bibliographie critique des "Divers travaulx" d'Euchaire Rösslin (1536) à l'"Apologie de Louyse Bourgeois sage femme" (1627)* (Geneva: Droz, 2007).

3. See *MM*, 150: "I will now offer clear instruction for all women who are midwives and assistants, so that they may learn the rules that must be observed in the parturition of the fetus; for surely, due to the ignorance of these midwives, many children and their mothers either die or endure hardship." According to Monica H. Green, the *Rosegarden for Pregnant Women and Midwives* (1513) by the German physician Eucharius Rösslin "solidified the rhetoric of midwives' ignorance that the Dominican preacher Thomas of Cantimpré had first introduced three hundred years earlier," and it is only in the fifteenth and especially the sixteenth century that midwives move from being seen as sometimes incompetent to being dangerous and ignorant. Green, *Making Women's Medicine Masculine*, 306.

4. *MM*, 59.

Notwithstanding the probable illiteracy of fifteenth-century midwives,[5] and the fact that the text suggests a primarily male readership,[6] Savonarola's *Mother's Manual* at least helped create an expectation that midwives and women in general would be able to access this new obstetrical literature. It presents, in fact, the image of a "female textual community," and an authoritative social voice; sometimes the author's own male voice seeks to disrupt this imagined community, while at other times it seems to participate in or enable it.[7] There is no evidence that Savonarola fears competition with midwives or barber-surgeons, as might perhaps have been expected.[8] The academic and court physician plainly asserts

5. It should be clarified from the start that the midwives, nurses and, in general, the women of Ferrara whom Savonarola is addressing in the *Mother's Manual* could not possibly have read the text. The fabric of the treatise was composed using complex arguments and rhetoric, and it is highly improbable that "all women who are midwives and assistants" (*tute le donne obstetrice et astante*) could make any direct use of it; *MM*, 150. Women were generally illiterate into the nineteenth century, exceptions being noblewomen belonging to court circles or monasteries, who were by now able to read and write, as well as some few midwives from the sixteenth century onwards. The rhetorical and literary sophistication of the dedication leaves no doubt that the work was intended for male readers, not only due to the abundance of quotations and erudite allusions—whether of a medical, biblical or literary nature—and the digressions on morality, but precisely because this idealized dedication is a stylistic artifice which draws on distinguished precedents. Aristotle, for instance, dedicated part of chapter VII of *De historia animalium* to the *maia* (midwife, in Greek), and the ancient Greek physician Soranus wrote his *Gynaecia* (Gynecology. Latinized Greek title literally meaning *Women's things*, nature and diseases, not restricted to gynecology in the modern sense) for women; but by the fifteenth century, the awareness that midwifery was once a literate profession had been completely lost. On female "medical literacy," see Monica H. Green, "The Possibilities of Literacy and the Limits of Reading: Women and the Gendering of Medical Literacy," in *Women's Healthcare in the Medieval West: Texts and Contexts*, ed. Green (Aldershot, UK; Burlington, VT: Ashgate, 2000), 1–76. As for northern Italy in the fifteenth century, my examination of a large number of manuscript epistles preserved at Milan's State Archive has not allowed me to prove that Fraxina, the midwife active from at least 1493 to 1497, who served the most important noblewomen of the time and their households, was able to read. See Gabriella Zuccolin, "Gravidanza e parto nel Quattrocento: Le morti parallele di Beatrice d'Este e Anna Sforza," *Quaderni di artes* 2 (2008): 111–45.

6. The anticipated vernacular readership of the *MM* is in fact not exclusively male or female, but it envisages a spectrum from the *litteratus*, proficient in Latin, down to the midwife; the intended audience of the work includes nobles and middle-class laymen on the one hand, and practical physicians working as professionals along with less qualified figures, such as surgeons and empirics, on the other. On the developing interest in matters of generation by experts and laypersons throughout Europe in the thirteenth through fifteenth centuries, see the section in this Introduction on "Gynecology and Midwifery in the Middle Ages," at 15–20.

7. On the concept of textual communities within the specific field of "women's medicine," see Jennifer W. Hellwarth, "'I wyl wright of women prevy sekenes': Imagining Female Literacy and Textual Communities in Medieval and Early Modern Midwifery Manuals," *Critical Survey* 14.1 (2002): 44–63.

8. So established were the hierarchies of both medical learning and gender in fifteenth-century northern Italy that Savonarola's posture of superiority in dealing with these two categories of medical practitioners is unsurprising.

his dominance over the dangerous realm of the midwife: she is taught to call a university-trained doctor into the birthing room at the slightest sign of a complicated birth, and a surgeon for the thankless task of trying to save the mother by cutting the dead fetus into pieces. Savonarola may have had some "hands-on" knowledge of women's bodies and practical experience of birth, although his knowledge remains largely theoretical, as was the case for most fifteenth-century university-trained physicians. What is certain is that this physician had full authority in diagnosing and prescribing treatments for women's gynecological and obstetrical conditions. But since he acted vicariously in the vast majority of cases, not entering the birthing room, Savonarola probably felt—much earlier than other medical practitioners—that educating midwives had become a pressing social need in the setting of fifteenth-century Ferrara, ruled by the house of Este. This is why, as Riccardo Gualdo counsels, when reading Savonarola's text, we should always bear in mind the "presence of a double filter": an "operative" one, between physician→midwife→woman in labor; but also a "linguistic" one: between physician→male head of household→midwife→woman in labor.[9]

In many ways, the *Mother's Manual* cuts across the gender and linguistic divide between the medically-trained male professional and the traditionally unlearned female practitioner, giving a distinct voice to two newly visible categories of women at one time: the midwife and the birthing mother. Through engaging fictional dialogues (perhaps testimonies of real issues raised by women in the physician's daily routine),[10] Savonarola makes both of these figures supporting yet important actors in his own drama, one in which the so-called "masculine birth of gynaecology,"[11] but also the rise of a new literary genre, the obstetrical treatise addressed to women and midwives, had a role. While these (imagined?) female textual communities are possibly not representative of those who actually used this text, they do imply and envision—for the first time in Western Europe—a

9. Riccardo Gualdo, "La lingua della pediatria: Il trattato di Paolo Bagellardo dal Fiume," in Gualdo, ed., *Le parole della scienza: Scritture tecniche e scientifiche in volgare, secoli XIII–XV: Atti del convegno, Lecce, 16–18 aprile 1999* (Galatina: Congedo, 2001), 30.

10. Some instances from within the text: "But perhaps you will ask, *frontosa*: 'tell me now, why has nature given so much pleasure to the man in impregnating and conceiving, and so much pain to the woman in giving birth?'" (*MM*, 150); or again: "But *frontosa* may say, 'Oh my maestro, you provide sound and beautiful teachings on raising and caring for newborn babies. But who is able to observe these rules? Who will be able to observe so many of them? . . . So how is it that babies live when their caretakers fail to follow so many regulations?'" (*MM*, 181); "But it only makes sense that the midwife wonders and asks: 'Maestro, what can I do to improve the shape of the head? Teach me.'" (*MM*, 169). For other examples of real (and imagined) cross-gender dialogues involving midwives and learned physicians, see Jennifer Richards, "Reading and Hearing 'The Womans Booke' in Early Modern England," *Bulletin of the History of Medicine* 89, no. 3 (2015): 434–62. For the meaning of the term *frontosa*, see Note on the Translation, 53.

11. Green, *Making Women's Medicine Masculine*, viii, 27, 246.

potential and desired, if not actual readership. That female readership, seemingly invoked and feared at the same time, is one that professional male practitioners, but also elite laymen aiming to gain knowledge of women's reproductive potential, seek to oversee and control.[12]

Life and Works of Michele Savonarola

Michele Savonarola's precise date of birth is unknown, although scholars point to 1385 as the likely year.[13] We know he was born in Padua to a family that made its fortune in the wool trade. Giovanni, his father, called a *lanarius* (wool trader) in the surviving documents, travels as far as Apulia and invests his capital in land tenures and business activity. Giovanni's links with men of the Carrara court, the chancellery, and the University of Padua help to shed some light on Michele's early education. His relationship with the well-known humanist Giovanni Conversini (1343–1408), who perhaps had the young Michele among his private pupils,[14] is

12. For the historical context of the *MM*, see the section in this Introduction on "Gynecology and Midwifery in the Middle Ages," at 15–20.

13. The following biographical sketch and discussion of Savonarola's work mainly draws on information collected at the turn of the twentieth century by Antonio Segarizzi, *Della vita e delle opere di Michele Savonarola, medico padovano del secolo XV* (Padua: Gallina, 1900), and more recently by Tiziana Pesenti Marangon, "Michele Savonarola a Padova: L'ambiente, le opere, la cultura medica," *Quaderni per la storia dell'Università di Padova* 9–10 (1977): 45–102; and Antonio Samaritani, "Michele Savonarola riformatore cattolico nella corte estense a metà del secolo XV," *Atti e memorie della deputazione provinciale ferrarese di storia patria* 3, no. 22 (1976): 44–85. Lynn Thorndike discusses some aspects of Savonarola's scientific thought in chapter 46, "Michael Savonarola," in *A History of Magic and Experimental Science* (New York: Columbia University Press, 1934), 4:183–214. The outline of Savonarola's unique bilingual production along the lines of the Pseudo-Aristotelian *Secretum secretorum* is based on Jole Agrimi's early insight and on subsequent work on Savonarola by Chiara Crisciani and Gabriella Zuccolin; see Agrimi, review of Michele Savonarola, *Libreto de tute le cosse che se magnano: Un'opera di dietetica del secolo XV*, ed. Jane Nystedt (Stockholm: Gotab, 1982), in *Aevum* 58 (1984): 358–65; Crisciani, "*Historia* ed *exempla*: Storia e storie in alcuni testi di Michele Savonarola," in *Il principe e la storia: Atti del Convegno, Scandiano, 18–20 settembre 2003*, ed. Tina Matarrese and Cristina Montagnani (Novara: Interlinea, 2005), 53–68; Crisciani, "Histories, Stories, *Exempla*, and Anecdotes: Michele Savonarola from Latin to Vernacular," in *Historia: Empiricism and Erudition in Early Modern Europe*, ed. Gianna Pomata and Nancy G. Siraisi (Cambridge, MA: MIT Press, 2005), 297–324; Crisciani, "Michele Savonarola medico: Tra università e corte, tra latino e volgare," in *Filosofia in volgare nel Medioevo: Atti del Convegno della Società italiana per lo studio del pensiero medievale (S.I.S.P.M.), Lecce, 27–29 settembre 2002*, ed. Nadia Bray and Loris Sturlese (Louvain-la-Neuve: Fédération internationale des instituts d'études médiévales, 2003), 433–49; and Zuccolin, *Michele Savonarola "medico humano": Fisiognomica, etica e religione alla corte estense* (Bari: Edizioni di Pagina, 2018). For further bibliography, see Crisciani and Zuccolin, eds., *Michele Savonarola: Medicina e cultura di corte* (Florence: SISMEL, Edizioni del Galluzzo, 2011).

14. Savonarola's choice of opening his treatise on gout, *De gotta* (see *Works by Michele Savonarola*, #11) with a story about "A Spider and the Gout" (a story of Horatian origin, later developed by Petrarch and

likely at the root of the future physician's pedagogical interests, observed in the whole of Savonarola's work.[15] The educational values that underpin his medical texts and, rejecting medieval practices, adopt the gentler methods of Quintilian— the irreplaceable role of parents, the insistence on the persuasive qualities of the teacher—are shaped by the pedagogical theories advanced by the humanists Pier Paolo Vergerio (1370–1444), Guarino Veronese (1374–1460), and Vittorino da Feltre (1378–1466), all former students of Giovanni Coversini.[16]

Savonarola enrolled in the faculty of Arts and Medicine of the University of Padua, which was then in its heyday, enlisting some of the most distinguished professors of the day, and graduated in 1413, having studied with, among others, Giacomo della Torre da Forlì, Galeazzo Santasofia, and Blasius of Parma (who taught philosophy and astrology until 1411).[17] He appears to have been tied less to these primarily theoretical authors, however, than to Antonio Cermisone, a model of extraordinary practical ability and professional creativity, who is affectionately recalled countless times in his medical works with such titles as "excellent teacher" and "father" par excellence (*praeceptor splendidus* and *pater*).[18] Savonarola could not have studied with the thirteenth-century professor Peter of Abano (ca. 1250–1315), but he frequently cites the latter's *Conciliator differentiarum quae inter philosophos et medicos versantur*, the fundamental text on which Savonarola bases his theoretical knowledge of medicine. Nor did he did meet the much younger Niccolò Leoniceno (1428–1524) who, unlike Savonarola, reacted

---

then by Giovanni Conversini) might be in itself another small confirmation of a tight relation between the two, beyond confirming the physician's wide variety of literary interest. See Riccardo Gualdo, "Le cure e i bagni del principe nelle opere di Michele Savonarola," in *Gli umanisti e le terme: Atti del convegno internazionale di studio, Lecce, Santa Cesarea Terme, 23–25 maggio 2002*, ed. Paola Andrioli Nemola, Olga Silvana Casale, and Paolo Viti (Lecce: Conte, 2004), 196.

15. A further note on pedagogy: Savonarola's exceptional—for his time—long life (he died aged eighty-one in 1466) also allowed him to oversee the early education of his famous granchild Girolamo Savonarola (1452–1498), with whom Michele shared the family house in Ferrara for fourteen years. See Roberto Ridolfi, *Vita di Girolamo Savonarola*, 6th ed. (Florence: Le Lettere, 1997), 3–4.

16. Savonarola later lived in Ferrara in the same years as Guarino's residence there, but the relationship between the two, although marked by the humanist's high opinion of the Paduan physician, was superficial. For the humanist educational program, see *Humanist Educational Treatises*, ed. and trans. Craig Kallendorf (Cambridge, MA: Harvard University Press, 2002), whih includes a translation of Vergerio's *De ingenuis moribus* at 2–91, as well as pedagogical works by humanists Leonardo Bruni, Aeneas Sylvius Piccolomini, and Battista Guarino, son of Guarino Veronese.

17. For Savonarola's Paduan masters, see his encomium of Padua, the *Libellus de magnificis ornamentis regie civitatis Padue* (see *Works by Michele Savonarola*, #18), at 25–29, 33, 37, 40, 43.

18. The lessons of Antonio Cermisone—whose *Consilia* (especially the *Consilium contra pestilentia*) Savonarola regularly referenced and whose medical expertise he often placed before that of the great master Avicenna—were largely delivered outside the classroom. Cermisone taught Savonarola by way of example, practice and live discussion of professional and deontological medical issues. Cermisone only began to teach at the university in 1413, the year Savonarola took his medical degree.

against astrology and the dominance of Avicenna, turning instead to Hippocrates. Savonarola never was, as Leoniceno would be, a "physician-philologist," someone who set out a new method of scientific research.[19]

At Padua, Savonarola absorbed a tradition of medical learning which was both practical and formed by a naturalistic understanding of science averse to logical interests. At the same time, he developed profound links with Paduan humanism, the culture of rhetoric and the liberal arts. His work depicts, in fact, the complex totality of the Paduan dialectic of humanism on the one hand and medical and philosophical thought on the other.[20]

After finishing his studies, Savonarola practiced medicine in Padua for some twenty years, during which his professional skill won him fame and distinguished clients, before returning to the university in 1433 for a brief stint as a professor. During the years when he was primarily a practitioner, he not only concerned himself with social diseases, such as plague or fevers, which affected a large population, but also displayed the commercial mindset he shared with his father and others of his family.[21] In his *Practica maior* (*Great Compendium of Practical Medicine*), for instance, Savonarola declares that a treatment is to be preferred to the extent that it

---

19. For the Italian philosopher, astrologer and physician Peter of Abano, see Jean-Patrice Boudet, Franck Collard, and Nicolas Weill-Parrot, eds., *Médécine, astrologie et magie entre Moyen Âge et Renaissance: Autour de Pietro d'Abano* (Florence: SISMEL, Edizioni del Galluzzo, 2013). Leoniceno, the prototype of the "medical humanist," was one of the first Renaissance scholars to apply humanistic philology and ideological criticism to ancient medical texts. See the bibliography listed in Paul F. Grendler, *The Universities of the Italian Renaissance* (Baltimore, MD: Johns Hopkins University Press, 2002), 324.

20. His friend Sicco Polenton praises him with these words: *diligentiam laudo tuam quod non, utique plerique solent, Galieno et Avicene solum, sed, cum datur otium, antiquitati, eloquentiae ac omni virtuti studes. Legisti enim apud Ciceronem, puto, eum qui nesciat historias puerum sempre esse* ("I praise your diligence because you do not apply yourself only to Galen and Avicenna, as many do, but you also commit yourself to the study of antiquity, eloquence, and every moral virtue, in your leisure time. I believe you read in Cicero that he who does not know history, always remains a child"). Sicco Polenton, *La Catinia, le orazioni e le epistole di Sicco Polenton*, ed. Arnaldo Segarizzi (Bergamo: Istituto italiano d'arti grafiche, 1899), letter #19, at 119.

21. Savonarola pairs the teaching and practice of medicine with the same business his brothers were pursuing. They continued to boost the father's activity in wool trade and increased the real estate of the family. Savonarola, too, invested in lands and houses, joined the wool guild, and practiced money-lending. The social investment of Savonarola's family seems to mirror the same pragmatic attitude as does its economic activity: Michele is a doctor, his brother Niccolò is a lawyer, and his other brother Ludovico is *doctor in Sacra Pagina* (master of sacred theology). It is hard to imagine a more effective ascent towards the intellectual aristocracy of the city than this safe stance of the three Savonarola brothers towards the three faculties of the University of Padua.

guarantees *magnum introitum* (greater income) and that the practice of medicine aims to achieve *lucrum et gratiam* (profit and favor).[22]

After a full career in Padua as a practicing physician and professor, Savonarola pursued a further one at the court of Ferrara under the patronage of the Este rulers. In September 1440, he was called to Ferrara by the Marquis Niccolò III of Este (who would die a year later) as court physician, a position held until then by Ugo Benzi. In September 1439, even before Savonarola arrived in Ferrara, Guarino Veronese had commended the physician's scientific and professional cordiality and dedication.[23] On January 28, 1443, Leonello of Este, illegitimate son of Niccolò and the new marquis of Ferrara (until his sudden death in October 1450), conferred Ferrararese citizenship on Savonarola and all his descendants, asserting once again the physician's scientific excellence, trustworthiness and piety. In June 1450, in order to preserve the health of a by then elderly Savonarola, he restricted the latter's service as court physician to his own care and that of his close relatives; at the same time, he assigned to Savonarola some fiscal proceeds (the so-called "tenths") of the village of Sant'Elena, located near Rovigo between Padua and Ferrara. In conferring the donation certificate upon him, Leonello recalls why his father Niccolò had called Savonarola a decade earlier: "he greatly honored medical science by his exceptional intelligence, his foresight and skill in caring for human bodies, and by the many volumes and books he wrote,"[24] words testifying that the fame the court physician possessed was based on a sound scientific production as well as on his professional skill and human qualities.

In 1452, Savonarola formally requested Pope Nicholas V (1447–1455) to allow him to enter the Gerosolimitan Order, an unusual request made because he had a wife and children (eight of them!), which should have prevented him from taking vows. At the end of the same year, after having obtained the papal dispensation from vows and the concession of wearing the habit, Savonarola also obtained from the pope the right to dispose of his property in a will. In 1461, Borso of Este, another illegitimate son of Niccolò, younger brother of Leonello and new marquis of Ferrara, granted Savonarola the rich fief of Medelana. It should be remembered that Savonarola was also a businessman, and that he had been called to Ferrara for these skills as well as for the professional and scientific credentials as a physician and renowned university professor. At court he served more as a banker than as

---

22. Michele Savonarola, *Practica maior* (Venice: Giunta, 1559), for example at fols.142r and 247v. For other editions, including the 1479 *editio princeps*, see *Works by Michele Savonarola*, #6.

23. In a letter addressed to Count Ludovico of San Bonifacio, Guarino wrote: "Humanity and graciousness dwells in him" (*is est humanitatis et urbanitatis hospitium*). Guarino Veronese, *Epistolario di Guarino Veronese*, ed. Remigio Sabbadini (Venice: A spese della Società [di storia veneta], 1915–1919), 2 (1916): 362.

24. Quoted in Segarizzi, *Della vita e delle opere di Michele Savonarola*, at 11–12: *suo ingegnio singulari, sua in curandis humanis corporibus providentia et arte, suisque voluminibus et libris, quos plures condidit, medicine disciplinam maxime illustravit.* The English translation in the text is the editor's.

a doctor: he performed the first function throughout his stay in Ferrara, together perhaps with teaching,[25] whereas he abandoned the second just ten years after his arrival in the city. It has been suggested that the Este donations were granted in recognition of his fiscal services more than for his professional and academic achievements. Apparently Savonarola was called to Ferrara both because of his scientific prestige and because of his commercial skills and interests—for, as it seems, the austere and pious physician was open to the pursuit of personal profit. It is likely that the Este repaid Savonarola for the hefty loans he made them with land assets offering a lower return.

Savonarola's last years were dedicated to writing, his literary activity no doubt intensifying in response to the dynamics of the court environment. His date of death is as uncertain as that of his birth but it can be placed with some precision between March 8 and July 28, 1466.

The thirty-one works that constitute Savonarola's textual production are presented under the heading *Works by Michele Savonarola* that forms the first section of this volume's Bibliography. The works, numbered consecutively, are divided into five sections detailing medical works composed in Padua; medical works composed in Ferrara; and, also composed in Ferrara, historical works, courtly works, and religious works. For each work, full references to manuscripts or first editions are provided together with a concise alphabetical listing by author and date of the most relevant secondary literature (fully referenced in the general bibliography). Also indicated are the addressees of the works, where present, and the language chosen by Savonarola, signalled by the letter L for Latin and V for Vernacular. Some treatises bearing Latin titles were in fact written in the vernacular.

The kaleidoscopic spectrum of Savonarola's work illustrates three features of fifteenth-century medicine. The first is the growing importance, inside and outside universities, of practical medicine and the consequent development of "practical" medical genres—health regimens, advice (presented in *consilia*), collections of medical recipes, and monographic treatises on such matters as thermal baths, on food, on poisons, etc. The second is the development of courtly medicine, requiring increasingly diverse competencies, including in the related disciplines of astrology, alchemy and physiognomy, as well as politics and history. The third, not the least of these, is the increasing number of vernacular translations of medical and scientific texts and of works composed directly in the vernacular.

It is striking that Savonarola's production changes notably in quantity and quality when he moves from Padua to Ferrara in 1440, and thus from a strictly

---

25. Samaritani, "Michele Savonarola riformatore cattolico," 40, reports that Savonarola's university activity at Ferrara is documented, as promoter of degrees, from April 6, 1446 to January 20, 1466. This does not in itself imply that Savonarola has actually also taught up to this date, but it indicates that his presence at the medical faculty in Ferrara does not ends after 1450, which is the date given by Segarizzi in his biography, *Della vita e delle opere di Michele Savonarola*.

academic context to a courtly one. In Padua, he composed medical treatises exclusively written in Latin; in Ferrara, he composed works written in Latin, or in double redaction (in both Latin and the Italian vernacular), or solely in the vernacular (which often deal not only with medical, but also with historical, ethical, political and religious subjects). Composing Latin and vernacular redactions of the same work was not unusual in Italy at the time, nor was it uncharacteristic for Savonarola. Setting aside the double redactions (*Works by Michele Savonarola*, ##7 and 20), many of Savonarola's vernacular works—for example, to consider medical subjects only, the *Mother's Manual* itself, as well as the texts on plague, gout, and dietetics (##13, 9, 11, and 12 respectively)—have in fact a Latin counterpart among his academic works. Several of Savonarola's moral and political writings, as well, testify to his bilingual approach. Savonarola's bilingualism means that the author becomes, in a sense, a translator, a compiler, a commentator on himself, giving the historian a wonderful perspective on the transmission of knowledge and the relation between different languages and types of sources and audiences within the mind of a single individual.

The analysis to be presented in this volume of Savonarola's vernacular *Mother's Manual* will tangentially examine the corresponding Latin chapter on gynecological topics in Savonarola's *Practica maior*, the source from which Savonarola draws for the vernacular work. But the complex intertwinings of the Latin and the vernacular in Savonarola's bilingual production, and the possibilities of comparison within it, are not limited to this specific work. Simultaneously interrogating Latin and vernacular textual traditions is essential, as will be seen, for a thorough analysis of the pedagogic project for the court modeled by Savonarola in all of his Ferrarese works.

The growing prominence, noted earlier, that was given to the practical purposes of medicine resulted in a broadened audience for Savonarola's work, one not exclusively academic. In many of his treatises, not only those medical in nature, he addressed the Este princes along with the nobles and citizens of Ferrara, thus presenting a unified pedagogical program that transcended traditional disciplinary boundaries. It is true that Savonarola's Latin medical treatises, more valued apparently by posterity than his other literary products, were quickly printed and reprinted (see *Works by Michele Savonarola* ##2, 3, 4, 6, and 10 for multiple incunables and sixteenth-century editions), while his writings on social, moral, and political matters survive in unique manuscript dedication copies for the Este patrons. Yet these latter, constituting the bulk of Savonarola's Ferrarese writings from 1440 onwards, must not be ignored: for they constitute a set of instructions on good governance for his Este patrons—in effect, an extensive *speculum principis*, or "mirror for princes," as the medieval genre of advice-books for rulers was called. And it is no coincidence that these works were created in a chronological order corresponding to the order of subjects of the Pseudo-Aristotelian *Secretum secretorum* (*Secret of Secrets*), "the best known of that large family of works in which the man of the study takes upon himself the task of telling the man of affairs what he should do."[26] Of course, Savonarola's pedagogical program for the Este court is also influenced by contemporary humanism and interwoven with religious discussions that are unrelated to the *Secretum*. Still, the similarity between the topics addressed in this ancient work and the subjects of many of Savonarola's treatises is striking—an impression reinforced by Savonarola's frequent quotation of the *Secretum*.[27]

A brief summary follows of some of the correspondences between the *Secretum secretorum* and Savonarola's works. The first book of the *Secretum* deals with the moral and political education of the prince, while Savonarola devoted four of his Ferrarese works to this subject (see *Works by Michele Savonarola*, ##20, 21, 22, and 23). Of these, two (##21 and 23) are composed in Latin; a third (#22), expressly critical of courtly vices and misbehavior, in the vernacular; and the fourth and most important work (#20), in double redaction.[28]

26. Robert Steele, Introduction to his edition of Roger Bacon, *Secretum secretorum cum glossis et notulis* (Oxford: Clarendon Press, 1920), ix. On the circulation of this popular work, allegedly written by Aristotle to advise Alexander the Great on a number of matters related to good government (actually a kind of encyclopaedic *speculum principis* of Arabic origins compiled around the ninth century), see Mario Grinaschi, "La diffusion du 'Secretum secretorum' ('Sirr-al'arsār') dans l'Europe Occidentale," *Archives d'histoire doctrinale et littéraire du Moyen Âge* 47 (1981): 7–69; Agostino Paravicini Bagliani, *Medicina e scienze della natura alla corte dei Papi nel Duecento* (Spoleto: CISAM [Centro Italiano di studi sull'alto Medioevo], 1991); Stefano Rapisarda, "Appunti sulla circolazione del 'Secretum secretorum' in Italia," in Gualdo, *Le parole della scienza*, 87–105; Steven J. Williams, "The Early Circulation of the Pseudo-Aristotelian 'Secret of Secrets' in the West: The Papal and Imperial Courts," *Micrologus* 2 (1994): 127–44, reprinted in Williams, ed., *The "Secret of Secrets": The Scholarly Career of a Pseudo-Aristotelian Text in the Latin Middle Ages* (Ann Arbor: University of Michigan Press, 2003), 109–40; Williams, "Giving Advice and Taking It: The Reception by Rulers of the Pseudo-Aristotelian 'Secretum Secretorum' as a 'Speculum Principis,'" in *Consilium: Teorie e pratiche del consigliare nella cultura medievale*, ed. Carla Casagrande, Chiara Crisciani, and Silvana Vecchio (Florence: SISMEL, Edizioni del Galluzzo, 2004), 139–56; and Williams, "The Vernacular Tradition of the Pseudo-Aristotelian 'Secret of Secrets' in the Middle Ages: Translations, Manuscripts, Readers," in *Filosofia in volgare nel Medioevo: Atti del Convegno della Società italiana per lo studio del pensiero medievale (S.I.S.P.M.), Lecce, 27–29 settembre 2002*, ed. Nadia Bray and Loris Sturlese (Louvain-la-Neuve: Fédération internationale des instituts d'études médiévales, 2003), 451–82. These contributions show how the *Secretum* circulated in the Latin West responding to scientific and philosophical interests common to both the papal and the imperial courts of Frederick II. In northern Italy, manuscript copies of the *Secretum* were owned by the cities of Padua, Mantua, Bologna, Milan, Venice as well as Ferrara. These studies also show that selective Italian translations of the text (privileging the scientific, dietary and practical parts rather than the philosophical ones) were more successful than complete versions. Finally, the set of interpolations present in hundreds of manuscripts of the *Secretum* suggest that parts of it were circulated even as single sheets.

27. For exact quotes from Savonarola's texts, and the presence of the *Secretum* in medieval inventories of the Este library, see Zuccolin, *Michele Savonarola "medico humano,"* 79–90.

28. This last work, *Del felice progresso di Borso d'Este/De felici progressu* [. . .] *Borsii Estensis*, develops and molds together the typical themes of the prince's journey toward knowledge and virtue, and the

The second book of the *Secretum* is recognized as a classic *regimen sanitatis* (rules for health), which attempts to regulate the so-called "six non-natural
things,"[29] accompanied by a list of illnesses and cures concerning the head, eyes,
chest and male genitals. Many of Savonarola's works address the same matters,
constituting in effect a series of *regimina sanitatis*: one, the *Mother's Manual*, intended for pregnant women, wet nurses and children (in the vernacular); one
for people affected by plague (in double redaction); one for those suffering from
gout (in the vernacular); one focused on dietetics (in the vernacular).[30] As for the
Secretum's section on illnesses and cures, the entire *Practica maior* of Savonarola,
listing diseases from head to toe and including a classic *regimen sanitatis*, performs the same function.[31] Also worth mentioning, although different in genre,
is Savonarola's massive Latin *De balneis* arguing the therapeutic role of thermal
baths, both for healthy or unhealthy individuals.[32]

---

pedagogy of good government: it consists of a *speculum principis* paired with an historical chronicle,
one *laudatio urbis* (encomium of the city), and one *disputatio artium* (competition between the arts).
See *Works by Michele Savonarola*, #20, for the manuscript preserving the Latin version of the text and
for the modern edition of the vernacular version. See also Maria Aurelia Mastronardi, " . . . *Redeunt
Saturnia regna*: Città ideale ed età dell'oro nella Ferrara estense," *Annali della facoltà di lettere e filosofia dell'Università degli studi della Basilicata* 8 (1998): 153–81; Zuccolin, *Michele Savonarola "medico
humano,"* and Zuccolin, "Princely Virtues in 'De felici progressu,'" for a comparison between the set of
princely virtues proposed by Thomas Aquinas and Giles of Rome and that developed by Savonarola.

29. On medieval health regimens, see Pedro Gil-Sotres, "Els '*regimina sanitatis*,'" in Arnaldus de
Villanova, *Regimen sanitatis ad regem Aragonum*, ed. Luis García Ballester, Juan A. Paniagua, and
Michael R. McVaugh (Barcelona: Publicacions i edicions de la Universitat de Barcelona, 1996),
17–110; and Marilyn Nicoud, *Les régimes de santé au Moyen Âge: Naissance et diffusion d'une écriture
médicale en Italie et en France, XIIIe–XVe siècle* (Rome: École Française de Rome, 2007). The so-called
res non naturales, or "non-natural things," are a Galenic set of physiological, psychological, and envi-
ronmental conditions held to affect health (the quality of air and places, exercise and rest, sleep and
waking, food and drink, excretion and repletion, and the passions of the mind). This category must be
understood in relation to the categories of the naturals (*res naturales*) and the unnaturals (*res contra
naturam*), which refer to innate human physiology and anatomy, and to diseases respectively. On the
non-naturals, see Luis García Ballester, "On the Origin of the 'Six Non-Natural Things' in Galen," in
*Galen und das hellenistische Erbe: Verhandlungen des IV. Internationalen Galen-Symposiums veran-
staltet vom Institut für Geschichte der Medizin am Bereich Medizin (Charité) der Humboldt-Universität
zu Berlin 18.–20. September 1989*, ed. Jutta Kollesch and Diethard Nickel (Stuttgart: Franz Steiner,
1993), 105–15; Saul Jarcho, "Galen's Six Non-Naturals: A Bibliographic Note and Translation," *Bulletin
of the History of Medicine* 44 (1970): 372–77; and Lelland J. Rather, "The 'Six Things Non-Naturals': A
Note on the Origins and Fate of a Doctrine and a Phrase," *Clio medica* 3 (1968): 3373–47.

30. See *Works by Michele Savonarola*, ## 13, 9, 11, and 12 respectively.

31. See *Works by Michele Savonarola*, #6, for multiple editions.

32. As was the case for the *Practica maior*, this work on thermal baths was an editorial success (see
Works by Michele Savonarola, #10, for the *editio princeps*, many other sixteenth-century editions, and
the first critical edition), and gained the first position in the well-known 1553 collection of thermal
works *De balneis omnia quae extant* (Venice: Giunta, 1553).

The third book of the *Secretum* deals with alchemy, positing the harmonious correspondence between stars, planets, vegetables, minerals, animals, and man himself. Corresponding to this text is Savonarola's treatise on the marvellous virtues of grape-spirit (seen as the quintessence, the elixir of long-life, the result of the alchemical process of distillation of terrestrial elements endowed with celestial virtues), likely to appeal to noblemen and rulers interested in the mysterious art of alchemy.[33]

The last book of the *Secretum* focuses on astrological physiognomy, a subject Savonarola addresses in one of his most interesting and still unpublished treatises, the *Speculum physionomie* (*Mirror of Physiognomy*): a Latin work filled with vernacular quotations from the astrologer Cecco d'Ascoli's encyclopedic poem *Acerba*.[34] Savonarola presents physiognomy as a kind of knowledge that is not only useful as an "art of good government" but also as philosophical and civic ethics, a science of human passions in their complex relationship to vice and virtue. The treatise emphasizes the social role of the physician, one that Savonarola performs in giving advice to the prince on childrearing and on choosing ministers, faithful counselors, and reliable servants. He performs this role as well in offering advice that might be called eugenic: the choice of the best wife to guarantee the birth of healthy and possibly male offspring; sexual advice on the best time and methods of coitus; and how to model and shape the newborn's cranium so as to improve the infant's intellectual capacities.

In addition to the works surveyed that correspond to the themes of the *Secretum*, mention should also be made of Savonarola's well-known history of Padua (in Latin); the unfortunately lost work on the history of Ferrara (in the vernacular, judging by the surviving title);[35] and his many devotional and pastoral works. In this last category are two vernacular texts of instructions for a good Christian confession, one addressed to noblemen, and the other to the Carthusian monks of Ferrara. It must be viewed as highly unusual (perhaps even audacious?) that a layman, indeed a physician, presumes to instruct religious men on their confessorial duties![36]

Evidently, the *Secretum secretorum* provided Savonarola with a template of topics that should be addressed by the physician advisor to a prince. Savonarola, of course, is not the only one to understand his role as court physician along those lines. Although he may be considered "an atypical Renaissance physician" as does

---

33. See *Works by Michele Savonarola*, #7.

34. See *Works by Michele Savonarola*, #8, and related bibliography. Scholars have not agreed on the meaning of the title *Acerba*, which if derived from the Latin *acerbus* might mean "a collection of unripe things"; but if from *acerva*, "collection" or "miscellany."

35. See *Works by Michele Savonarola*, ##18 and 19.

36. See in the Bibliography the entire fifth section (on *Religious Works*) of the *Works by Michele Savonarola*, especially ##28 and 29.

Ynez V. O'Neill,[37] given the wide range of topics, literary genres, and large number of works that Savonarola wrote, in a deeper sense he is a *typical* representative of a new profession, spreading in Italy, it seems, before the rest of Europe: the court physician.[38] Recognizing the importance of this new type is essential for a correct assessment both of late medieval medicine and the court as a non-academic site of culture. The prominence of the court physician, furthermore, undermines the now outdated assumption of an irreconcilable dichotomy between scholasticism and humanism.[39] Indeed, academic physicians in this period, though trained in scholastic disciplines, often engaged in the broader humanist culture. Savonarola's connections with famous humanist educators, as has been seen, may explain his interest in pedagogical problems. Moreover, physicians conceived of medicine as a science containing everything needed to promote human well-being, including political advice, especially if the subject of their care was the prince.[40] Court physicians emerged, in short, as a new type of professional figure entrusted with a diverse set of responsibilities that were not confined to matters of a medical nature; for they also functioned as political counselors, reliable diplomats, financial advisors, and conscientious tutors, capable of guiding others in economic, political, astrological, meteorological, cosmetic, culinary, musical, and, as has been seen, even religious matters.[41]

37. See Ynez V. O'Neill, "Giovanni Michele Savonarola: An Atypical Renaissance Practitioner," *Clio Medica* 10 (1975): 177–93.

38. Among recent studies see Elisa Andretta and Marilyn Nicoud, eds., *Être médecin à la cour: Italie, France, Espagne, XIIIe–XVIIIe siècle* (Florence: SISMEL, Edizioni del Galluzzo, 2013); Jean-Patrice Boudet, Martine Ostorero, and Agostino Paravicini Bagliani, eds., *De Frédéric II à Rodolphe II: Astrologie, divination et magie dans les cours, XIIIe–XVIIe siècle* (Florence: SISMEL, Edizioni del Galluzzo, 2017); and Marilyn Nicoud, *Le prince et les médecins: Pensée et pratiques médicales à Milan, 1402–1476* (Rome: École Française de Rome, 2014).

39. That is to say, between a scholastic and a humanist Aristotelianism, and the equally dated and partially misleading assumption of the non-academic nature of the latter kind of Aristotelianism. Among many relevant titles see Luca Bianchi, *Studi sull'aristotelismo del Rinascimento* (Padua: Il Poligrafo, 2003); Paul Oskar Kristeller, "Umanesimo e Scolastica a Padova fino al Petrarca," *Medioevo* 11 (1985): 1–18; Charles B. Schmitt, *Aristotle and the Renaissance* (Cambridge, MA: Harvard University Press, 1983); and Schmitt, *La tradizione aristotelica: Fra Italia e Inghilterra* (Naples: Bibliopolis, 1985).

40. Among such court physicians note may be made of Guido Parato, Giovanni Matteo Ferrari da Grado, and Benedetto Reguardati at the Sforza court of Milan; Pantaleone da Confienza in Piedmont for the Savoy; and Ugolino da Montecatini and Pierleone da Spoleto in Medici-ruled Florence.

41. The pedagogic polyvalence of Italian late-medieval physicians was also the result of a series of unique circumstances specific to the Italian context: in Italian universities, differently from elsewhere in Europe, the medical curriculum was unified with the study of the liberal arts in a joint and unique faculty (the faculty of arts and medicine). In Italy, medicine (along with law) became in fact the culmination of secular education, and its curriculum started to incorporate "lay" disciplines such as physiognomy, astrology and alchemy. This allowed learned Italian physicians to master comprehensive philosophical competencies that made them attractive, if not essential, to rulers. The strong alliance

Returning to the *Mother's Manual*, it can now be seen more clearly how and why the main aim of Savonarola in this work—to provide hygienic rules surrounding the act and the function of procreation—blurs into a more pedagogical and moral objective, also offering instructions on the best way to manage family life, emphasizing the need to procreate responsibly and to give each child a good upbringing. By providing a new context for the topic of procreation, no longer confined to medical issues but broached together with more general social, family-oriented and also political concerns, Savonarola the moralist often gets the better of Savonarola the physician, allowing us to read this gynecological-pediatric treatise as a special sort of those *libri della famiglia* that gained huge popularity during the Italian Quattrocento.[42] In other words, as will be seen, this work serves also as a guide to married life, an aid to women's fertility, a prescription for the responsible management of birth, and a presentation of the best possible care of the newborn.

Gynecology and Midwifery in the Middle Ages

Thanks to recent, pioneering scholarship, much more is known now than even three decades ago about the history of gynecology, midwifery, and medical texts on women's bodies and diseases in the medieval and early modern period.[43] Much

---

between the arts and medicine had an enormous impact on the development of the career of Italian physicians and, from an epistemological perspective, it granted a philosophical status to medicine, which proved to be seminal for the coalescence of Aristotelianism and medical research.

42. Notably, the *Libri della famiglia* (*On the Family*) by Leon Battista Alberti, written around 1430, where the treatment of sexual issues is overloaded with stronger social values, due to the central role assigned to the family microcosm; see the edition of Francesco Furlan (Turin: Einaudi, 1994). Also see the *Booklet on the Pursuit of Good Birth Conditions* studied by Gianfranco Fioravanti: "Un trattato medico di eugenetica: Il 'Libellus de ingenio bonae nativitatis,'" *Mediaevalia* 21 (2002): 89–111.

43. To cite but a few studies: Ron Barkaï, *A History of Jewish Gynaecological Texts in the Middle Ages* (Leiden: Brill, 1998); José Pablo Barragán Nieto, editor of Albert the Great [pseud.], *El "De secretis mulierum" atribuido a Alberto Magno: Estudio, edición crítica y traducción* (Porto: Fédération internationale des instituts d'études médiévales, 2012); Chiara Beneduce, *Natural Philosophy and Medicine in John Buridan: With an Edition of Buridan's "Quaestiones de secretis mulierum,"* PhD diss., Radboud Universiteit, Nijmegen (Zutphen: Koninklijke Wöhrmann, 2017); Evelyne Berriot-Salvadore, *Un corps, un destin: La femme dans la médecine de la Renaissance* (Paris: Champion, 1993); Joan Cadden, *Meanings of Sex Difference in the Middle Ages: Medicine, Science and Culture* (Cambridge: Cambridge University Press, 1993); Costanza Gislon Dopfel, Alessandra Foscati, and Charles S. F. Burnett, eds., *Pregnancy and Childbirth in the Premodern World, European and Middle Eastern Cultures, from Late Antiquity to the Renaissance* (Turnhout: Brepols, 2019); Mary E. Fissell, "Introduction: Women, Health, and Healing in Early Modern Europe," *Bulletin of the History of Medicine* 82 (2008): 1–17; Fissell, *Vernacular Bodies: The Politics of Reproduction in Early Modern England* (Oxford: Oxford University Press, 2004); Monica H. Green, "Books as a Source of Medical Education for Women in the Middle Ages," *Dynamis* 20 (2000): 331–69; Green, "From 'Diseases of Women' to 'Secrets of Women':

is also known of the activity of women in generic medical practice across the same periods.[44] Nonetheless, it appears to be the case that in Europe, from the seventh century (and likely before) to the thirteenth, there is no identifiable profession of midwifery, nor any attempt to define a standard knowledge expected of midwives before the fifteenth century. Before Savonarola's *Mother's Manual*, no medieval text focuses in such a detailed and monographic way on obstetrics, nor were midwives ever identified as the intended readers of any of the works, in Latin or the vernacular, on women's medicine. Even when such works were addressed to female audiences, as were many of the vernacular translations of the Trotula texts,[45] "female audience" meant a generic address to women, not specifically to midwives. The absence of professional "literate" identity for midwives is explained by the fact that midwifery was not yet a recognized profession: although the care of uncomplicated births was in the hands of women, female midwives did not hold

---

The Transformation of Gynecological Literature in the Later Middle Ages," *Journal of Medieval and Early Modern Studies* 30 (2000): 5–39; Green, *Making Women's Medicine Masculine*; Green, "The Possibilities of Literacy"; Green, "The Sources of Eucharius Rösslin's *'Rosegarden* for Pregnant Women and Midwives' (1513)," *Medical History* 53 (2009): 167–92; Nick Hopwood, Rebecca Flemming, and Lauren Kassell, eds., *Reproduction: Antiquity to the Present Day* (Cambridge: Cambridge University Press, 2018); Helen King, *Midwifery, Obstetrics and the Rise of Gynaecology: The Uses of a Sixteenth-Century Compendium* (Aldershot, Hampshire, UK; Burlington VT: Ashgate, 2007); Helen King, *The One-Sex Body on Trial: The Classical and Early Modern Evidence* (Farnham, Surrey, UK; Burlington, VT: Ashgate, 2013); Margaret L. King, "Concepts of Childhood: What We Know and Where We Might Go," *Renaissance Quarterly* 60, no. 2 (2007): 371–407; Britta-Juliane Kruse, *Verborgene Heilkünste: Geschichte der Frauenmedizin im Spätmittelalter* (Berlin: Walter de Gruyter, 1996); Hilary Marland, ed., *The Art of Midwifery: Early Modern Midwives in Europe* (New York and London: Routledge, 1993); Romana Martorelli Vico, *Medicina e filosofia: Per una storia dell'embriologia medievale nel XIII e XIV secolo* (Milan: Guerini e associati, 2002); Lianne McTavish, *Childbirth and the Display of Authority in Early Modern France* (Aldershot, Hampshire, UK; Burlington, VT: Ashgate, 2005); Jacqueline Musacchio, *The Art and Ritual of Childbirth in Renaissance Italy* (New Haven: Yale University Press, 1999); Katharine Park, *Secrets of Women: Gender, Generation, and the Origins of Human Dissection* (New York: Zone Books, 2006); Worth-Stylianou, *Pregnancy and Birth*; and Worth-Stylianou, *Les traités d'obstétrique.*

44. See Susan Broomhall, *Women's Medical Work in Early Modern France* (Manchester: Manchester University Press, 2004); David Gentilcore, *Healers and Healing in Early Modern Italy* (Manchester: Manchester University Press, 1998); Green, "Books as a Source of Medical Education"; Margaret Pelling, *Medical Conflicts in Early Modern London: Patronage, Physicians, and Irregular Practitioners, 1550–1640* (Oxford: Clarendon Press, 2003); Gianna Pomata, *Contracting a Cure: Patients, Healers, and the Law in Early Modern Bologna* (Baltimore, MD: Johns Hopkins University Press, 1998); Alisha M. Rankin, *Panaceia's Daughters: Noblewomen as Healers in Early Modern Germany* (Chicago: University of Chicago Press, 2013); and Adrian Wilson, *The Making of Man-Midwifery: Childbirth in England, 1660–1770* (London: UCL Press, 1995).

45. Even Trota's Latin *Treatments for Women*, composed in twelfth-century Salerno by a woman for women, was a training handbook on women's medicine in general, and did not deal only with obstetrics.

a monopoly over complicated births in the Middle Ages (as previously thought), because they did not yet exist as a class—or rather, they no longer existed, for there had been such a profession in antiquity.

In order to appreciate the central importance of Savonarola's work, attention must turn back to ancient times, when the duties of literate—that is to say, learned and professional—midwives encompassed gynecological as well as obstetrical care. Although the Hippocratic author of *Diseases of Women I,* addressed other male physicians like himself, the Greek *Gynecology* of Soranus of Ephesus (late first—early second century CE) was principally intended for a female group of practitioners, as were the Latin renderings of this work authored between the fourth and sixth centuries by the north-African writers Theodorus Priscianus, Caelius Aurelianus, and Muscio. Roman inscriptions, funerary epitaphs, laws, and other such records, testify to the existence of midwives and to their responsibilities, which were never restricted to obstetrics. Setting aside the issue of "audience" for a moment, and focusing instead on the content of works on women's medicine, it must be stressed that these works presented physicians, surgeons, and generic female audiences with material on *both* obstetrics (i.e., fertility, childbirth, and the care of the newborn) and gynecology (i.e., all of women's other conditions, such as menstrual disorders, uterine suffocation or prolapse, cancers, and lesions).

Although gynecology and obstetrics were always paired, however, in these ancient medical works (as they were as in the twelfth-century Trotula texts), gynecology and the theory of generation were perceived as two very different matters. The author of *Diseases of Women I,* for example, also wrote a treatise on the *Nature of the Child,* which never circulated together with the former work. Soranus devoted his *On Seed* to the speculative topic of generation, never suggesting that it should be read alongside his own practical *Gynecology.* The Pseudo-Galenic *De spermate (On Sperm),* similarly, or other embryological works, rarely circulated together with gynecological.

But by the time the Trotula texts were composed in southern Italy in the twelfth century, and midwives—although not literate—were starting to emerge again as specialist birth attendants, the separation between the two textual traditions of gynecological and generational texts began to blur. Collections of manuscripts juxtaposing texts on women's medicine (like the Trotula ensemble) and works displaying strong, though not strictly medical, interest in reproduction, embryology, and pregnancy multiply all over Europe. Meanwhile, on the level of medical practice, most aspects of gynecology, including the treatment of infertility, menstrual dysfunctions, uterine conditions, and such, had already passed into the province of male practitioners, physicians as well as surgeons. Medical advice on how to treat cases of retained placenta, serious hemorrhages, or other obstetrical complications appear in many general medical handbooks. The first surgical writing of the Latin West to incorporate detailed obstetrical instruction, including sections on how to extract a dead fetus from the mother's body (and conversely on how to birth a live child from a dead mother), is the *Inventarium sive Cirurgia magna* (*Inventory, or Great [Work on] Surgery*) by Guy de Chauliac (1363); but instructions for an embryotomy procedure were already present in *Surgery*, a work by al-Zahrāwī (tenth century, Latinized as Albucasis), which was translated into Latin before 1187 and often copied together with the well-known series of sixteen fetus-in-utero figures that had originally accompanied Muscio's *Gynecology*.[46] Albucasis' *Surgery* is only one example of a larger process, since scientific and medical writing as a whole was transformed by the introduction of Latin translations of Arabic texts into the West. Chapters on women's medicine are included in the most important Arab encyclopedic works later used as university texts, such as Avicenna's *Canon medicinae* (*Canon of Medicine*) or Rhazes's *Liber ad Almansorem* (*Book Dedicated to al-Mansur*). The late medieval followers of these Arabic authors composed many *Practicae* (*Compendia of Medical Practice*) themselves, such as Bernard de Gordon's *Lilium medicinae* (*Lily of Medicine*) or, indeed, Savonarola's *Practica maior*, which devoted ample sections to the diseases of the generative organs, both male and female. Whereas the participation of men in the field of gynecology expanded, the regulation of midwifery increasingly reinforced the notion that the expertise of midwives was limited to uncomplicated births, and did not extend to women's overall health.[47]

46. For an English translation of this text, see Lesley Bolton, "An Edition, Translation and Commentary of Mustio's Gynaecia," PhD diss., University of Calgary (Prism: University of Calgary's Digital Repository, 2015), <https://prism.ucalgary.ca/handle/11023/2252>. On Muscio's text in the Middle Ages, see Ann E. Hanson and Monica H. Green, "Soranus of Ephesus: Methodicorum Princeps," in *Aufstieg und Niedergang der römischen Welt: Geschichte und Kultur Roms im Spiegel der neueren Forschung*, vol. 2, part 37.2, ed. Wolfgang Haase and Hildegard Temporini (Berlin and New York: Walter de Gruyter, 1994), 968–1075.

47. Beginning in the fourteenth century, midwives in Paris came under the control of bishops and local parish priests, as attested by the earliest legislation known, a statute from the Paris archdiocese dated 1311. They had to swear an oath and were instructed to perform emergency baptisms. How much this kind of ecclesiastical scrutiny was replicated elsewhere in Europe is not clear. For England, no record exists before the sixteenth century. In Germany and the Low Countries, municipalities took the task of supervising and appointing midwives, but formal licensing practices are not known until the fifteenth century. For Spain and Italy, no regulation at all has been attested prior to the sixteenth century. See Monica H. Green, "Bodies, Gender, Health, Disease: Recent Work on Medieval Women's Medicine," *Studies in Medieval and Renaissance History* 2 (2005): 1–49; Green, *Making Women's Medicine Masculine*, 137; Fiona Harris-Stoertz, "Midwives in the Middle Ages? Birth Attendants, 600–1300," in *Medicine and the Law in the Middle Ages*, ed. Wendy J. Turner and Sara M. Butler (Leiden and Boston: Brill, 2014), 58–87; Ginger L. Smoak, "Midwives as Agents of Social Control: Ecclesiastical and Municipal Regulation of Midwifery in the Late Middle Ages," *Quidditas: Online Journal of the Rocky Mountain Medieval and Renaissance Association* 33 (2012): 79–96; and Kathryn Taglia, "Delivering a Christian Identity: Midwives in Northern French Synodal Legislation, c. 1200–1500," in *Religion and*

It is in this context that Savonarola's mid-fifteenth-century work is to be recognized as notably innovative and original. The *Mother's Manual* inaugurated a new approach in women's medicine, which had a dual aspect: first, in covering fertility issues and childbirth, and also childcare and generation, it addresses the interests of both practitioners and patients, midwives and birthing mothers, professionals and nonprofessionals; and second, by limiting its scope to obstetrics, and excluding medical topics not associated with childbirth (menstrual disorders, womb afflictions, etiological matters), it defines gynecology as something outside of women's competence, participating in what Green has called "the masculine birth of gynecology."[48] Together, therefore, with the emergence of obstetrical literature—that is, of works mainly focusing on childbirth—the birth of gynecology as a specialized field defines the transition to early modernity. Savonarola's work, in sum, separated gynecology from obstetrics and instructed laypersons on the culture of reproduction, while at the same time contributing to the growing perception of the midwife's ignorance.

Within this context, as well, may be viewed the process of vernacularization, and the structuring of gender categories. For men, vernacular texts like the *Mother's Manual* and its epigones, addressing not only physicians, barber-surgeons, and apothecaries, but also educated gentlemen, expanded both professional and lay audiences. But even as they lessened the gap between the two categories of "professional," and "lay," they reinforced the gender division between medical practitioners. Yet for women, who were for the greater part illiterate, these texts at least suggested the expectation that professional midwives and laywomen in general might access this new obstetrical literature—in which case, these vernacular texts played a significant role in the creation of a new audience.[49] Whether or not such a new audience materialized is hard to determine, given the inherent limitations of the possible sources (ownership notes, textual annotations, inventories, wills, and such) for a tracking of gendered reception—not only for this but also for similar texts, even at a later date and after the invention of print. Indeed, even if the recent explosion of studies on women's literacy and habits of reading makes clear that literacy does not necessarily mean "medical literacy," and that women's access to the literate culture of medicine may have been very low, yet the practices of reading aloud, and listening to information delivered orally, had great significance for female audiences.[50]

Medicine in the Middle Ages, ed. Peter Biller and Joseph Ziegler (Woodbridge, Suffolk, UK; Rochester, NY: York Medieval Press, 2001), 77–90.

48. Green, *Making Women's Medicine Masculine*, 165.

49. Green, *Making Women's Medicine Masculine*, 164.

50. Adrianna E. Bakos, "A Knowledge Speculative and Practical: The Dilemma of Midwives' Education in Early Modern Europe," In *Women's Education in Early Modern Europe: A History, 1500 to 1800*, ed. Barbara J. Whitehead (New York: Garland, 1999), 225–50; Judith Bryce, "Les livres des Florentines:

The extent to which female audiences—either laywomen or professional midwives—read, or heard, Savonarola's text is therefore as yet unclear. What is crystal clear, however, is Savonarola's utter confidence, conveyed in his *Mother's Manual*, that the treatment of gynecological and obstetrical conditions is "no job for a woman,"[51] but rather the responsibility of men like himself—his fifteenth-century northern Italian colleagues, other court physicians among them, who were involved in gynecological practice, the treatment of fertility issues, and, in sum, all major aspects of women's healthcare.[52]

Summary and Analysis of the Mother's Manual

The *Mother's Manual* is divided into three "treatises," each dealing with a different stage of the reproductive process. The first deals with conception, and offers guidelines for pregnant women; the second deals with the birth of the infant and post-partum conditions; and the third deals with the care of the newborn up to the age of seven.

Before proceeding to a discussion of these three treatises, it should be determined to what extent the content of the vernacular *Mother's Manual* corresponds to the gynecological chapter (chapter 21) of Savonarola's Latin *Practica maior* upon which it is based.[53] It is significant that the topics discussed in the

---

Reconsidering Women's Literacy in Quattrocento Florence," in *At the Margins: Minority Groups in Premodern Italy*, ed. Stephen J. Milner (Minneapolis: University of Minneapolis Press, 2005), 133–61; Julie D. Campbell and Anne R. Larsen, eds., *Early Modern Women and Transnational Communities of Letters* (Farnham, Surrey, UK: Ashgate, 2009); Margaret W. Ferguson, *Dido's Daughters: Literacy, Gender, and Empire in Early Modern England and France* (Chicago: University of Chicago Press, 2003); Green, "The Possibilities of Literacy"; Paul F. Grendler, *Schooling in Renaissance Italy: Literacy and Learning, 1300–1600* (Baltimore, MD: Johns Hopkins University Press, 1989); Hellwarth, "'I wyl wright of women prevy sekenes'"; Peter M. Jones, "Medical Literacies and Medical Culture in Early Modern Vernacular Medicine," in Irma Taavitsainen and Päivi Pahta, eds., *Medical Writing in Early Modern English* (Cambridge: Cambridge University Press, 2011), 30–43; Anne-Marie Legaré and Bertrand Schnerb, eds., *Livres et lectures des femmes en Europe entre Moyen Âge et Renaissance* (Turnhout: Brepols, 2007); Helen Smith, *"Grossly Material Things": Women and Book Production in Early Modern England* (Oxford: Oxford University Press, 2012); Helen Smith, "More Swete vnto the Eare/Than Holsome for ye Mynde: Embodying Early Modern Women's Reading," *Huntington Library Quarterly* 73, no. 3 (2010): 413–32; Edith Snook, *Women, Reading, and the Cultural Policy of Early Modern England* (Aldershot, Hampshire, UK; Burlington, VT: Ashgate, 2005); and Whitehead, *Women's Education in Early Modern Europe*.

51. *MM*, 136.

52. Examples would be the two court physicians to the Visconti lords of Milan: Antonius Guainerius, who dedicated his *Treatise on the Womb* to the Duke Filippo Maria, and Giovanni Matteo Ferrari da Grado, who wrote various gynecological *consilia*.

53. For a detailed comparison of the topics dealt with, readers are referred to the synoptic table in the appendix of Gabriella Zuccolin, "Nascere in latino ed in volgare: Tra la '*Practica*' e il 'De regimine,'"

first part of that chapter (sections 1–22, out of a total of 42), devoted to womb afflictions and menstrual disorders, are not included in the vernacular treatise at all, consistent with the author's stated intention to present medical precepts selectively:

> Here I also want to remind you of what is said about pregnancy: that it is a natural infirmity . . . when these conditions go beyond the natural, that is when they are not usual in nature, these conditions may become serious and require urgent care, and it will be necessary to consult a practicing physician, because this kind of treatment is no job for a woman or a layman.[54]

Savonarola makes the point about selectivity still more clearly at the beginning of the fourth chapter of Treatise Three of the *Mother's Manual*, devoted to the treatment of the most common childhood illnesses:

> If I wished to describe all the possible ailments that could afflict a child, I would need to translate all of medicine into the vernacular, and this would not only be impractical for women, but also for those who are illiterate. Moreover, it would be a huge burden for me; and besides, it might result in more deaths than recoveries, because novices would recklessly attempt to practice medicine solely by following recipes, as the charlatans do who do not fear God, not understanding the rules that teach how these recipes should be applied.[55]

It is because of Savonarola's deliberate selectivity that the Latin discussions in the *Practica* dealing mainly with the etiology of ailments, or with problems that were infrequently encountered, or that were not of a kind commonly experienced by pregnant women, are missing from the vernacular *Mother's Manual*. On the other hand, the *Mother's Manual* includes discussions completely absent from the *Practica* of such common ailments as nausea, vomiting, or constipation, or of matters that are not strictly medical. Evidently, then, the *Mother's Manual* is not a literal translation into the vernacular of chapter 21 of the Latin *Practica*. Not only is there a reworked organization of topics discussed, as these are changed in line

---

in Crisciani and Zuccolin, *Michele Savonarola*, 137–210. Here the indexes of the two sections of the *Canon* that Avicenna devotes to gynecology, obstetrics and pediatrics are set side by side with the index for chapter 21 of the *Practica* (which, in turn, uses the *Canon* as its main source) and the whole of the *DRP*.

54. *MM*, 136.

55. *MM*, 190–91. Here and henceforth, the term "recipe" in Savonarola's work refers to the components of a prescribed medication.

with the expectations of a variety of users and readers, but entirely new sections are included that relate to the sexual and moral conduct of lay readers.

But more significantly for the relationship between the Latin *Practica* and the vernacular *Mother's Manual*, demonstrating that the latter is not a mere simplification and translation of the former, is the absence in the *Practica* of any discussion of the care and upbringing of children—that is to say, of the whole third treatise of the *Mother's Manual*.[56] Lacking any counterpart in the *Practica*, this original treatise on childcare, pediatrics, and pedagogy finds its closest models in the Latinized works of the Arabic authors Rhazes, both the *De curis puerorum* (*On the Treatment of Small Children*) and the *Regimen infantis* (*On the Regimen of Children*) included in his *Book Dedicated to Al-Mansur*, and the ubiquitous Avicenna, who devoted to childcare and pediatrics one section of his *Canon*. Savonarola's announces at the end of chapter 21 of the *Practica* that he would be dealing with such subjects, but the promise is kept only in the *Mother's Manual*, written directly in the vernacular.[57] In doing so, he implicitly confirms the existence of a tight link between the two works, and illustrates the complementarity of Latin and vernacular traditions in Quattrocento Italian medicine.[58]

Indeed, Savonarola sometimes blurs the line distinguishing between the two. In the vernacular *Mother's Manual*, erudite quotes (in Latin), technical instructions, and medical rules that are set forth using a learned terminology without making much allowance for lay readers—rather, expecting them to be able to follow complex scientific arguments—are combined with a profusion of precepts with a moral-pedagogical intent, animated by a highly rhetorical and emotive tone. The narrative fabric of the book, with its interweaving of disseminative and

56. Features common to many vernacularizations of medical texts include the extension of the original Latin text, at times by a substantial amount, and a tendency to interpret the content while organizing it in a different manner. These characteristics are pointed out by Maria Luisa Altieri Biagi, "Forme della comunicazione scientifica," in Alberto Asor Rosa, *La letteratura italiana*, vol. 3: *Le forme del testo*, 2: *La prosa*, 891–947 (Turin: Einaudi, 1984); Luke Demaitre, "Medical Writing in Transition: Between Ars and Vulgus," *Early Science and Medicine* 3.2 (1998): 88–102; and Irma Taavitsainen and Päivi Pahta, "Vernacularisation of Medical Writing in English: A Corpus-Based Study of Scholasticism," *Early Science and Medicine* 3, no. 2 (1998): 157–85.

57. Savonarola, *Practica maior*, VI, ch. 21, rubr. 42 (fol. 274rb): *Et spero in sui clementia tractatum edere specialem de regimine infantium et cura suarum aegritudinum, pro quibus omnibus Deo semper laus* (And with his mercy I hope to write a separate treatise on the care of children and their ailments, for all of which may God be praised).

58. The originality of the treatise on the care and upbringing of children marks the *MM* as a didactic work, and confirms the existence of a specific form of literature related to medicine, designed to be read in the vernacular, addressing medical professionals, who may thereby extend their knowledge. Nonetheless, this aim coexists with the aim of dissemination, which is observed wherever Savonarola addresses non-academic readers. Indeed, the *MM* lies midway between a disseminative work and a technical handbook. Of course, as a vernacular work, it assumes different reading approaches from those typical of the professional use of a Latin *Practica*, meant to be read section by section.

high-level didactic aims, is meticulously manicured: the author accompanies the reader with paternal concern through the pages of the text, orchestrating his shifts from technical-didactic to moral-pedagogical content in a masterly fashion. Only a reading attentive to this "doubling" of genre, which translates into a plurality of intentions, audience, and language registers, permits the recognition of the work's full originality.[59]

When dealing with the *Mother's Manual*, therefore, it is necessary to transcend those arbitrary confines separating Latin from vernacular medical works, and, in line with recent scholarship on late medieval and Renaissance multilingualism in the sciences, to adopt a more flexible approach.[60]

Treatise One: From Conception to Pregnancy

The first treatise of the *Mother's Manual* is devoted to the many practical and theoretical problems connected with procreation and conception.[61] The ample space that Savonarola devotes to these subjects (five chapters, corresponding to over a third of the book), together with his substantial development of ideas that were implicit or even absent in his Latin *Practica*, testifies to their importance.

With a paternal stance, Savonarola dwells for entire pages on the right age to conceive, condemning the custom of marrying young people off too quickly, and warning that pregnancy is unadvisable at too early an age. This becomes an opportunity to introduce his theory of the progressive physical and spiritual decay of humankind:

> That it has become normal today for young boys to marry young girls is one of the reasons why our lives are so brief—as it has caused the decline of human nature from the greatness it had attained in the past, when people lived longer and healthier lives.[62]

This conviction is a key idea which frames the whole of the *Mother's Manual*: it appears not only at the beginning of this first treatise, but is taken up again at the end, to justify the need to start educating one's children properly and in a timely

---

59. See Altieri Biagi, "Forme della comunicazione scientifica," 897.

60. See Maria Luisa Altieri Biagi, *Guglielmo volgare: Studio sul lessico della medicina medievale* (Bologna: Forni, 1970); Maurizio Dardano, "I linguaggi scientifici," in *Storia della lingua italiana*, vol. 2: *Scritto e parlato*, ed. Luca Serianni and Pietro Trifone (Turin: Einaudi, 1994), 497–551; and Mirko Tavoni, "Il Quattrocento," in *Storia della lingua italiana: Il Quattrocento*, ed. Francesco Bruni (Bologna: il Mulino, 1992), 29–34.

61. Treatise One thus corresponds to sections 22–27 of chapter 21 of the *Practica maior*.

62. *MM*, 60.

fashion.[63] Savonarola specifies two reasons why humankind has been brought so low. The first explanation is astrological, but as humans cannot influence what is determined by heavenly bodies, the author omits any further discussion. The other reason, that of the sexual habits and life choices made by individuals and families, allows the physician to advise and interact with his readers, alerting them to the problems of premature conception. Having children before eighteen years of age in the case of women, and twenty-one in that of men, is unadvisable for physiological reasons: at those ages, the quality of both the male's sperm and the woman's menstrual blood is insufficient.

Especially interesting to modern readers, Savonarola also describes in explicitly socio-political and economic terms the consequences of early marriage. The social consequences that premature conception can have—the greater chance of the young mother dying or birthing weak or sick children—legitimize the intervention of the physician in a field which would normally lie totally outside his competency. Savonarola rails against the law that established the minimum age for marriage at twelve years of age for women, and fourteen for men, and he directly addresses the legislators, advising them to raise these age limits, giving the argument that such action, by promoting the greater health and strength of men of military age, would enhance the capacity of the state to defend itself in times of war. Only healthy individuals, neither too old nor too young, will give birth to healthy and capable defenders of their homeland.[64] Savonarola offers another non-medical argument in persuading fathers to prevent their daughters' early pregnancy, which may lead to an early death in childbirth: they would risk both cutting short the lives of the girls, and losing the money spent on their dowries.[65]

Savonarola regularly enjoins his readers to conduct their sexual behavior in line with Christian teachings, terrifying them with epithets meant to arouse the fear of God, while at the same time, in the guise of a confidant, offering guidance that might seem almost comic today. Non-procreative sex is for "scoundrels" (*ribaldoni*). A man who insists on lying with women, perhaps even with virgins, despite his advanced age, is nothing but a "wretched old man" (*vecchio sagurato*). Those who have sexual intercourse even though they are feverish are defined as "absent-minded beasts" (*smemorati bestiali*). Those who do so right after dinner should not be surprised "to wake up with the taste of rotten eggs in [their] mouth, a gaunt face, and bags under [their] eyes."[66] Anyone who has sexual relations while

---

63. "And if ever it were necessary to begin early, now is the time, because our generation has declined so much compared to the past, so that children who are three years old at the present are as astute as five- and six-year-olds used to be, and those who are five behave like seven- or eight-year-old children. We certainly see that life spans are getting shorter now than they were long ago." *MM*, 211.

64. *MM*, 70.

65. *MM*, 71.

66. *MM*, 73.

drunk is a "filthy ruffian" (*rofianazo lordo*), and irresponsible besides, because he might generate another drunkard. It is better to avoid having sex when it is too hot or too cold. Above all, men are cautioned to avoid any kind of contact with menstruating women, as this might generate leprous children or monsters—not to mention the still more serious possibility of unleashing the wrath of God (even the Old Testament states this prohibition).[67] Savonarola is realistic and knows how hard it is to behave correctly, and so employs proverbs and evocative images to persuade his readers.

In using this frank language in these passages, and employing a colloquial tone, Savonarola is pursuing a deliberate rhetorical and literary strategy. He is especially cautious when tackling the subject of procreation, aware that such discussion might offend the sensibilities of some readers. After explaining his use of the vernacular, he also defends himself from possible attacks on his standing as a good Christian; he takes refuge in the argument that the ultimate goal of his work is to serve the greater good, to which, by dealing when necessary with intimate and obscene matters in accessible language, he was even willing to sacrifice his professional reputation. At the same time, remarking on the levity with which he sometimes approached these topics, Savonarola sets his perceived reader at ease:

[I]n writing this, I have often burst out laughing, because these things can certainly sound humorous. But on the other hand, I have thought about the glorious fruit born of this act, and this is why I have not refrained from writing about it, and I have felt comfortable proceeding with my writing.[68]

When writing about "sordid topics" (*cosse sordide*), Savonarola continues, it is sometimes necessary to use "sordid words." Hinting at the sensuality, frivolity, and provocativeness typically attributed to women by a whole stream of literature—certainly not restricted to medical writings—he finally urges young women not to be ashamed of hearing things from his work that they would not be unwilling to do in the real world.

A scientific explanation of the mechanism of procreation follows, with a digression on the opposing theories of generation held by philosophers, on one hand, and physicians, on the other. Those theories revolve around one "great question": whether the woman's seed, or semen, as some supposed existed, has

---

67. Couples who repeat this behavior are actually reproached only in the third and last treatise: "This is why the Old Testament instructs *do not approach the menstruating woman*." *MM*, 192, quoting Ezekiel 18:6.

68. *MM*, 92.

any role in the procreation of the fetus.[69] The great attention Savonarola pays to this longstanding debate is significant, especially in light of the small space the author devotes to the same subject in his Latin *Practica*.[70] Although the practical nature of the *Mother's Manual* does not allow him to dwell too much on theoretical disputes, he cannot resist writing about a subject deeply interesting for both professional and lay readers, and to illustrate the debate with statements inherited from ancient discussions as well as more recent accounts.[71] His elucidation of the embryological doctrines from the medical and philosophical standpoints is swift but comprehensive. What role can female seed have in conception if trustworthy mothers declare that they have never felt anything akin to the emission of such a secretion during the sexual act, and since it seems obvious that "it is possible for a woman to get pregnant without feeling any pleasure"?[72] How then can one explain that some children look like their mothers? And why do bastards sometimes look more like their putative fathers than their real ones?

Savonarola plainly sets out the divergent Aristotelian and Hippocratic-Galenic positions with regard to procreation while also tending, as is typical of fifteenth-century medicine, to re-evaluate the utility of Galenism and to abandon overly rigid Aristotelian doctrinal positions.[73] He clearly presents the threefold

69. *MM*, 90. On the theme of generation and conception, the medieval world inherited from antiquity two conflicting schools of thought. In the revised Arabic version of this theory, Avicenna—while maintaining an Aristotelian framework—manages to reconcile the Hippocratic-Galenic doctrine (which holds that the so-called female seed, or semen, plays an active role in generation) with the Aristotelian theory (which assigns an active and formal role to the male semen only, while women's menstrual matter plays a passive role).

70. See *Practica maior*, VI, ch. 21, rubr. 22 (fol. 262vb): *nec in hac magna discordia inter philosophos et medicos me hic non interpono, tum quia inutilis esset nostro proposito haec disceptatio, tum quia non sum tanti ut de his iudicium faciam aliud ab eo, quod visum est magno medico Galieno et sequacibus* (nor so I want to be involved in this great controversy between philosophers and physicians, both because this digression would be useless for our purpose, and because I am not able to make a judgment different from the opinion of the great physician Galen and his followers).

71. How should one explain the case reported by Averroes concerning those young girls who became pregnant while bathing in a place where some boys had previously been disporting themselves? What about the case, reported by Gregory, concerning the mother who was made pregnant by her own little son? Should we believe Marsilio Santasofia, who assures us he has seen a little girl of only eight years of age pregnant? Then, what about Niccolò Pallavicini, a nobleman one hundred years old who made his wife pregnant, and it was, moreover, a boy child? See, e.g., *MM*, 64.

72. *MM*, 66.

73. When explaining the theory of embryology according to Aristotle, Savonarola specifies more than once that he is "speaking according to the philosophers"; he then explains the medical theories regarding this subject clearly and convincingly, stressing that we should consider "the teachings of doctors to be for the most part true and rarely fallacious." *MM*, 62.

function of the supposed female sperm,[74] maintaining that only if the woman, as well as the man, is emotionally involved in the sexual act can it lead to a successful conception. At this point, the author introduces a guide to sexual intercourse, urging that attention must be paid to the woman's timings, holding that the expulsion of her seed, if not strictly necessary to conception, is nonetheless highly desirable to achieve pregnancy.[75] Even if erotic advice was not unheard of in medical literature, the advice given in the *Mother's Manual* seems not to be intended only to educate physicians and obstetricians.[76]

Another recurrent theme is the need to condition women's (and men's) imagination about the fetus, supported by a famous passage from Avicenna, which Savonarola faithfully translates without acknowledging him, thus mixing yet another source into his vernacular account.[77] The author then details the early phases of the development of the embryo. Brief definitions in Latin, taken word

74. These functions are: 1. to participate in the conception; 2. to allow a better reception of the male sperm, and 3. to give pleasure to the woman. Savonarola also deals here with the Avicennian distinction between menstrual blood, female seed and another lubricating fluid: *alguady*. Such distinction is totally absent from the *Practica*, where this term does not appear even once, nor is any detectable effort on the author's part to try to clarify the thinking on this point.

75. "The couple should touch one another, especially the man should touch the woman, touching her and rubbing her pudenda with his fingers: because this is the exterior place where a woman receives the most pleasure, because of its proximity to the neck of the uterus, where women achieve great pleasure; and as a result of this rubbing, women are more easily stimulated to spermatize. Afterwards, they should continue to delay intercourse, and he should touch with his hands her breasts and lightly rub her nipples, kissing her cheeks, mouth, and other parts, and he should touch her especially the area under her abdomen, while bringing closer his penis, but not penetrating her just yet, continuing to hold off. All of these things should be done to stimulate the woman to spermatize." *MM*, 91.

76. As Claude Thomasset reminds us, between the thirteenth and fourteenth centuries in particular "si produce uno sviluppo considerevole dell'arte erotica." Thomasset, "La natura della donna," in *Storia delle donne in Occidente: Il Medioevo*, ed. Christiane Klapisch-Zuber (Bari: Laterza, 1994), 56–87. Even if they cannot be considered organic monographic treatises, it is worth remembering that Mondino dei Liucci wrote some *Consigli per restare incinte* (*Advice on How To Get Pregnant*) in the vernacular, and Marsilio Santasofia composed a *Consiglio per generar fiole* (*Advice on Conceiving Girls*). See Aldo Pazzini, *Crestomazia della letteratura medica in volgare dei due primi secoli della lingua* (Rome: Università degli studi di Roma, Scuola di perfezionamento in storia della medicina, 1971), 14. These works could also be considered in the light of the commentaries on sections of Avicenna's *Canon* by the same authors; see Romana Martorelli Vico's edition of Mondino dei Liucci, *Expositio super capitulum de generatione embrionis canonis Avicennae cum quibusdam quaestionibus* (Rome: Istituto storico italiano per il Medioevo, 1993), and Tiziana Pesenti Marangon, *Marsilio Santasofia tra corti e università: La carriera di un "monarcha medicinae" del Trecento* (Treviso: Antilia, 2003).

77. Avicenna, *Liber de anima*, in the edition of Simone Van Riet: *Liber de anima, seu Sextus de naturalibus: Édition critique de la traduction latine médiévale*, vol. 2 (IV–V) (Louvain: Éditions Orientalistes; Leiden: Brill, 1968), 64. This passage about the power of the imagination gives the example of the man who calmly walks along a narrow beam if it is laid on the ground, whereas if it is suspended over deep waters and he thinks he is going to fall, he will. See also *MM*, 91.

for word from the corresponding section of the *Practica maior*,[78] serve to specify the differences between *conception, generation* and *impregnation*, and clarify the etymology and meaning of the words *embryo, infant, secundine, pregnant* and *gravid*.[79] Yet another Latin quotation, one absent from the *Practica*, is taken from Galen's *On Semen*, and serves to justify the complex description of three blisters, which would become the heart, the brain and the liver of the future individual.[80] Also absent from the *Practica*, not surprisingly, is the question of how the Virgin Mary became pregnant with the Son of God—a matter Savonarola declares he has included particularly to satisfy the curiosity of devout readers.[81]

Savonarola then presents prevailing theories of astral influence as a cause of and condition for conception, and of planetary movements on the development of the fetus.[82] At this point, he turns quickly to what actions men and women must take to attain a successful pregnancy: that is, to conceive a healthy child, a boy if possible, and to recognize whether the desired pregnancy has been achieved. Here, as he begins the book's most practical part, the addressee also seems to change: no longer does Savonarola write only for the young husband or his noble partner (despite his declaration that he is writing precisely so that the man is not deceived by his partner), but also for the professional physician, and, through him, the midwife. Indeed, the concise list of signs of a cold or hot womb, the nine signs of impregnation, the nine signs of a dead fetus, and the notes on the molar pregnancy with which the first treatise of the *Mother's Manual* ends mirror exactly the contents of the Latin *Practica*. In contrast, those sections of the *Practica*

78. See *Practica maior*, VI, ch. 21, rubr. 22 (fol. 262vb).

79. *MM*, 77–78.

80. *MM*, 84.

81. *MM*, 87–88. The physician's response is the traditional one, which asserts that the ultra-pure blood of the Virgin Mary provided the matter needed for the fetus, and that the Holy Spirit replaced the male seed's *virtus informativa*, or "informing power." For a detailed examination of this topic, see Maaike Van der Lugt, *Le ver, le démon et la Vierge: Les théories médiévales de la génération extraordinaire: Une étude sur les rapports entre théologie, philosophie naturelle et médecine* (Paris: Les Belles Lettres, 2004).

82. *MM*, 88–89. On planetary influences over the stages of gestation, and particularly on the theory about the likely death of the eight-month child, which falls under the rule of cold and dry Saturn (whereas the seven-month child, ruled by the Moon, can often survive), see Charles S. F. Burnett, "The Planets and the Development of the Embryo," in *The Human Embryo: Aristotle and the Arabic and European Traditions*, ed. Gordon R. Dunstan (Exeter: University of Exeter Press, 1990), 95–112; Ann E. Hanson, "The Eight Month's Child and the Etiquette of Birth: Obsit Omen!" *Bulletin of the History of Medicine* 61 (1987): 589–602; and Liana Saif, "The Universe and the Womb: Generation, Conception, and the Stars in Islamic Medieval Astrological and Medical Texts," *Journal of Arabic and Islamic Studies* 16 (2016): 181–98. The earliest account of astral influences over fetal development in the Western Middle Ages is provided by Constantinus Africanus (eleventh century), who relied on Arabic sources. The *Prose Salernitan Questions* repeated that account, which then became widely held throughout the Middle Ages and popularized by such works as Vincent de Beauvais' *Speculum naturale* and *De secretis mulierum* by Ps.-Albert the Great.

examining the causes of sterility, of superimpregnation, and of multiple births, all matters specifically the concern of the professional physician, are not included in the vernacular *Mother's Manual*, where they are replaced by brief comments.[83]

Furthermore, while omitting from the *Mother's Manual* some discussions found in the *Practica*, Savonarola also adds others to the former that are not included in the latter, and fundamentally rearranges the order of topics treated. Addressing himself directly to the citizens of Ferrara, he shows his familiarity with their eating habits and their most common illnesses, and offers little slices of everyday life, as well as autobiographical anecdotes that witness his strong professional involvement with the city in which he had then been living for twenty years. Showing his awareness of the social environment, as well, Savonarola's recipes for medications and the ingredients that he recommends are differentiated according to social status, between those conceived for *poverete* (poor women) and those suitable for nobles.

Some examples follow of the rearrangement of topics, and the selection of themes, in the vernacular *Mother's Manual* relative to the Latin *Practica*. The signs that reveal whether a woman is actually pregnant as presented in the *Mother's Manual* follow the paragraph on *signa* ("signs") at section 22 of the Latin chapter, but the *a capite ad calcem* ("from head to toe") order in which they are given in the *Practica* is abandoned in the *Manual*. In the Latin version, the first thing considered is the expectant woman's headaches, problems with the sight, pulsations of the neck, the enlargement of the breasts, and the nausea typical of the early period of pregnancy. Only later does Savonarola consider the retention of menstrual blood, the possible perception of the simultaneous emission of male and female seed, the closing of the neck of the womb that the obstetrician can verify manually, and the quality of urine, which he analyzes in great detail.[84] In the *Mother's Manual*, instead, the symptoms are presented in the order of how obvious and important they are or, in effect, in chronological order of appearance—an arrangement harder to remember, perhaps, but intuitively much easier to understand. The first sign: upon paying a little attention, both partners will feel that they have emitted their respective semen simultaneously; the second sign is the retention of menstrual blood; the third, which according to Galen is un-

---

83. Although the causes of multiple births are not explained in full, Savonarola blames women for not avoiding sexual intercourse when already pregnant, which was thought to be such a cause, and blames them once again using the argument of pleasure—that is, that the sensation of pleasure a woman feels in intercourse results in increased coital movements and in the opening of the already pregnant womb, which should remain closed. He makes this argument even though, as he admits, women might be forced to lie with their husbands. The effect of these statements was to cast a much greater moral and biological responsibility for twinning on women. On medical theories and moral implications connected to twin births in the Middle Ages, see Gabriella Zuccolin, *I gemelli nel Medioevo: Questioni filosofiche, mediche e teologiche* (Pavia: Ibis, 2019).

84. *Practica maior*, VI, ch. 21, rubr. 22 (fol. 263vb).

mistakable, is the closing of the neck of the womb. Other symptoms follow, and particular stress is placed on the instruction that the expectant mother should refrain from coitus. After discussing the "internal" signs of pregnancy, Savonarola deals with the "external" ones, a distinction absent from the *Practica*: here he notes the possibility of diagnosing pregnancy by examining the urine, and suggests recipes, this time in the vernacular, which can be used to confirm the diagnosis.[85]

The first treatise of the *Mother's Manual* ends with notes on molar pregnancies and on the method of determining if the fetus in the womb is dead. The physician does not discuss the causes of these accidents, nor does he assign specific sections to these topics. Nonetheless, given the practical nature of this part of the *Mother's Manual*, and the importance of detecting fetal deaths quickly so as to save the mother, Savonarola does include the list of symptoms that announce that these phenomena have occurred.

Treatise Two: From Pregnancy to Childbirth

The first chapter of the second treatise, taking up one-third of the whole, and entitled "On the regimen of pregnant women with regard to the six non-naturals," offers guidelines for diet, exercise, and sexual practices to be followed during pregnancy.[86] Prescriptions are given both in Latin and in the vernacular, and are divided into those for the rich, who can "afford the expense," and those for the poor. Despite the attention paid to poor and peasant women (*poverete* and *rusticane*), the intended addressees of the regimen are rather the noble court ladies and the rich wives of the citizens of Ferrara with whom Savonarola deals with on a daily basis.[87] The pregnant woman is advised to eat at least three times a day, and the foods suggested, including capons, pheasant, partridge and other luxury meats, are the most expensive on the market.[88] Forgetting for a moment

---

85. *MM*, 95–99.

86. The corresponding section in the *Practica*, *De regimine pregnantium et earum appetitu*, is no more than two columns long and is organized in a very different way. See *Practica maior*, VI, ch. 21, rubr. 28 (fols. 269vb-270ra).

87. An example of these elite women is the Marchioness of Monferrato, who used to regularly lose her baby during the fifth month of pregnancy due to her excessive idleness (*MM*, 121–22). In the following chapter, Savonarola addresses rich and "delicate" women, who risk having a very painful delivery because they continuously use "fragrant things by mouth"—a comment following the line that the uterus is naturally attracted by fragrances: "O rich and refined *frontosa*, know that the use of fragrant things by mouth makes your delivery difficult, because the womb is naturally attracted to good odors, and draws itself upwards when these are used" (*MM*, 150). Later, he is careful to exclude noble ladies (*madone segnoresse*) from his reproval of those who do heavy work although childbirth is imminent (*MM*, 148).

88. "Therefore you, *frontosa*, who are rich and privileged, when you are pregnant, you should seek such meats and other foods that generate good blood." *MM*, 111.

the true social condition of most of his fellow citizens, Savonarola comments ironically: "O *frontosa*, who would not want to get pregnant and be treated to such dishes?"—and is bold enough to suggest that meats less suitable for the delicate stomachs of pregnant women should be gifted to the physician.[89] Savonarola also repeats the amusing anecdote regarding the widespread consumption in Ferrara of oysters, a well-known aphrodisiac, and the clever response he gave to Marquis Niccolò who asked him mischievously how useful they were.[90]

Savonarola's classification of what the expectant mother may and may not eat and drink follows the pattern used in the *Libreto de tute le cosse che se magnano comunamente* (*Small Book on All Things Commonly Eaten*), the book on dietetics he had written for Borso of Este.[91] To drive home the dangers of eating certain foods, Savonarola invokes Avicenna, quoting directly in Latin, and calls repeatedly for moderation.

Having dealt with food and drink, Savonarola moves onto the other five so-called non-naturals: exercise and rest, including bathing; sleeping and waking; excretion and repletion, this last section providing advice on "evacuation by medicine, by mouth, by clyster [enema], or by bloodletting," and the strong interdiction of sexual intercourse. The list ends with some notes on the emotional state of the pregnant woman,[92] and advice on the quality of air and places. In the last words of the chapter, Savonarola expresses his compassion for pregnant women who have to do heavy work while fasting, or bent over while sweeping churches or suffering in the fields under the summer sun—and who in doing so risk committing the mortal sin of miscarrying "by your own negligence":[93] a miscarriage that

89. "You may eat quail, but in small amounts and seldom. Quail meat is difficult to digest and it makes the pregnant woman susceptible to fever; rather, when you have some quail, repay your physician by sending him some as a gift." *MM*, 111.

90. "Now, there are some idiots who like this type of seafood, especially oysters, claiming that they keep their cocks hard when they need to be. O stupid fools! Oysters may make your poles perk up, but they don't bring with them the flour to bake the bread. I will recall here what I said to Marquis Niccolò on this subject when he asked me about oysters, knowing well the reason for his question. I responded to him: 'an oyster is a baker who orders others to bake bread, but if there is no flour, the order is placed in vain.' You know what I mean, frontoso." *MM*, 112.

91. *Libreto de tute le cosse che se magnano comunamente*: See *Works by Michele Savonarola*, #12. The corresponding list of forbidden and recommended foods in the *Practica* is instead very limited. The following sections in the *Mother's Manual* do not appear in the Latin treatise: on bread; on the meat of quadrupeds and bipeds; on fish, crustaceans and seafood; on fruit, roots, seeds, types of grain, leafy vegetables, *agrumi* (that is, garlic, onions, leeks, shallots); on milk and cheeses; on oil and animal fats; on spices, and, to top it all off, on honey and sugar. *MM*, 109–19.

92. "It is best if the pregnant woman stay clear from anger, deep sadness, fear, and similar emotions, especially in the first month, because the fetus can be debilitated through her weakened spirits caused by fear, anguish, or sadness." *MM*, 125.

93. "O impoverished pregnant *frontosa*, who, in the country, must bear the sun and the summer heat, I have great compassion for you. I remind you of these things for your benefit, so that you may take care

would endanger the body and soul not only of the woman but also of the child, a terrible crime for which they would have to answer on Judgment Day.[94]

The second chapter of Treatise Two of the *Mother's Manual*, *Of the conditions or states common to pregnant women*, divided into fifteen subsections, corresponds to thirteen sections of the *Practica*.[95] The comparison between the two presentations is complex, since Savonarola utilizes a greater variety of communicative techniques in the vernacular text than in the Latin, which is characterized by communicative linearity, and chooses different topics and orders the subject matter differently in the two works. As the content of this chapter is reviewed, the treatment of material in the *Mother's Manual* will be related to corresponding sections of the *Practica*.

The second chapter presents the essential obstetrical information that parturient mothers and midwives need to know.[96] Here Savonarola provides women and midwives with the necessary instruction to help the mother while she is giving birth. But the physician must always be in charge, in order to prevent unskilled women or empirics lacking a thorough doctrinal background from endangering the lives of the future mothers, perhaps by using medicines that are too strong, or carrying out difficult operations beyond their expertise. As before, Savonarola omits some important information, devoting most of the discussion to those accidents that are defined as natural and common to many pregnancies, pregnancy

---

of yourself as best you can, because it is certainly a great sin to miscarry by your own negligence, and if this occurs, you may certainly expect punishment and retribution." *MM*, 126. And a few lines earlier: "This is why, *frontosa*, you who so devoutly bend down each day to sweep the church floor, beware of fasting too often when pregnant, and especially from the end of the third to the ninth month, because the more the fetus grows, the more it wants to eat; and let the friars say what they will, they who often preach without any discernment." *MM*, 123.

94. In the section regarding precautions to take against miscarriage Savonarola writes: "Therefore, be very careful, *frontosa*, not to allow yourself to have a miscarriage through your carelessness. Because if this happens, then two souls die together, yours and that of your child, and God will ask you for an explanation on the day of judgment. If you are found guilty, you may then expect great punishment for your soul beyond anything you have received on earth." *MM*, 139. Attention to the woman's diet and overall health even when the child is born justifies a further reference to Judgment Day, on which the nursing mother will be held responsible for the death or any illnesses of her child due to her negligence in feeding: "O *frontosa* who pays no attention to these things, you must remember that when you are the cause of great harm to your child and even his death, as is often the case, you will be held responsible on Judgment Day. Therefore, *frontosa*, be careful, and do what you can to not cause your child such harm, and such harm to yourself, insofar as you are responsible for both your own soul and body, and your child's." *MM*, 193.

95. See *MM*, 126–63; *Practica maior*, VI, ch. 21, rubr. 29–41 (fols. 270r–274r).

96. The fifteenth subsection deals with the loss of appetite of the pregnant woman, gassiness, nausea and vomiting, heart palpitations, blood discharges, miscarriage prevention, constipation and suffocation, labor and birth, and finally with some common postpartum complications, like hemorrhages and fever.

itself being defined as a natural condition (*infirmità naturale*). Not only do pregnant mothers have a disordered appetite, craving or rejecting certain foods, but few expectant mothers avoid chronic vomiting, especially during the first months of pregnancy—a disorder described in a mere twelve lines of the Latin *Practica*, but which in the *Mother's Manual* merits a long and thorough explanation. It is in this section that the clinical history is told of Savonarola's daughter-in-law,[97] and the special technique is described that Giacomo della Torre used to cause therapeutic vomiting.[98] It also supplies a list of the injurious secondary effects that vomiting may have, and details ways to protect the patient from these: by binding one's eyes, eating cooked apple, chewing mint, and other remedies.[99]

In the section of the *Mother's Manual* on the prevention of miscarriage, Savonarola gives as the first cause of a spontaneous abortion the taking of overly strong medicines, and as the second, a bad constitution of the uterus. He omits from the vernacular work, understandably, a discussion of the right times for bloodletting the pregnant woman and the ways this should be carried out. As phlebotomy could only be safely performed by an expert physician, a discussion of that procedure would have no place in the *Mother's Manual*. Notwithstanding that, Savonarola cannot help but include a hint to a piece of information so important as the cause of the successful outcome of the pregnancies of the (previously) unfortunate Marchioness of Monferrato, who used to regularly lose her babies during the fifth month.[100] It was precisely thanks to bloodletting that the noblewoman at last gave birth to those children from whom "descends the present-day Marquis of Monferrato."[101]

97. "My daughter-in-law in numerous pregnancies has been variously afflicted. In some pregnancies, she was vomiting until her second month, at times until her third month, at times until her last month, and in her last birth, even though she was carrying a boy, she was vomiting even on the day of her labor." *MM*, 133.

98. "These women can try to vomit by drinking a large carafe of sweet wine all at once—as prescribed by Giacomo da Forlì, my mentor, who reigns sovereign over the discipline of medicine." *MM*, 135.

99. A question (dense with practical consequences) that is not even raised in the *Practica* provides an opportunity in the *Mother's Manual* to resolve a long-debated issue: that is, understanding why and to what extent "vomiting is beneficial for pregnant women." *MM*, 134–39.

100. See note 87 on page 30 of this Introduction and *MM*, 121–22 and 140.

101. *MM*, 121 and 140. This same information appears in the corresponding section of the Latin *Practica*; see *Practica maior*, VI, ch. 21, rubr. 30 (fol. 270va): *Et credo quod domina Marchionissa de Monte ferrato ob hanc causam abortiebatur. Et quidam medicus cognoscens causam phlebotomavit et foetus ad lucem venit, ante autem semper faciebat mortuos, et sic filiis carebat* (And I believe the Marchioness of Monferrato used to miscarry for this reason. And a certain physician, knowing this reason, drew out her blood and she gave birth to a child, whereas before she always used to miscarry and had no children). In rubric 30 of the Latin chapter 21 alone, this therapeutic technique is suggested six times, whereas there are no such discussions in the *Mother's Manual*.

In the same way, Savonarola restricts the discussion of the preternatural causes of miscarriage to professional physicians, including it only in the *Practica*. He does, however, make the expectant woman knowledgeble (*docta*)—and with her, other nonprofessionals, including surgeons, empirics, and midwives, as well as kinsmen and nobles, both male and female—of the *signa* of miscarriage, which announce the possibility of an untimely end to the pregnancy. Savonarola is also reticent in the *Mother's Manual* regarding the issue of the dead fetus, which is dealt with fully in the *Practica*'s section 41, *On the regimen of the dead fetus*. He writes in his conclusion to the paragraph in the *Mother's Manual* devoted to the delivery:

> Now, I have said "if the fetus is alive", because when it is dead, labor becomes even more difficult, . . . and often a surgeon must pull out the fetus using cutting tools and hooks. The birthing attendant can at first be of great assistance, of course, keeping the parturient upright. . . . However, if the attendant's hands, and the lavage, and the greasing or the smearing, do not help, then it is necessary to turn to the practicing physician.[102]

With the same circumspection as in the section on the prevention of miscarriage, although Savonarola does not include in the *Mother's Manual* any discussion of the cause of infant stillbirths, he scrupulously reports the nine signs of the dead fetus, so that even without the assistance of an expert physician, birth attendants may recognize the dreadful thing that has happened.[103]

In a society in which women were effectively abandoned to their own devices at the delivery of an infant, it was absolutely necessary to provide clear rules to follow. That necessity explains the high level of detail in the sections on labor, childbirth, and the expulsion of the afterbirth which constitute the heart of the obstetrical instruction Savonarola provides in the *Mother's Manual*. Savonarola describes a birthing-chair designed to facilitate parturition, and drew it in the margins of the original manuscript of the work, unfortunately lost.[104]

---

102. *MM*, 159. A more detailed discussion of removal of the dead fetus is found in *De regimine foetus mortui* in the *Practica maior*, VI, ch. 21, rubr. 41 (fol. 274ra), altough, even in the discussion of this topic in Latin, Savonarola states that he omits many particular extraction techniques, since they are surgical.

103. The list is given at the end of chapter 5 of Treatise One, after the more reassuring enumeration of *signa* indicating pregnancy and the possible sex of the baby. See *MM*, 107.

104. The sketch of the chair is missing in all the three extant manuscript copies of the *DRP*. Its textual description does not coincide with the drawing of the primitive chair (or better, of the "Y" shaped birthing stool) printed in some editions of the *Practica maior* (e.g., Venice, 1547 and 1559; the editions of 1486, 1497 and 1561 do not present any drawing), and it resembles most the kind of birthing chair printed and described in Rösslin's *Rosegarden*. See *MM*, Figures 1 and 2 at 154.

Having dealt with conditions of pregnancy, Savonarola proceeds to discuss the delivery of the infant and care of the mother. The apparent symmetry between the section devoted to the care of postpartum fever in the *Mother's Manual* and rubric 36 of chapter 21 in the Latin *Practica*, titled *De regimine febrium earum* (*On the Regimen of Their Fevers*), is deceptive, resting only on a similarity of headings. Fevers, which are discussed in a medical genre of practical monographs—of which Savonarola's own *Practica canonica de febribus* (*Canonical Practice on Fevers*) is one—should always be treated solely by the physician, if and when they need to be treated. The only discussion of postpartum fever in the *Mother's Manual*, in contrast, is the recommendation to seek the services of a professional as soon as the temperature rises inordinately, or remains high after the normal few days of post-delivery fever, one reason being, as Savonarola points out, that bloodletting may be required.[105] Indirectly confirming what was said earlier regarding phlebotomy (although in this case the veins from which blood should be let are indicated), the instruction is unequivocal that no one other than the physician can decide whether or not to proceed with this treatment.[106]

The brief discussion in the *Mother's Manual* of the accident classified as number fifteen (*Treatment for the dislocation of the sacrum*) deserves a special note, as no counterpart for this discussion is found either in Savonarola's *Practica* or in Avicenna's *Canon*. In this case, the vernacular treatise has been extended beyond what is stated in Latin medical texts, owing to Savonarola's clinical experience occurring some time after he wrote the *Practica* (by 1446) but before he wrote the *Mother's Manual* (by 1460). He could hardly pass up on an opportunity to document one of his own clinical successes![107]

Returning to the delivery itself, Savonarola lists eight general reasons for a difficult delivery, expounding each one in detail:

[F]irst, labor may be difficult because of the pregnant woman; second, because of the fetus; third, because of the uterus; fourth, because of the afterbirth; fifth, because of the organs near the uterus; sixth,

105. "At times the parturient may come down with a fever. But if this is the case, her care should be left to the physician, especially when her fever lasts long or when it is high. . . . And the cure is to bleed the woman from the large veins in her legs or from under her knees. Go to the physician for this treatment." *MM*, 162.

106. In the Latin *Practica*, in contrast, the statement is made first and foremost that bloodletting is advisable, and where to let the blood and why; there follows a list of all the substances and compounds which can help to bring down the temperature. See *Practica maior*, VI, ch. 21, rubr. 36 (273vb).

107. "Sometimes after labor a woman's sacrum [the bone at the base of her spine connecting to the pelvis] does not return completely to the joint, making her cry constantly. I was called to deal with such a case, and investigating the cause of the pain, I made the following correct judgment: I had the midwife relocate the bone with her hands, and the pain ceased immediately. Therefore, *frontosa* midwife, pay attention and learn about this kind of relocation, and make note of it." *MM*, 163.

because of the improper hour; seventh, because of the fault of the midwife, that is, the birth attendant; and eighth, from any other exterior cause, such as, for example because of the cold or something similar.[108]

As Savonarola advises mothers and midwives, he pays great attention to the atmosphere of solidarity and trust that must be created during the delicate time of delivery. He writes, for instance, of the comfort that should be offered the mother in childbirth:

> If she is weak and sickly, her expelling power is weakened. If it is her first birth, or if she is frightened and has lost her vigor and courage, her expelling power may also be weakened. This is why the women by her side should comfort her and give her courage.[109]

He also expresses concern for his readers, sometimes giving them some respite from the most technical passages, and sometimes persuading them to read attentively, as what they will learn will benefit them:

> It seems to me, *frontosa*, that you must be very eager to learn about this, and that you are desirous to be instructed on these things more than others, for these are the most important things for a pregnant woman to know, that is, all the things that will relieve her anxiety and bring her ease. This is why I want to make sure that I am clear and thorough in this chapter above all others, and I hope also to include advice here for pregnant women that is very useful and agreeable and likely to bring them great satisfaction. [110]

Savonarola presents a heartwarming image in these pages of a woman devoting all her thoughts to her child: she is a mother *zilosa dil feto suo*, a phrase that can be translated as "concerned about," or "zealous for," or "enthusiastic for her fetus."[111] His words attest to the close attention he pays to women's concerns, and show him to be an affectionate, fatherly physician, who reaches out to his young fellow citizens. One example: when he imagines a woman asking him a more than justified question (why has nature given so much pleasure to the man in impregnating and conceiving, and so much pain to the woman in giving birth?),

108. *MM*, 146.

109. *MM*, 146.

110. *MM*, 146.

111. *MM*, 86.

he has no answer to give, but still expresses his full solidarity.[112] Another: when he advises women in labor to scream and shout to lend a bit of drama to the act of delivering their child, even when unnecessary, solely for the benefit of the men of the household, who might treat their wives better in recognition of all their suffering.[113]

The third and last chapter of Treatise Two, *On the regimen of the woman who has given birth*,[114] consists of only a few pages in which Savonarola directly addresses the midwife, delegating to her the task of caring for the new mother, who is still weak and convalescent. The midwife should see that the mother is not overfed, and should carefully watch over every aspect of her life—a concept Savonarola expresses by means of an adroit simile: "Therefore, the wisdom of the midwife should be helmsman of this vessel, at times raising and at times lowering the steering arm."[115]

Treatise Three: From Birth to Childcare

Treatise Three on pediatrics and pedagogy (which is divided into five highly detailed chapters) can be considered almost a separate work from the first two treatises of the *Mother's Manual*, and it has attracted the interest of those historians of medicine and science who specialize in the history of pediatrics.[116] The first three of these chapters, dealing with childcare and devoted primarily to training

112. "And holding the opinion that man experiences greater pleasure in generation than woman . . . , I leave that question unanswered, so that the audience may have reason to dispute among themselves. Yet it seems that God has punished women much more than men, for God said to Eve *you will bear your children in pain*, because since God created woman more fragile than man, sin should not be imputed less to man than to woman." *MM*, 150–51.

113. "And know, *frontosa*, that screaming loudly in such a situation is very beneficial to you, which is why Avicenna says "do let her cry out"; and even if it does not hurt so much, I recommend that you scream loudly, so that your pain is believed, your husband and family will feel compassion for you, lighting a great fire for you, and serving you capons, sweets, and excellent wines." *MM*, 156.

114. *MM*, 163–65.

115. *MM*, 164. In contrast, in the last part of the more somber and technical Latin chapter bearing the same title, *De regimine enixae*, in the *Practica maior*, VI, ch. 21, rubr. 42 (fol. 274rb), the author describes all the symptoms pointing to an imminent postpartum death.

116. See the fundamental study by Philippe Ariès of the medieval child as a historical and social subject: *L'enfant et la vie familiale sous l'ancien régime* (Paris: Plon, 1960; rev. ed. Paris: Éditions du Seuil, 1973); English translation by Robert Baldick, *Centuries of Childhood: A Social History of Family Life* (New York: Alfred A. Knopf, 1962). For an overview of the numerous lines of subsequent research on that subject, see King, "Concepts of Childhood." On Quattrocento northern Italy in particular, see Giiuliana Albini, "I bambini nella società lombarda del Quattrocento: Una realtà ignorata o protetta?" *Nuova rivista storica* 68 (1984): 611–38. For medieval medical texts containing notes on childcare, see Luke Demaitre, "The Idea of Childhood and Child Care in Medical Writings of the Middle Ages," *Journal of Psychohistory* 4 (1977): 461–90; Gualdo, "La lingua della pediatria"; Danielle Jacquart,

midwives, are entitled *What the midwife should do with the newborn child*; *On the regimen of children regarding the six non-naturals*; and *Of the reduced production of milk and its treatment*.[117] The fourth chapter, *On the treatment of small children*, is a self-standing section on pediatrics, in which childhood diseases are listed following the classical order *a capite ad calcem* (from head to toe).[118] The fifth and last chapter, *On how to care for the well-being of the soul and body of the child*,[119] is a digest of moral and pedagogical teachings, not only for children, but also for mothers and, especially, fathers, expounding their moral and ethical duties as Christians, and detailing their most serious educational mistakes. This last section in particular marks a shift in the *Mother's Manual* from a didactic and specialist stance to a more moralistic and prescriptive one. Savonarola the physician alternates with Savonarola the pedagogue: the former intent on initiating midwives in the rudiments of practical medicine, and the latter, on promoting Christian principles. The dialectic of these two voices invites the interpretation of the treatise on two different levels. This analysis will work backwards, starting with the ethical and pedagogical discussion appearing mostly in the fifth chapter. The pedagogical chapter in this third treatise can be set within that surge of humanistic awareness in pedagogy mentioned earlier, deriving from the rediscovery of Quintilian's innovative teachings and the educational theories that were developed at the same time by thinkers including Vittorino da Feltre, Pier Paolo Vergerio and, in Ferrara itself, Guarino Veronese. In Savonarola's instructions are found clear echoes of the attention to teaching principles based on persuasion, dialogue, and the knowledge of Scripture that characterize the humanists' works.[120] Savonarola had written on this subject before, as he informs us in the *Mother's Manual*, speaking of a pedagogical treatise of which nothing was known up to now.[121] Furthermore, the moral advice he gives to fathers, mothers, teachers,

---

"Naissance d'une 'pédiatrie' en milieu de cour," *Micrologus* 16 (2008): 271–94; and Silvia Nagel, "*Puer e pueritia* nella letteratura medica del XIII secolo," *Quaderni Fondazione Feltrinelli* 23 (1983): 87–107.

117. *MM*, 165, 173, and 187.

118. *MM*, 190.

119. *MM*, 211.

120. Vergerio, in his *De ingenuis moribus* (1400), had stressed the importance of teaching children not to talk too much; Guarino recommended moderating use of the spoken word in his notes on teaching, which were collected by his son and published in the mid-fifteenth century under the title *De ordine docendi ac studendi*. On this topic, see Luigi Piacente's edition of Battista Guarini, *La didattica del greco e del latino: De ordine docendi ac studendi e altri scritti* (Bari: Edipuglia, 2002).

121. "Children must, therefore, be pushed to acquire good habits, so that they can acquire good virtues, something that everybody can acquire and make his own, as I have demonstrated in that little book *De non dictandis filiis*." *MM*, 215. Cited in *Works by Michele Savonarola*, #27. See Pesenti, "Michele Savonarola a Padova," 50, and Samaritani, "Michele Savonarola riformatore cattolico," 59. For my hypothesis on the exact title of this lost work, see *MM*, 215, note 319.

nursemaids, and young children in the *Mother's Manual* is consistent with those of his writings of a specifically moral, religious and devotional nature, such as the *Confessionali* (*Handbooks for Confession*) I and II, *De cura languoris animi ex morbo venientis* (*On the Cure of Sadness Deriving from Illness*), the advice *Ad Laurentium adolescentem* (*To the Adolescent Lorenzo*), or the allegorical tale *De nuptiis Battibecco et Serrabocca* (*On the Wedding of Bickering and Shutmouth*), which assails the vices and defects of courtiers.[122]

In these works, Savonarola the strenuous defender of the moral life takes precedence over the physician, regaling the reader with portents of the prospect of eternal damnation and digressions on the love of God, delivered with a rhetorical gusto more reminiscent of texts like the fifteenth-century *Prediche volgari* (*Vernacular Sermons*) of San Bernardino da Siena than a specialized medical regimen.[123] In pursuing his moralist mission, Savonarola employs a wide range of derogatory epithets (as he does in other contexts), not refraining from railing against those parents "with demonic and wicked morals" (*di mal costumi indiavolati acerbissimi*),[124] quite unfit for the educative duties they should be performing.[125] In addition to fathers, other targets of Savonarola's reprimands are, again, the rich ladies and noblewomen of Ferrara, who can afford the luxury of having their children wet-nursed (a practice the physician sees as diabolic) so as not to ruin their lovely breasts, while complaining about all the bother of breastfeeding—but who then, when invited to balls or parties, soon forget how tired they are. As Savonarola writes: "Certainly every mother should breastfeed her child when possible and not fear the burden, just as she doesn't fear the burden when she goes out dancing, for in that she takes great pleasure."[126] In addition to medical arguments for maternal breastfeeding, which are established galenic *topoi*,[127]

---

122. See *Works by Michele Savonarola*, respectively ##28, 29, 30, 31, and 22. On these texts in general, also see Samaritani, "Michele Savonarola riformatore cattolico."

123. In his sermons, Bernardino does not only preach Christian doctrine but also has much to say about women, condemning the indolence, the excesses, and the other shortcomings of wives. See Bernardino da Siena, *Prediche volgari sul Campo di Siena 1427*, edited by Carlo Delcorno, 2 vols. (Milan: Rusconi, 1989).

124. "O father, O mother, you with demonic and wicked morals, what sort of models will you be for your children and what terrible vices will they inherit from you?" *MM*, 216.

125. "Of course, I also condemn those good-for-nothing slacker fathers—they should be stoned!—who do not esteem holy matrimony and lie with wretched women and so give birth to wretched children. O my dear children, how much grace you receive from God when you are born of a legitimate marriage and of proper parents who take good care of you!" *MM*, 215.

126. *MM*, 180.

127. "Oh gentle and delicate *frontosa*, who possesses so many of these qualities, how can you not want to breastfeed your child, taking into consideration the quality of his care, his good health and wellbeing, and even your own health and longevity? By not breastfeeding, you will get pregnant again very quickly, and then for most of a year you will have a disordered appetite, stomachache, backache, and

there are also ethical and religious reasons, which Savonarola finds to be even more important. Savonarola deems refusing to breastfeed not only unnatural and counterproductive both for mother and child, but also contrary to Christian principles: it is disgraceful, to say the least, and is set against the divine example given to us by the blessed Virgin, who deigned to nurse the incarnate son of God.[128]

Discussing child welfare gives the author the opportunity to emphasize the ethical and nurturing qualities that all the figures surrounding the child, apart from its parents, should possess: the priest must be discreet and admonishing; a teacher can only inspire respect if he is old, which means he will be prudent. Branching out into the field of financial management and careful handling of the family's assets, Savonarola recommends investing in the future of the child by engaging a good tutor, no matter what the cost, so as not to risk having a son who ends up throwing away on prostitutes and gambling the money his parents have saved for his education.[129] Finally, the choice of the wet nurse is critical: she should not only be young (but not too young), strong and healthy, a woman who has suffered no miscarriages and is not, herself, pregnant but, above all, she has to be well-mannered and of sound principles, preferably a widow who no longer

---

similar ailments, and the number of your childbirths will multiply. And remember that every birth is a great blow to your own life, shortening it, and often causing poor health, and since your life is affected in this way, you often die younger because of frequent pregnancies." *MM*, 175. On these galenic *topoi*, see Demaitre, "The Idea of Childhood," 474. On Savonarola's advocacy of maternal breastfeeding, see Maaike Van der Lugt, "Nature as Norm in Medieval Medical Discussions of Breastfeeding and Wet-Nursing," *Journal of Medieval and Early Modern Studies* 49, 3 (2019): 563–88.

128. "*Frontosa*, I have known many who have not wanted to breastfeed in order to conserve the beauty of their breasts and to be able to show them off in public, like those women who keep their breasts beautiful so as to display them to admirers. I want to remind you that your milk is best for your child, especially as you would give it to him with greater care than does a hired wet-nurse: and consider how much more you would love the child you have breastfed compared to the one you have not breastfed, and also, accordingly, how much more you will be loved by the child you have breastfed. . . . I would also like to remind you that God gave you breasts like other animals so that you might nourish your children. And as we will later explain, bad nourishment spoils the baby's constitution. *Frontosa*, you should always keep before your eyes the humble virgin mother of the son of God, who breastfed her own son and took such great care of him. . . . O wretched woman, who has bestowed more love on her lovers than on her own children, I can say with certainty that you have given the devil much pleasure, and also, that your failure to breastfeed is frowned upon by medicine. If you are rich and noble, keep a maid with you to help you with the tasks you fear you cannot manage if you are breastfeeding your child." *MM*, 176.

129. "For if you are not diligent from the start in your search for the appropriate tutor, it then follows that once they are grown, children who have been badly reared will run after prostitutes and gamble, causing you great pain and suffering, and you will spend much more money for them than if you had found a good and moral tutor from start." *MM*, 215.

has a sex life.[130] A wet nurse who leads a healthy life can be identified by her complexion, among other things. If it is good, then her milk will be of good quality.[131] Of course, the quality of the milk depends, first and foremost, on the kind of food eaten: this is why Savonarola offers so much dietary advice and so many prohibitions for mothers and wet nurses, who are directly charged with a moral responsibility for improving their milk by appropriate eating habits.[132] In the light of the foregoing, it would constitute a serious threat to the health of the child if the choice of a wet nurse fell, for financial reasons, on nurses who are "impoverished women" (*poverete*), who "eat and drink whatever they can."[133]

Savonarola's emphasis on the care of children in their early years is more than justified: this is the period when the foundation for future physical, psychological, and moral health are laid out. In line with Aristotelian ethical principles, which—following Avicenna—Savonarola reaffirms, it is during childhood that the *habitus fixus* is acquired, that predisposition to virtue which becomes a stable feature of moral character in adulthood. Indeed, the passions of the soul, such as rage, fear

130. "Good and praiseworthy manners" provide the fifth characteristic to look for in a nurse, according to Savonarola. Finally, she must not be either choleric or melancholic. If she is, she may actually refuse to give her breast to a newborn baby squalling for food, with disastrous consequences: "she should not be choleric—that is, she should not be quick to anger, so that she does not spoil the blood; also she should also not be very melancholic or capricious, for if she were, she might decide, either because of the baby's crying or for other reasons, to withhold milk from him, not being his mother, or not to soothe him or to ease his discomfort. O *frontosa* mother, fierce harridan, moderate, moderate your anger and disdain for your reasonless baby, and make sure to soothe your baby as much as your duty calls you to do." *MM*, 175.

131. The concept is better stated by Savonarola's direct source, Avicenna, in his *Canon medicinae*, ed. Giovanni Costeo and Giovanni Paolo Mongio (Venice: Giunta, 1608), Lib. I, fen 3, doctr. 1, c. 2 (p. 165): *Secundum mores vero suos consideratur, quoniam ipsam oportet omnium bonorum morum et laudabilium esse, quae tarde a malis animae passionibus patiatur, sicut ira, tristitia et timore et reliqua ab istis. Omnes enim istae corrumpunt complexionem, et fortasse a lactatione abstinebit: et propter hoc prohibuerunt quidam, ne stolida lactet. Et praeter hoc totum malitia morum ipsius eam perducet ad hoc, ut infantis parvam habeat sollecitudinem, et ei parum blandiatur* (The wet nurse should be judged on the basis of her character, since it is necessary that she be of good and praiseworthy habits, one who calmly bears the bad passions of the soul, like anger, sadness, fear, and the like. For all these passions spoil the complexion, and perhaps she must refrain from breastfeeding: and, because of that, some forbid the dull-minded wet nurse to breasfeed. Moeover, a wicked character will lead her to not take prompt care of the child and to not soothe him). The term "complexion" (Latin *complexio*, Greek κρᾶσις, also known as temperament) refers to the natural balance of the four basic humors (blood, phlegm, yellow bile or choler, and black bile or melancholy), and the four qualities associated with them (hot, cold, dry and wet), within the body as a whole or within one particular part. Affections of the soul (emotions, passions) were thought to disrupt this precarious balance.

132. Here Savonarola introduces one of his pertinent analogical arguments, comparing the quality of the nurse's milk to the food and good wine that every respectable husband should always make sure he has at home. *MM*, 179–80.

133. *MM*, 179.

or sadness, which have been induced in the child by bad parents or teachers, can lead to a deterioration of bodily complexion, and thus, given the interdependence of body and soul, to a deterioration in both the physical and mental health of the individual.[134] Moreover, as noted earlier, the fifth and last chapter of Treatise Three of the *Mother's Manual* resumes the theme of the progressive moral and physical deterioration of the human race with which Savonarola opened his first treatise, bringing it full circle. This argument, by itself, fully justifies the author's insistence on the early education of children.

To return to the first four chapters of Treatise Three, which set forth important precepts on childcare and pediatrics that are not discussed in the *Practica maior*, Savonarola introduces authoritative texts from the medical pediatric tradition. These include Rhazes's *On the Treatment of Small Children*; the *On the Regimen of Children* from treatise 4 of the *Book Dedicated to Al-Mansur* also by Rhazes; and, of course, Avicenna, who devotes four chapters to the subject in the *Canon* (Book I, fen 3). Savonarola's work is strikingly faithful to the *Canon*, even to the point of inconsistency, as when he states, as Avicenna did at the end of his chapters on pediatriccs, to devote a further chapter to the upbringing of boys and girls up to the age of fourteen, without then fulfilling his stated intent: "At the end of this book, where we will deal with behavior for children until the age of fourteen, we will discuss the accidents of the soul, such as anger, sadness, happiness, fear, and similar things."[135] Savonarola also makes careful use of Rhazes. When listing the most common childhood illnesses, despite proposing an order different from that followed by both Rhazes and Avicenna, he writes that "I promised to include at the end of this section a treatment for children about which Rhazes wrote a few brief pages . . . "[136]

As Savonarola extends the spectrum of works to which he refers, his citations of the *auctores* (authoritative writers), both ancient and modern, physicians and surgeons, are increasingly frequent.[137] Only in Treatise Three, furthermore, does Savonarola make specific references to other works he himself has written, both medical and non-medical.[138] Also notable is the greater freedom Savonarola

---

134. *MM*, 211–12.

135. *MM*, 186. Savonarola's intended chapter would correspond Avicenna's chapter on the years seven to fourteen, the *De regimine adolescentium communi*, the chapter that opens the second *doctrina* of the third *fen* of the first book of the *Canon* (which follows the four chapters devoted to children of up to seven years of age). This inconsistency was already noted by Gualdo, "La lingua della pediatria," 29.

136. *MM*, 195.

137. He gives, for instance, for the treatment of milk crust, the solution drawn from Guglielmo da Saliceto in addition to the treatments recommended by Avicenna and Rhazes; *MM*, 195.

138. He refers not only to the *Practica maior*, as he did in the first and second treatises, but also to his own works on fevers (*Canonical Practice on Fevers*), on worms (the *De vermibus*), and his lost work on children's pedagogy discussed earlier (*On What Should Not Be Prescribed to Children*). See *Works by Michele Savonarola*, respectively ##2, 4, and 27, and note 121 for the work on pedagogy.

allows himself in these pediatric passages than in the treatises on conception and pregnancy, acknowledging, for example, the significance of what he calls *pratica comuna*, or "common practice." He not only considers valid the practical knowledge possessed by ordinary women, whose knowledge is gained by experience and transmitted orally, but uses it at times to confirm the recommendations of the authorities.[139]

Savonarola also sketches the desirable physical characteristics of the midwife: she should, for example, have the nail on her little finger cut short, because she will be using this finger to free the throat of the new born baby from organic residues, whereas the nail of the index finger should be "long and sharp, like the finger of a harpist,"[140] so that it can be used if necessary to pierce the amniotic sac. Savonarola's critical description of some birth attendants reveals a different reality than the ideal wet nurse envisioned by medical professionals: Savonarola complains of nurses with rotten teeth who pre-chew the baby's food, infecting them with the serious maladies, or whose hands are so rough they cannot feel the temperature of the water, and scald the newborn with red-hot baths.[141] Worse, he is aware of some women working in the Slavic territories within the Venetian domain, whom he calls "women possessed by the devil" (*femene indiavolate*), who cast magic spells to cause the milk of nursing mothers to run dry. Savonarola only tells this tale, he writes, to satisfy the reader's curiosity: "And this anecdote is most certainly true. I have told it not because it has anything to do with medicine, but because it tells of an amazing and diabolical act, as well as for the pleasure of the reader."[142]

This passage prompts a small foray into the field of magic, and Savonarola's approach to it.[143] In the *Mother's Manual*, he avoids comment on these matters,

---

139. In his *Practica maior*, Savonarola admitted that "in diverse regions and cities women have invented diverse methods, which are not possible for me to enumerate" (*in diversis regionis et civitatibus diversa habent ingenia mulieres ipsae quae a me enumerare non est possibile*). *Practica maior*, VI, ch. 21, rubr. 32 (fol. 272ra). Or again, at fol. 272rb: "and some women, such as the Greeks, have a seat made in this manner" (*et quedam mulieres ut grecae habent sedem hoc modo factam*). See also *Practica maior*, VI, ch. 21, rubr. 7 (fol. 257ra): "and Avicenna determined, in his second [book] of the *Canon*, as I have learned from experienced women, that sheep dung is an efficacious remedy" (*et est expertum Avicenna secundo Canonis, idem ab expertis mulieribus habui fortius operari stercus ovis*).

140. *MM*, 155.

141. "But take note, *frontosa* who has an old mother who has rotten teeth and whose breath often stinks, do not allow her to pre-chew the food for your child. And also when you are ill, do not prechew it for him; but have someone else do this for him, some young healthy maiden." *MM*, 183. "Do be careful, *frontosa* with thick-skinned hands, that you are not fooled when you test the bath water. Have the attendant with thin-skinned hands test it too, because many children in my experience have been scalded." *MM*, 167.

142. *MM*, 188–89.

143. Following Albertus Magnus and Peter of Abano, Savonarola believed that natural substances such as plants, stones or metals, possess occult physical properties, which are occult only because

offering only a few succinct remarks on the properties of stones, plants, and substances that he considers occult but natural; and these are reported because the *pratica comuna* makes use of them, or because that is what "the authorities say."[144] In the *Practica*, in contrast, he abandons his reluctance to divulge potentially dangerous knowledge, and frequently mentions magical practices. When dealing with sterility issues, for instance, he states that there are times when conception is prevented by evil spirits, and that the only way to evade them is to get a new bed or even move house, and to sprinkle everything with dogs' blood.[145] Savonarola is careful to state that these are methods, together with prayers and the invocations of saints, which lie outside his art (*extra artem*), but the fact remains that, in the *Practica*, though not in the *Mother's Manual*, he misses no chance to bring them up.[146]

Some further comment should be made on women's medical practice, which was not confined merely to the sphere of pregnancy and uncomplicated births, nor did it wholly lack rational foundation. On the contrary, women with medical roles were legally licenced and officially recognized by government documents. The delegitimization of women as medical practitioners, which was achieved by a gradual cultural, ideological, juridical and social marginalization,[147] does not

---

not completely known to us, yet these properties are natural and fit perfectly into the natural order of things, a position he clearly expresses in his alchemical *Libellus de aqua ardenti* (*Small Book on Grape Spirit*). See *Works by Michele Savonarola*, #7. In the Renaissance, medical practices based on natural magic and astrology were popular, as physicians, responding to a variety of pressures, were open to alternative solutions and approaches.

144. For example, he writes: "The authorities say that holding a magnet tight in the left hand makes labor easier; or you may also tie a string of corals to the right thigh"; *MM*, 158. And again: to make sure the baby does not fall prey to attacks of "falling sickness," i.e., epilepsy, it may be useful to "keep some root of peony, or emeralds, tied close to his collar; coral tied to the neck of the child is also useful, and this is common practice. Also useful is the pulverized bone of the head of a man given to him in his food or with wine or sugar." *MM*, 210.

145. See *Practica maior*, VI, ch. 21, rubr. 24 (fol. 267r): *impeditur autem conceptio cum fascinationibus, et maleficiis* (for conception is prevented with incantations and curses). Savonarola follows this statement with a note that the previous chapter (ch. 20), devoted to the male genitals, offers many of these sorts of solutions. In sections 30 and 32 of ch. 21, respectively on the prevention of miscarriage and on birth complications, Savonarola stresses the benefits deriving from stones and substances with special properties for an easy and painless delivery (magnets, corals, the hooves of asses or horses), and testifies to the usefulness of amulets and seals, which must be accompanied by the recitation of prayers and praises to God and the Virgin.

146. *Practica maior*, VI, ch. 21, rubr. 32 (fol. 273r): *Agnus Dei ex cera nova alba et balsamo et chrismate a papa consacratum, cum super se habuerit mulier et huiusmodi, quae cum sint extra artem relinquo* (for the woman to have on her an "Agnus Dei" [seal] made of new white wax and balm and holy oil blessed by the pope, and similar things that I omit because they fall outside the art [of medicine]).

147. The historical and textual case of Trota/Trotula and the legal cases of Jacoba Felicie (as well as Perretta Petone, Jeanne la Poqueline, and Isabelle Estevent) are emblematic for different reasons.

negate Savonarola's own frequent references in his work to women's expertise.[148] Nor does it prevent him from sanctioning some forms of apprenticeship and technical training for these women practictioners, similar to the institutional forms of transmission of medical practice among men. Although a wet nurse must be, above all, young, healthy, and of good character, a good midwife excels not solely for these qualities but especially for her prudence and practical skills which, over time, make her *docta*, or expert, in the full sense of the term. For Savonarola, a competent female practitioner is almost a teacher, or physician, who passes on to her students practical information and skills that will be useful to them in real situations, and techniques and treatments to remember and execute out when necessary:

> Now take note, *frontosa*, how much prudence and agility of hands the midwife or nurse must possess, and how strong she must be to handle the child. This means that when she is old and her hands tremble, she can no longer perform this job; however, she can still teach her job to others. But heaven help those of us who wind up in the hands of a nurse who is too old, who is often the cause of the death of our children or of their difficulties of body and soul. Since we surely want our children to be raised by the most expert nurses, every experienced midwife, as if she were a doctor (*come doctore*), should mentor apprentice midwives and teach them all they know.[149]

The same reasoning that leads to the recommendation that one should preferably consult an older physician, with lengthy experience,[150] is thus applied also to the physician's female counterparts—without prejudice but, on the contrary, recognizing a common heritage of practical knowledge, accumulated experience, and the ability to teach and transmit valuable learning.

For more on these and other female practitioners, see Green, *Making Women's Medicine Masculine*, 120–45, 296–97.

148. As an example, Savonarola is keen to report the lexicon used by women: e.g., *maestreto* is the term women use for the umbilical cord; *sgramolato* the adjective they use to refer to the baby suffering from the spasm of the jaws. *MM*, 165, 196. Whether or not Savonarola approves of their medical practices does not alter the fact that he observes and describes them, and that they often provide an opportunity for debates between physicians and nonprofessionals. Among other examples: "Once the umbilical cord is detached, the common practice is to apply a bit of flour to the navel.... Some women use crushed coal; but myrrh is better, or dragon's blood." *MM*, 166. And explicitly, referring to binding the head of newborn babies, which Avicenna strongly advises: "I am well aware, *frontosa*, that some people will object to my writing things that are against common practice; but I am guided by reason and moved to write as authorized by respected and honored philosophers." *MM*, 171.

149. *MM*, 170.

150. "I advise the wet nurse to consult an old physician, not a young one." *MM*, 205.

Afterlife of the Text

The original text of Savonarola's *Mother's Manual* survives in only three fifteenth-century manuscript copies,[151] and did not make the transition into print until Belloni's 1952 edition. This seems to suggest that the work did not enjoy great popularity, especially when compared to the physician's Latin medical production, and that it had no influence north of the Alps. As Savonarola himself was aware, the choice of writing in the Italian vernacular, and not subsequently translating the vernacular work into Latin, is partly to blame for its limited circulation. But, as said earlier, he rhetorically waives any rights to the fame that a Latin version of the *Manual* might have procured him in order to benefit his fellow female citizens, adding that women living north of the Alps (*le ultramuntane*) "who are unfamiliar with the vernacular used in this volume, will be able to have it translated with great ease."[152]

The possibility cannot be ruled out that such a translation once existed, but there is no evidence of this today. Yet the limited circulation of the *Mother's Manual* did not prevent Savonarola's gynecological and obstetrical knowledge from having an important afterlife. His Latin *Practica maior* (on which, again, the vernacular *Mother's Manual* is based) found its way to Germany and underlies Eucharius Rösslin's 1513 German midwifery bestseller *Der swangern Frauwen und Hebammen Rosegarten* (*Rosegarden for Pregnant Women and Midwives*).[153] Probably no other book had a more profound influence on the practice of midwifery during the sixteenth and seventeenth centuries than did the *Rosegarden*, which went through at least sixteen editions in its original version, was revised in three different German versions, was printed multiple times, and was translated

---

151. See *Works by Michele Savonarola*, #13, citing manuscripts in the Vatican, Venice, and Reggio Emilia.

152. *MM*, 58.

153. See Green, "The Sources of Eucharius Rösslin's '*Rosegarden*,'" and the bibliography therein. Also see Green, *Making Women's Medicine Masculine*, 247–48, 269–73, and 301–20. Rösslin's *Rosegarden* was first published in Strasburg in 1513: *Der swangern Frauwen und hebammen Rosegarten* (Strasburg: Martin Flach, 1513); facsimile reprint edited by Huldrych Martin F. Koelbing (Zurich: Verlag Bibliophile Drucke von J. Stocker, 1976). An anonymous Italian version was published in Venice in 1538: *Libro nel qual si tratta del parto delhuomo, e de tutte q[ue]lle cose, che cerca esso parto accadeno, e delle infermita che po[sso]no accadere a i fanciulli, con tutti i suoi rimedii posti particolarme[n]te* (Venice: Giovanni Andrea Valvassori, 1538). In the Uppsala Universitetsbibliotek copy of this very rare edition that I consulted, some handwritten annotations on the first page ("Cette version Italienne, d'après la version Latine, est rare et inconnue aux Bibliographes") confirm the impression that the circulation of this Italian edition of Rösslin's work must have been very limited. Useful among a multitude of other translations is the modern English version: *When Midwifery Became the Male Physician's Province: The Sixteenth-Century Handbook* The Rose Garden for Pregnant Women and Midwives, ed. and trans. by Wendy Arons (Jefferson, NC : McFarland, 1994).

into at least eight different languages: Czech, Danish, Dutch, English, French, Italian, Latin, and Spanish. Many of these translations, moreover, went through their own multiple editions.[154]

In a fascinating narrative, Monica Green establishes that the gynecological and obstetrical chapters of Michele Savonarola's *Practica*, and not Muscio's *Gynecology*, must be recognized as the key source for the *Rosegarden*, which in turn became the foundational text of early modern European obstetrical literature.[155] It will suffice here to briefly summarize Green's findings to establish that through Rösslin's unacknowledged deployment of Savonarola, the obstetrical practices of fifteenth-century northern Italy served as the basis not only for German-speaking territories, but indeed for all of western Europe.[156] This textual influence was mediated by a 1494 German manuscript, now in Hamburg, titled *Von Kranckheiten, Siechtagen und Zuval der Swangern und geberenden frowen und ihrer neugebornen Kinderen* (*On the Sicknesses, Illnesses, and Accidents of Pregnant and Laboring Women and Their Newborn Children*), which has been identified as the ultimate source of Rösslin's printed text.[157] In her detailed contribution on the

154. Emmerik Ingerslev writes that "it is on the whole doubtful whether any other medical work has been translated into as many European languages as this little book . . . which was intended to improve the miserable state of the art of midwifery of that day." Ingerslev, "Rösslin's 'Rosegarten': Its Relation to the Past (the Muscio Manuscripts and Soranus), Particularly with Regard to Podalic Version," *Journal of Obstetrics and Gynaecology of the British Empire* (part 1), 15 (January 1909), 1.

155. The well-known woodcuts depicting fetus-in-utero illustrations that appear in the *Rosegarden* are not discussed here, because their iconographic debt to the fetal images found in Muscio's *Gynecology* (which were often attached to Albucasis's *Surgery* or were otherwise circulating independently of Muscio's work) has been established by medical historians.

156. Unsurprisingly, Savonarola himself heavily relies on previous sources, especially on Avicenna's *Canon* as has been seen repeatedly, as well as (as originally noted by Ingerslev, "Rösslin's 'Rosegarten'") on the fourteenth-century academic and court physician from Naples, Francesco da Piedemonte (Pedemontanus, Pindemonte), whose activity is documented until 1320, and whose obstetrical instructions are unacknowledged by Savonarola. A Venetian edition of Piedemonte's *Complementum in opera Mesue* (1541) names him as *lettore in gymnasio patavino* (teaching at the University of Padua) although this activity is not confirmed by Paduan archival records. A close reading and comparison between Savonarola's and Piedemonte's obstetrical chapters is the subject of a forthcoming article of mine, drawing on Piedemonte's work in the *Supplementum in secundum librum Compendii secretorum medicinae Io. Mesues medici celeberrimi, tum Petri Apponi Patavini, tum Francisci de Pedemontium medicorum illustrium*, contained in vol. 2 of Mesue's *De medicamentorum purgantium delectu, castigatione et usu, Libri duo.* [. . .] *quod nomine Supplementi in Mesuen* [sic] *inscriptum est* (Venice: Giunta, 1623); especially fols. 15vb–18rb (on breasts and breastfeeding), and 89vb–103ra (on female genitalia). At this point it can be stated that the differences between these two sets of chapters by far outreach their undeniable similarities, suggesting the extreme "heaviness" of Savonarola's layer of authorship.

157. Ms. Hamburg, Staats- und Universitätsbibliothek, cod. med. 801, an. 1494: 9–130. For the specific differences between the Hamburg manuscript and the *Rosegarden*, see Britta-Juliane Kruse, "Neufundeiner handschriftlichen Vorstufe von Eucharius Rößlins Hebammenlehrbuch 'Der schwangeren Frauen und Hebammen Rosengarten' und des Frauenbüchleins Ps.-Ortolfs," *Sudhoffs Archiv* 78

sources of the *Rosegarden*, Green explains why Muscio's Latin *Gynecology* should be excluded as Rösslin's main source, notwithstanding the availability of the whole Muscian work in Germany from the second half of the fifteenth century. Through four thematic examples from the *Rosegarden*,[158] and (for Rösslin's text) through the discussion of the non-correspondence between the fetal images of mispresentations and their explanations, Green demonstrates that both German works, the *Kranckheiten* and the *Rosegarten*, "are little more than an abbreviated and somewhat rearranged translation of Savonarola's Latin."[159]

Moreover, even if there is no evidence of a direct influence of Savonarola's *Mother's Manual* on the *Rosegarden*, it can at least be conjectured that Rösslin might have known about the existence of such a work, which is specifically written for a female audience of laywomen and—for the first time since the age of Muscio—also for midwives. It might be knowledge of these previous works that inspired Rösslin to address his own work to the same audience. He could not have been so inspired by the anonymous author of the *Kranckheiten* (the underlying source of the *Rosegarden*) who did not address his work to women, as noted by Britta-Julliane Kruse; and the only other printed German text dealing with similar topics before 1513, the *Frauenbüchlein* (Augsburg, c.1495), also anonymous, was addressed to pregnant women, but not to midwives.[160]

Although it is unlikely, therefore, that Savonarola's *Mother's Manual* made its way to Germany before Rösslin published the *Rosegarden*, Savonarola's *Practica* may well have done so. Green points out the frequency of personal exchanges between northern Italian and German medical professors and students, especially from the fifteenth century onwards; knowledge of Savonarola's work could well have been transmitted by such a path. For example, the Munich physician and translator Johannes Hartlieb (d. 1468), who had announced his plan to translate

---

(1994): 220–364. The Hamburg manuscript incorporates some pediatric material in its final part (this section on childcare is taken from Bartholomeus Metlinger's *Kinderbüchlein*, first printed in Ausburg in 1473). Therefore, the presence of this same pediatric and non-obstetrical material in the last section of the *Rosegarden* is also not to be considered the result of an original choice by Rösslin.

158. These relate to difficult deliveries, the obstetrical chair, some causes of difficult labor, and menstrual retention and exccessive menstrual flow. See Green, "The Sources of Eucharius Rösslin's 'Rosegarden,'" 183–89.

159. Green, "The Sources of Eucharius Rösslin's 'Rosegarden,'" 187. At 188, Green is more indulgent, in observing that such editing devices like the substitution of one of Savonarola's personal and amusing anecdotes with a local German episode, shows Rösslin's "astute eye for nuanced adaptation."

160. Kruse, "Neufundeiner handschriftlichen Vorstufe," 231. See also Kruse, *Verborgene Heilkünste*. Kruse also discovered the manuscript version of the *Frauenbüchlein* (Women's Booklet), which predated the 1495 edition, and seems to be another adaptation, very brief in this case, of Savonarola's Latin obstetrics intended for a lay audience of women. Kruse notes the difficulty of fully ascertaining the exact lines of affiliation between this text (both in manuscript and print), the Hamburg manuscript (*Kranckheiten*), and the *Rosegarden* with regard to Savonarola's chapters.

Muscio's *Gynecology* into German,[161] not only studied in Padua in the same years in which Savonarola was teaching there, but also took his medical degree with Antonio Cermisone and Bartolomeo Montagnana, who were Savonarola's close acquaintances.[162] Hermann Schedel (1410–1485), a physician from Nuremberg, made his own copy of Savonarola's *Practica* when he was a student in Padua around 1442, thirty-five years before the first edition of that work, printed in 1479.[163] Moreover, two more printed editions of Savonarola's *Practica* appeared before the end of the fifteenth century (Venice 1486 and Venice 1497), making it even more likely that by the 1490s this work by Savonarola was easily obtainable in Germany. The *Practica maior* was not Rösslin's only source: although most if not all the references to Avicenna within the *Rosegarden* seem to be directly lifted from Savonarola, Green noted the novelty of references to Albert the Great and to the *Trotula*, mediated by Gilbertus Anglicus in one instance, as signs of the German author's originality.[164]

Green concludes her study of, effectively, the importation of northern Italian obstetrical practices into Germany, and hence all of Europe, by listing some possible candidates who could claim responsibility for the complex work of the translation and adaptation of Savonarola's obstetrics into German. It must have been someone very likely older than the then young and inexperienced aphotecary Eucharius Rösslin, who was in his twenties at the time of the possible appearance of this adaptation—an adaptation which must predate even the 1494

161. Hartlieb translated into German both the Ps.-Albertus Magnus *Secrets of Women* and, as a companion volume to this text, the *Trotula* ensemble, but his goal of translating Muscio's work was not fulfilled. See Green, *Making Women's Medicine Masculine*, 178–81 and 212–14, and Green, "The Sources of Eucharius Rösslin's '*Rosegarden*.'"

162. Cermisone (ca 1360–1441), as has been seen, was Savonarola's preceptor, whom Savonarola, with filial admiration, remembered numerous times as a father, and not just as a teacher. Montagnana (1380–1452) was Savonarola's colleague and near-contemporary. The fact that he does not appear in Savonarola's list of distinguished Paduan physicians in his *Libellus de magnificis ornamentis regie civitatis Padue* can perhaps be ascribed to professional rivalry.

163. See Green, "The Sources of Eucharius Rösslin's '*Rosegarden*,'" 183, and note 39 for the reference to Schedel's manuscript. Hermann's cousin, Hartmann Schedel (1440–1516), himself a medical student in Padua, who like his cousin demonstrated a deep interest in the culture of reproduction, wrote a prologue to Hermann's collection of Cermisone's *Consilia*, and himself collected 156 *consilia* by Montagnana. These manuscripts are now Munich, Bayerische Staatsbibliothek, Clm 207 (*Antonii Cermisoni consilia* [. . .] *cum prologo Hartmanni Schedelii et effigie Cermisoni ab Hermanno Schedelio Paduae collecta et conscripta*), and Munich, Bayerische Staatsbibliothek, Clm 25 (*Bartholomaei de Montagnana consilia*).

164. Green, "The Sources of Eucharius Rösslin's '*Rosegarden*,'" 189. Here the reference is to the German author of the Hamburg manuscript, not to Rösslin himself, who in his turn can be instead "credited with very little originality." Green, 192.

Hamburg manuscript, as that version is unlikely to have been the original of the *Kranckheiten*.[165]

Whoever that person was, this story underscores the importance of interrogating what was really new in women's medicine in the first age of print, in order to show how much the earliest phase of printed vernacular medical culture owes to late-medieval learning. The link beween late medieval manuscript culture and Renaissance print culture is much tighter than it seems: both the continued circulation and the wealth of manuscript material on women's medicine, gynecology and obstetrics after 1475, that is, after the invention of movable type, surely deserve deeper studies.

The circulation of the *Mother's Manual* was not boosted by the printing press, and it never gained popularity. Still, it inaugurated a textual tradition that would characterize every single midwifery text for at least two centuries: one in which the female midwife is subordinate to the physician or surgeon; in which the separation of gynecology from obstetrics is reinforced (in continuity with the medieval tradition); and in which lay readers, notably together with midwives, are invited to manage a full-rounded culture of reproduction. Their concern was no longer limited to the procreative function, but had broadened to include a pedagogical, ethical, and political dimension. Such topics as sexuality, the female anatomy, pregnancy, and childcare had always generated a strong general interest—not confined to physicians and specialists—and could not fail to attract readers in a society which based its social order on the continuity of family lineage.[166]

---

165. The candidates are: 1. a certain otherwise unknown Constantine Rösslin, perhaps an older relative of Eucharius, who owned the Hamburg manuscript; 2. Bartholomeus Metlinger, the author of the German *Kinderbüchlein* (Augsburg, 1473)—which was inspired by, but not dependent from, the Latin *Libellus de egritudinibus infantium* (Padua, 1472) by Paolo Bagellardo da Fiume—and which was incorporated into the Hamburg manuscript; 3. Bartholomeus Scherrenmüller, a German court physician active until at least 1493, who claimed to have translated a text—now lost—bearing this title: *Wie sich die kindendenn frawenn in dem geberen der kind halten sollent* (*How Pregnant Women Should Comport Themselves in Bearing Their Children*). Green, "The Sources of Eucharius Rösslin's '*Rosegarden*,'" 190–91, considers Scherrenmüller to be the most likely candidate, as "the text in the Hamburg manuscript may, therefore, be Scherrenmüller's 'lost' text."

166. Although the traditional works on this subject—the gynecological section of the Hippocratic corpus, the biological works of Aristotle, Galen's gynecological writings, the various works of gynecology by Soranus, Celsus and the Salernitan School, the formidable body of Arabic treatises on the topic and their medieval counterparts—were, at least in principle, reserved for professionals, the great medieval encyclopedias allowed information about these subjects to spread to a much larger group of the educated public. Attention should be paid not only to the Latin, but also to the vernacular textual traditions, e.g., the *Sidrac*, the dialogue *Placide et Timeo*, the *Composizione del mondo* by Ristoro d'Arezzo or the *Acerba* by Cecco d'Ascoli. Mention should also be made of the sections of the *Divine Comedy* and the *Convivio* (*Banquet*) that Dante Alighieri devoted to the topic: *Divine Comedy, Purgatorio* 25:37–75, and *Banquet*, IV, ch. 21. Theologians were also deeply interested in the subject: the *De animalibus* by Albert the Great and the *Summa theologica* by Thomas Aquinas, just to mention

Savonarola is responding to the need for medical information that he perceived to exist among fathers and husbands from the wealthier social classes. Being sensitive to stimuli he detected outside the academic sphere, deriving from the professional, urban, and court context in which he was immersed, the physician amiably includes in his treatise autobiographical anecdotes and little slices of daily life in Ferrara or Padua, which take their place alongside philosophical digressions, proverbs, and rhetorical intrusions and asides of all descriptions. His main concern, which was typical of court literature of the time, is to capture his readers' imagination by any device that might delight and intrigue them. This engagement with his audience differentiates Savonarola's text from Rösslin's *Rosegarden*, and also from the first Italian midwifery texts composed after Savonarola's, authored by Giovanni Marinelli and Scipione Mercurio, dated 1563 and 1595 respectively.[167]

It will be necessary to wait until the beginning of the seventeenth century for the publication of the first female-authored text on women's medicine (after the twelfth-century Salernitan Trota), when, between 1609 and 1626, the French midwife Louise Bourgeois publishes her *Diverse Observations*. But more than another century and a half separates this text from the first Italian midwifery handbook authored by a woman, the *Breve compendio dell'arte ostetricia* by Teresa Ployant (1787)—and she, too, was a Frenchwoman by birth, although practising in Naples.[168] Thus, at least in Italy, more than three centuries divide the first invocation by Savonarola of the midwife as a desired and potential, if not actual,

---

the main works, display detailed annotations on female physiology and on matters connected with procreation and generation.

167. This is true, notwithstanding the greater amount of gynecological and obstetrical material contained in these two Italian later works. Rudolph M. Bell writes in his *How To Do It: Guides to Good Living for Renaissance Italians* (Chicago: University of Chicago Press, 1999), 24, that "authors such as Giovanni Marinello simply copied Savonarola's pregnancy guide in their own printed books," but upon examination, no direct correspondence to Savonarola is found within these texts. See Giovanni Marinelli, *Le medicine pertinenti alle infermità delle donne* (Venice: Francesco de Franceschi Senese, 1563); and Scipione (or Girolamo) Mercurio, *Della comare o riccoglitrice* (Venice: Giovan Battista Ciotti, 1595).

168. Louise Bourgeois, *Observations diverses sur la stérilité, perte de fruict, fœcondité, accouchements et maladies des femmes et enfants nouveaux naiz* (Paris: Saugrain, 1609), first of many subsequent editions. The work is now also available in English translation: Louise Bourgeois, *Midwife to the Queen of France: Diverse Observations*, trans. Stephanie O'Hara, ed. Alison Klairmont Lingo (Toronto: Iter Press; Tempe, AZ: ACMRS, 2017). For Ployant, see Teresa Ployant, *Breve compendio dell'arte ostetricia di Madama Teresa Ployant* (Naples: Vincenzo Orsino, 1787). On this midwife, born in Paris but Italian by adoption, see Nadia Filippini, "Levatrici e ostetricanti a Venezia tra Sette e Ottocento," *Quaderni storici* 20.58 (1985): 149–80. The first academic establishment of obstetrical studies as an autonomous field in Italy dates back to 1761, with the institution, in Padua, of the chair *De morbis mulierum, puerorum et artificium*, later named *Ad artem ostetriciam, ad morbos mulierum*, and finally simply *Ad artem ostetriciam* in 1785.

reader and recipient of a midwifery text, and the first midwife as *author* of her own professional handbook.

Note on Annotations to the Text

Although the *Mother's Manual for the Women of Ferrara* included in this volume is a translation of Luigi Belloni's 1952 edition of Michele Savonarola's *De regimine praegnantium* (based on the manuscripts Reginense Latino 1142 housed in the Vatican Apostolic Library, and the 1460 Marciano Italiano III 30 housed in Venice's Biblioteca Nazionale Marciana), I have reported in the notes the most significant textual variants identified by cross-checking Belloni's edition with the third surviving manuscript of the text, unknown to him, i.e. the Codice Turri C 12, housed in the Biblioteca Panizzi in Reggio Emilia.

Belloni did not include a critical apparatus of sources in his edition. This edition provides readers with full identification of all sources quoted by Savonarola in the *Mother's Manual*. Savonarola quotes from medical and philosophical authorities directly in Latin. The Latin quotations, which have been reported in the notes, are Savonarola's transcriptions of the manuscript texts he consulted, and are not exact quotations of the cited standard modern editions (although in most cases these quotations differ only slightly from these).

Any quotations from such works that are not cited from existing English translations are direct translations from Savonarola's Latin transcriptions. Any quotations from works cited in English translation are taken from the modern editions cited.

Note on the Translation, by Martin Marafioti

The *Mother's Manual for the Women of Ferrara* included in this volume is a translation of Luigi Belloni's 1952 edition of Michele Savonarola's *De regimine praegnantium*. Belloni based his edition on two of the three surviving manuscripts of the treatise, the Reginense Latino 1142 housed in the Vatican Apostolic Library, and the 1460 Marciano Italiano III 30 housed in Venice's Biblioteca Nazionale Marciana. The third manuscript, unknown to Belloni when he published his edition, is the Codice Turri C 12, housed in the Biblioteca Panizzi in Reggio Emilia.

My goal in this translation is to make Savonarola's treatise accessible to a wider audience—an audience not familiar with Quattrocento Italian (specifically, Paduan vernacular with Ferrarese inflections). In Savonarola's era, medical literature was almost exclusively written in Latin and only circulated in the domain of male intellectuals of an elite class. Savonarola's *Mother's Manual* is unique, bold, and even revolutionary in its use of the vernacular; its author decided to break with the orthodox practice and address a female, lay audience, unfamiliar with Latin. In the spirit of Savonarola, the English translation of this text will bring his words and ideas to a wider audience.

As you read this translation, you will find one word (and its variants) that has not been rendered into English: *frontosa* (in the feminine form), and *frontoso* (in the masculine), used both as an adjective and as a noun. Savonarola uses this term repeatedly in the *Mother's Manual*, but curiously, he does not use it in other vernacular works, or even its Latin variant *frontosus* in his erudite Latin works. *Frontoso* comes from the Latin *frons*, which means "forehead," so when the author addresses the reader as *frontosa* he evokes the image of a person holding their forehead high and proud, someone who is "shameless," "bold," and even "audacious," "brazen," or "impudent."[169] As it would have been cumbersome to present so many alternate translations for a single word, the term *frontosa* remains in the text in italics. Therefore, when Savonarola says *ascoltami frontosa*, he is actually saying "listen to me, O shameless, brazen, proud woman," "you who thinks she knows it all."

Savonarola's attempt to make the text more accessible to his contemporary female reader, or listener, required him not only to abandon the convention of writing in Latin, but also to adopt colloquial vernacular terms, evoke colorful, visual metaphors and proverbs, and make references to the popular culture with which fifteenth-century Ferrarese women would have been familiar. He also makes jokes and utilizes the double entendre (especially when discussing racy topics). Colloquial and culturally specific language can be difficult to translate, as often the reader does not have the same cultural awareness or references as the audience for which the text was written. As an American-born scholar of Italian medieval literature, I found it necessary to recruit the assistance of native speakers of Italian (especially those familiar with northern dialects), and historians of medicine to help me understand and elucidate the meanings of numerous terms and sayings in the text. I would like to extend my deepest gratitude to Valeria Finucci, Roberta Ricci, Guido Giglioni, Roberto Poma, Monica Green and of course, Gabriella Zuccolin, editor of this volume, for their patience and insight into the world of Savonarola.

---

169. This word was not commonly used in the fifteenth century. Savonarola borrows the term from Augustine's exegetical treatises devoted to the Psalms (*Enarratio in psalmum*). Curiously, we find this term used by Augustine in a psalm discussing a *peccatrice*, or "sinner" (Mary Magdalene). See TLIO [Tesoro della Lingua Italiana delle Origini], *sub vocem* "frontoso," for other medieval vernacular attestations of this word.

A MOTHER'S MANUAL FOR THE WOMEN OF FERRARA

A Mother's Manual for the Women of Ferrara

To the Women of Ferrara

A true ingrate is one who forgets those benefits received by others. My dear ladies of Ferrara, since I have always greatly detested the vice of ingratitude and considered it an abomination, and as I do not desire to be considered an ingrate by you—who, I will never forget, have given me so much love and so many benefits—I have set out to compose this volume for your assistance, and I have dedicated it to you. Also, as you will see, I have made this great effort so that you may look upon me as a good father. This book is for you, my daughters, to accompany you in the attempts, risks, and mistakes you make in your pregnancies and in your parturition, hoping to benefit you and to make you as happy as you can possibly be. And in order to increase your happiness, I have also decided to include a section to help your children—the offspring to which you have bravely given birth—with advice that will assist in saving their lives. Therefore, considering that nothing is more valued and welcome than life, I have felt the need to satisfy you with this volume of mine, written to aid the life of both the mother and child, because of the many benefits and great love you ladies have shown me. I say this because it seems to me that my efforts could never merit the greatness of the benefits you have bestowed upon me.

Therefore, the awareness of all that you have done should, and with good reason, cause those to bite their tongues who reprimand me for writing in the vernacular, since they believe that such a work merits publication in Latin, and so be understood in other lands where Latin is spoken, and since Latin is typically used in this type of writing. However, my ladies, since I have decided to write this as a last will and testament in which you are the sole heirs, and since you are not proficient in Latin, it is necessary that I write in the vernacular tongue—not taking into account my honor and glory, but instead avoiding that abominable vice of ingratitude—considering also that my work will be easy to translate into Latin.[1] Therefore, my Ferrarese daughters, I have decided to reciprocate your favors with

---

1. See in this volume the Introduction, passim, for a full discussion of Savonarola's use of the vernacular in the *Mother's Manual*, and the relation between this vernacular work and his own Latin works and those by other authors. See also the discussion of women's literacy in the Introduction to this volume, especially at 19–20, which shows that the recent explosion of medieval and early modern studies on women's literacy, habits of reading, book ownership and production, although demonstrating an increasing level of access by women to the literate culture, does not alter the conclusion that women's access to the literate culture of medicine was limited: literacy does not necessarily mean "medical literacy." On this issue, see especially Green, "The Possibilities of Literacy"; Hellwarth, "I wyl wright of women"; Jones, "Medical Literacies and Medical Culture"; and Richards, "Reading and Hearing 'The Womans Booke.'"

my efforts. No one should wonder that I choose to settle this debt by writing in the vernacular, because if this work ever obtains some fame, it will boldly proclaim that women have always championed my reputation. Of course it is true that if I had been driven by fame and glory, I would have written this work in Latin. But instead, I have chosen gratitude over such glory and fame—for vainglory, ladies, as you well know, is a vice of which one can easily be accused, but it is not so easy to avoid—by giving more ample recognition of your many, many favors. It is important to note that northerners, who are unfamiliar with the vernacular used in this volume, will be able to have it translated with great ease. Therefore, my learned friends, I pray you kindly to indulge me and excuse me, and taking into consideration my gratitude to the ladies for whom I write, I pray that you forgive me for not having written this work in Latin. All of this I write in praise of God, the omnipotent father, whose son Jesus was born of the pregnant Virgin Mary.

Having explained my motivation for writing such a book, as well as my linguistic choice, I will now proceed to outline the structure of the work, which will be divided into three treatises.

- Treatise One, in which we will deal with impregnation, will begin by discussing the time, or better yet, the ideal age, for a woman to copulate with a man—that act essential for reproduction, that act without which no one can reproduce, even though Averroes wrote of some young virgins who became pregnant by bathing in the same water where some young boys had previously ejaculated.[2] And the reason I write about this is because pregnancy has its own very specific rules that must be obeyed so that it may be carried out in the most perfect way. We will discuss this topic for the benefit of mothers, fathers, and newborn infants, expanding upon the topic for the greater pleasure of the readers.
- Treatise Two of this guide to the prevention, care, and healing of disorders experienced by the pregnant woman will describe ways to facilitate parturition.
- Treatise Three will discuss the upbringing of children, from their birth to the age of seven, at which tender age the prevention, care, and healing of their infirmities can be treated by mothers rather than doctors. I will also

---

2. Averroes recounts the story of a girl (one girl, not more than one in the original source) who became pregnant after taking a warm bath in a tub filled with water in which men had recently ejaculated. Averroes uses this story to side with Aristotle against Galen in believing that male sperm is the only seed necessary for reproduction, whereas female ejaculation is totally unnecessary. See Averroes, *Colliget libri VII* (Venice: Giunta, 1562), II.10 (fol. 22vb): *Et vicina quaedam mea, de cuius sacramento confidere multum bene poteramus, iuravit in anima sua quod impraegnata fuerat subito in balneo lavelli acquae calidae, in quo spermatizaverunt mali homines, cum essent balneati in illo balneo* (And a neighbour of mine, whose oath we can fully trust, swore with all her heart that she was pregnant after bathing in hot water in which evil men had just ejaculated).

add moral guidelines that fathers and mothers should study diligently, observe, and ensure that their children follow for their moral well-being. Therefore, my ladies, through my book you will become both physical and spiritual healers for your children.

I will divide our volume into these three treatises. I hope that you, my Ferrarese ladies, as well as all Italian ladies, find this volume fruitful for yourselves and for your children, and I also hope that you will experience delight in reading this work.

Treatise One
The following will be the chapters of Treatise One of our volume:

- Chapter One: on the form of sexual intercourse to be most advantageously practiced according to one's age
- Chapter Two: on the time when the husband and wife should engage in sexual intercourse in order to achieve pregnancy
- Chapter Three: on pregnancy, and the rules that should be observed in order to achieve pregnancy
- Chapter Four: on the signs of pregnancy
- Chapter Five: on conceiving male and female infants, and the techniques to be followed so that one sex or the other is conceived, and on signs that reveal whether the fetus is male or female

Chapter One
On the form of sexual intercourse to be most advantageously practiced according to one's age

Regarding the topic of the first treatise, we can say with the authority of the great philosopher Aristotle that appropriate and honorable sexual intercourse (that is to say, within marriage and as commanded by God in Genesis 1) should be engaged in at an appropriate age for both men and women. This is a rule that was certainly followed more diligently in past generations than in the present one. For in the past, young men married young women, whereas now, young boys marry young girls, and greatly endanger their future progeny, as we will now explain. Also, nowadays, without shame or embarrassment, old women take young men for husbands, and old men, with a clear conscience, take young women. This new generation mixes the Old Testament with the New, without worries, so if these Christians [i.e. the young] become Jews [i.e. the old], too bad for them!

Furthermore, on age, on the authority of the Philosopher [i.e. Aristotle] and the consensus of physicians, I will say that the suitable age for both males and females to engage in intercourse is when they have reached the end of their physical growth: for females this is normally in their eighteenth year and for males in their twenty-first. When they have reached maturity, it is believed, the seed is well-formed and perfect and will produce perfect offspring: that is, whole and perfect progeny destined to live a long life. Since it is true that from weak principles descend weak effects, young people, who are weak and imperfect before they reach maturity, will produce weak and wretched children destined to live a short life, and in doing so these young couples defeat the principal goal of matrimony, which is to have robust, healthy, and long-lived children. That it has become normal today for young boys to marry young girls is one of the reasons why our lives are so brief—as it has caused the decline of human nature from the greatness it had attained in the past, when people lived longer and healthier lives. O wretched old man who steals a child bride, take heed, or you will give birth [not to a healthy infant], but a mandrake!

Furthermore, what I say using reason is also known through experience: young animals produce small and feebleminded offspring, as do those who are too old. These effects occur because of a defect in the sperm produced, since sperm is imperfect in young boys and girls as well as in the elderly. Now, before going on any further, I wish to remind you that I am addressing you as good, God-fearing Christians. I purposefully named this chapter "On the honorable and proper act of sexual intercourse" to exclude the scoundrels and the improperly married who do not desire any progeny at all, but only to find pleasure in shameful delights that are abhorred by God. Remember that when the sexual act is undertaken by those who fear God, it is blessed, and the offspring born into this world are honorable. Otherwise, the propagator and all his progeny are defiled. Therefore Christian, make certain that your coitus is honorable and appropriate, and blessed by God, and make certain to wait until your sperm is sound and fertile.

The sperm of the tender-aged male, that is, before a boy has reached the peak and perfection of his physical growth, lacks sufficient heat and is weak from excessive moisture; its power is blunted, and in this state, it cannot generate. Nor is the menstrual blood of a tender-aged female well-disposed to generate life (here I am speaking according to the philosophers), since at this stage, menstrual blood is not prepared to receive the form and image of the generating male. For it is the male's sperm that possesses generative power, and conditions and prepares the menstrual blood as matter for generation, which receives its likeness just as melted wax receives the imprint of a seal. Since the sperm of a young boy is not sufficiently hot, it cannot prepare the menstrual blood to receive the form of the body—for menstrual blood, to use a philosophical term, is the matter of everything.

At such an early age, menstrual blood impedes impregnation because it is too moist and not yet sufficiently concocted, nor hot; and hence for this reason it resists the activity of the male's seed, thereby losing heat and generative power. Even if it engenders, it produces a weak, small, and wretched fetus due to the lack of heat: a fetus with no opportunity to gain strength or grow in size.

As Albert the Great states, in *De animalibus* (*On Animals*) V:

> In the same manner, the disposition of the children of animals differs according to the age of the parents. The first seed that comes out of animals at the beginning of the age when coitus is possible is very mediocre, in so far as up to that point Nature has not yet placed much in the seed, and that which has been supplied has not yet ripened; and again because the pathways by which the seed passes to the genitalia have not yet widened, and because the seed itself has not yet reached its necessary maturity. Instead, it is at this point moist its heat not having yet risen, but is overcome by the excessive moisture. And because of these three causes, if it happens that a pregnancy should result, the child born will be weak, having a fragile body. This is seen frequently in humans and in quadrupeds and some kinds of birds.[3]

Having explained the theory of generation according to the philosophers, we will now discuss how doctors like Hippocrates and Galen maintain instead that a woman's sperm, along with her menstrual blood, contribute to generation as both active and passive principles. However, it is the man's sperm that contributes as the main active principle, by warming the woman's sperm, which by itself would not actively lead to generation.[4] This is why it is necessary that the virile sperm have much of the spirited heat, which cannot be achieved in a male who is too young.

However, according to the doctors, it is also true that a woman's sperm plays an important role in the formation of body parts, as dough does in baking a

---

3. In Latin in the text: *Eodem autem modo et filiorum animalium dispositio diversificatur secundum etatem parentum. Primum enim sperma quod ex animalibus exit in principio etatis coitus, modicum est valde, eo quod non adhuc natura multum ponit in semine, cum incrementum nundum ad plenum steterit: et iterum quia nundum adhuc vie non sunt ampliate, per quas ad inguina descendit: et quia ipsum sperma nundum adhuc debitam adeptum est maturitatem: sed est adhuc aqueum, cuius calor non est acutus, sed fractus in humido aqueo: ed propter istas tres causas, si contingat ipsam impregnationem fieri, nascitur partus debilis habens fragile corpus. Hoc autem, ut frequentius, apparet in hominibus et quadrupedibus et modis avium.* See Albert the Great, *De animalibus libri XXVI, nach der Cölner Urschrift*, ed. Hermann Stadler, 2 vols. (Münster: Aschendorff, 1916–1920), vol. 1, Lib. V, tract. 2, c. 1 (pp. 426–27).

4. See for instance Galen, *De usu partium corporis humani*, Lib. XIV, ch. 6–7, in *Claudii Galeni Opera Omnia*, vol. 4, ed. Karl Gottlob Kühn (Leipzig: Cnobloch, 1822), 158–75; and Galen, *De semine*, Lib. II, c. 1, in Kühn, *Opera omnia*, 4:593–610. Kühn, *Opera omnia*, will be cited henceforth as Kühn.

loaf of bread, while very little of the man's sperm is employed in the formation of body parts. In order to further elaborate on such matters, which I feel my readers would appreciate, I will proceed by saying that Nature creates five substances out of menstrual blood: the first and most pure, which tends to be white, generates, together with spermatic material, bones and nerves; the second type, less pure, generates the flesh and fat; the third nourishes the fetus in the womb; the fourth generates milk in the breasts for the future nourishment of the child; the fifth, impure and fetid, is kept in the body until the moment of parturition and is expelled during labor; and this type of blood cannot be drained without great danger to the fetus until the moment of birth.[5] We will elaborate on this in the following section.

We have stated why a young boy's sperm is not highly fertile; likewise, the sperm of drunkards, of the elderly, of those who copulate too much, of the weak, as well as of the man whose penis is too long, is not prolific. As Avicenna writes in his chapter on non-generating seed, *De spermate non generante*:

> the sperm of the drunkard, the decrepit, and the child, and of those who engage too often in sex does not generate; nor that of him whose members are weak, or whose penis is excessively elongated, so that the distance that the sperm has to travel is lengthened, which is why it arrives at the womb with its innate heat already diminished, and therefore, according to the opinion of many, it does not generate.[6]

We should always keep this in mind if we consider the teachings of doctors to be for the most part true and rarely fallacious: that sperm may be defective, either because it is too cold or too hot, too humid or dry. These are all conditions that make sperm non-prolific. Similarly, defective sperm from a parent who suffers from gout or leprosy produces infirm offspring—in other words, gouty children and lepers.

---

5. As does Avicenna, Savonarola attempts to reconcile the conflicting views of Galen and Aristotle as to whether female seed is necessary for procreation. Notwithstanding the somewhat conflicting citation of authorities, he ultimately sides with Galen's statement that female seed is essential to the formation of the fetus's body. Savonarola then lists five different types or states of menstrual blood, which, in his view, is mixed with the female seed, and can be thought of according to a hierarchical scale of purity and impurity. This blood is in turn responsible for the generation of the new baby's main organs, and for his fleshy and fatty parts; it nourishes the fetus within the mother's womb, and generates breast milk. The impure fifth part is expelled with the afterbirth. Even though Savonarola emphasizes the dangers of impure menstrual blood not used up in its earlier states, he clearly espouses the medical view, which mitigated against religiously-inspired fears about the evil powers of women's menses.

6. In Latin in the text: *Sperma ebrii, decrepiti et infantis et multi coitus non generat, et habentis membra debilitata. Et cum prolungatur virga valde, prolungatur spatium motus spermatis, quare venit ad matricem calore eius innato iam fracto, non ergo generat secundum plurimum.* See Avicenna, *Canon*, Lib. III, fen 20, tract. 1, c. 13 (p. 903).

But perhaps you might challenge me, *frontoso*: "Tell me master, does Gregory not tell in his dialogues of a nine-year-old son who impregnated his mother?"[7] Also Marsilio [Santasofia], the great doctor worthy of much respect, adds that he had come across in his practice a gravid eight-year-old girl. And in my time, Messer Niccolò Pallavicino, comrade of the duke of Milan, Gian Galeazzo [Visconti], tells of a man more than one hundred years old who impregnated his wife with a male infant.[8] And again I will restate Averroes' tale of the young boys who released their sperm into a tub of bathwater, and shortly after, a group of young girls who bathed in the tub became pregnant.

Following such stories, retold for my readers' delight, I recall next what Aristotle states. In response to the inquiry of why drunkards cannot emit sperm or get a woman pregnant, he notes: it is because as the vapors from the wine ascend to the brain, perturbing, altering, and extinguishing reason—as clouds block the light of the sun on earth—the spirits of the perturbed head and, most importantly spermatic matter, which descends from the brain and flows to the genitals to produce a fetus, because of these humid, undigested, and watery vapors, become non-prolific.[9] And even if this type of sperm generates, it produces a weak fetus, disposed to fall into a fit of apoplexy and die like an epileptic of a similar infirmity. Therefore, *frontose*, be careful not to allow yourselves to be taken by a drunken husband.

Considering what we have discussed, those who do not wish to create a family, and who abstain from sexual intercourse for many days in order to avoid this, should beware: because when they eventually partake in the act, they come with "good currency" and "really pay for it"; and the opposite of what they desire occurs [as they will immediately conceive]. But what has just been explained is true when they don't retain sperm far too long, since retaining it can be harmful, diminishing the intensity of the heat and weakening the spirits. Therefore, those who wish to impregnate their wives must act in a moderate way: in other words, coitus should not occur too often, nor should it be engaged in too seldom. I believe that the most common time frame is once every five days, at the appropriate moment, which we will discuss in the next chapter. However, it is also true that some may engage in the act more often, such as those who are by temperament

---

7. This anecdote cannot be found in Gregory the Great's *Dialogues*. According to a legend, Gregory himself was both the product of incest and a participant. Son of brother-sister pairing, he unwittingly married his mother. When the truth came out, he repented, and went on to become Pope. See Willem P. Gerritsen and Anthony G. Van Melle, eds., *A Dictionary of Medieval Heroes: Characters in Medieval Narrative Traditions, and Their Afterlife in Literature, Theatre and the Visual Arts* (Woodbridge, Suffolk, UK; Rochester, NY: The Boydell Press, 1998), 130–32.

8. The same examples are cited in Savonarola's *Practica maior*, tract. VI, c. 21, rubr. 23, fols. 264v–65r.

9. See Aristotle [pseud.], *Problems*, ed. and trans. Robert A. Mayhew (Cambridge, MA: Harvard University Press, 2011), III.4, 871a23–26 (p. 103); III.11, 872b15–25 (p. 109), and III.33, 875b39–876a14 (p. 135).

choleric, while others, who are melancholic, should do so less frequently.[10] I leave such decisions to be determined by attending physicians.

And regarding the length of the penis, I shall recall what Aristotle states in the second book of *On the Generation of Animals*. He says that when serpents copulate, they coil and they press against each other, shortening their length, so that the sperm dispersed from a shorter vessel retains its heat and so travels more vigorously and more directly.[11] And also take note, *frontoso*, that too great brevity of the penis may also prevent conception, as the doctors have affirmed. And this is because a very short penis cannot ejaculate the sperm far enough into that spot in the neck of the uterus where the woman receives pleasure, and where, from such delight, the uterus draws itself up on the sperm, absorbing it as the stomach swallows food.

Now on this topic I will present the following argument: if sperm emitted into a woman from a short penis does not impregnate, how is it that when sperm is ejaculated outside of her, it can impregnate? Well, *frontoso*, I am not sure what to think of the story I have told you from Averroes:[12] but certainly you will agree that a woman may be amazingly crafty. Now since Averroes claims that he was told [this story] by an old woman whom he trusted, but does not cite himself as eyewitness, we may infer from this that she tricked him, and that those young girls involved tricked the old woman, as they know well how to do, and that they were impregnated by sperm ejaculated inside of them and not outside their bodies.[13]

So if you ask about the length of the penis, I'll tell you that a handbreadth is what doctors claim is the most common size. If we revisit the story told by Gregory [the Great], it seems that this mother excused herself [for her own sexual misdeed] with a feeble excuse, as women often do, blaming her young child for impregnating her—a child who knew nothing about such business. O *frontosa*, if you can believe such a thing, I suggest you not keep your child too close to you while you sleep! Regarding Marsilio's tale, I believe it, as I do the story told by Messer Niccolò, considering the fact that the woman was noble and well-known.

10. When a medieval physician defines a particular individual as having a choleric, melancholic, phlegmatic, or sanguine temperament (or complexion), he is referring to the Hippocratic and Galenic derived humoral medical doctrine. According to this theory, each body has a natural balance of the four basic humors (blood, phlegm, yellow bile or choler, and black bile or melancholy), and an equally natural prevalence of one of these humours over the others. It is this prevalence that defines the individual temperament, to which different physical and character characteristics are linked, as well as different predispositions to health and disease. See note 131 in the Introduction to this volume (41).

11. See Aristotle, *On the Generation of Animals*, ed. Hendrik J. Drossaart Lulofs (Oxford: Clarendon Press, 1965), I.7, 718a17–34.

12. See *MM*, 58 and note 2.

13. In the original source Savonarola is referring to, there is not the old woman who acts as an intermediary between the story recounted by the young girls and what was told to Averroes, but only a woman who swears she got pregnant in this way.

We must remember that such things are possible, even though they occur very rarely; and that of those things that occur out of the ordinary, Aristotle says there can be no science.[14]

Concluding such a digression, and returning to our proposed topic, I intend to persuade you, using rational arguments, that young men and women should wait until the appropriate age to engage in coitus so that the result may be pregnancy and strong, robust, and long-lived progeny.

At this point, however, I would like to clarify a notion before it is too late to do so, in order to resolve a great doubt. This is regarding what we have said about the female's seed, that it necessarily contributes to the generation of the fetus, although many women find themselves pregnant who have never felt their own seed ejaculated at all, as I have been informed, and this is true. It is also important, however, to know that women produce something that is similar to sperm, but is not real sperm: a substance that doctors call *alguadi*, a substance which, when it is emitted by the uterus, gives pleasure, as does that substance that is discharged from a man's penis when he kisses or caresses a woman with his hands. This moisture is also *alguadi* and not sperm. Nature has given an increased quantity of this substance to the woman in order to give her pleasure and to render her more ready for coitus, so that she may be more prepared to generate children. In addition, this moisture helps to cool off a man's sperm when it is too hot, as happens in cholerics whose testicles are scorching hot. In addition, this moisture is useful in smoothing out the rough spots in the cervix, so that the man's sperm does not disperse, but instead descends evenly and as a mass down the uterus to the place of generation.

In addition to this lubrication, a woman also produces real sperm generated in her testicles, which are located outside of her uterus and attached to her exterior membrane. This real sperm is sent directly through her seminal tubes inside the uterus, and does not pass through the cervix, where there is the sensation of so much pleasure; instead, it is not felt, as in the esophagus when food that had been enjoyed when eaten descends to the stomach. And although as I have previously stated, this substance is a necessary and active contribution to generation, it is more passive than a man's sperm, since the spermatic members of the fetus are created by the man's sperm,[15] as Galen says, and Nature emits the female seed

---

14. See Aristotle, *Metaphysics*, ed. William D. Ross (Oxford: Clarendon Press, 1924), VI.2, 1027a19–26.

15. In expounding the medical theory of generation, in which both seeds contribute actively and passively to the formation of the fetus, Savonarola follows Avicenna in considering the male sperm responsible for the formation of the so-called "spermatic parts" of the fetus (bones, nerves, cartilage, and the main vital organs), which correspond to the noblest limbs. According to this medical tradition, conversely, female menstrual blood was held responsible for the formation of the "bloody parts" of the future individual, identified in the flesh and fat. The theory of (Aristotelian) philosophers assigned instead to the male semen a purely formal role, while the female menstrual blood was the only material element of the fetus. On these issues, see Karine Van 't Land, "Sperm and Blood, Form and Food.

where it needs to be [in the uterus] in order for the female to get pregnant, mixing it with the sperm deposited by the male.

Thus, it is possible for a woman to get pregnant without feeling any pleasure, since that moisture called *alguadi*, the source of her delight, does not always appear in the uterus because it is not necessary for pregnancy. It is also true that some women do experience pleasure when they become pregnant, having moisture in the uterus, which is the source of her delight.

Contrary to the opinion of philosophers, Galen adduces numerous explanations to prove that the woman's sperm contributes to the generation of the fetus. Among them, he argues that there is no other possible explanation for the resemblance of sons to their mothers. He says:

> this is why the seed of the man through its qualities does not overpower the seed of the woman, except in the place and determination of sex, and in all or many other members the qualities of the woman's seed win out; and for the opposite reason, it happens that the daughter is similar to the father.[16]

So briefly, we can summarize that both a man's and a woman's sperm contribute to generation, but generally it is a man's sperm that contributes much more than the woman's.

Now perhaps you may ask, *frontosa*, "how is this possible, since it is common knowledge that children more often resemble their mothers than their fathers, and we can see this from experience, too?" As I have previously stated, my response is that in the sperm of one and the other lies the generative power, called by doctors the generative spirit, which is composed of three spirits: the vital, which descends from the heart; the natural, produced by the liver; and the animal, born in the brain. This last spirit is the most noble of them all because it controls movement of the body and regulates the sensitive and intellectual cognition of the soul, which differentiates man from beast. This is why Plato deemed the brain nobler than the heart, from which the vital spirit descends, but which heart, according to Aristotle, is also the foundation of the natural and the animal spirits. It is on this point that these two most important philosophers do not agree; they do, however, agree that these three spirits contribute to the generation of the testicles, in which

---

Late Medieval Medical Notions of Male and Female in the Embryology of *Membra*," in *Blood, Sweat and Tears: The Changing Concepts of Physiology from Antiquity into Early Modern Europe*, ed. Manfred Horstmanshoff, Helen King, and Claus Zittel (Leiden and Boston: Brill, 2012), 363–92.

16. In Latin in the text: *eo quod sperma viri suis qualitatibus non vincit sperma mulieris nisi in solo loco et causa sexus, et in omnibus aut pluribus aliis membris vincunt qualitates seminis mulieris: et per oppositum accidit quod filia est similis patri.* See Galen, *De semine*, Lib. II, c. 2 (p. 610).

sperm is produced and in which they reside, with the capacity to generate and to imprint the parent's own likeness on the fetus.

Therefore, this animal spirit, which descends from the brain at the moment of impregnation, where the impression of the likeness of external things is engraved, especially in the first ventricle of the brain, where the faculty of fantasy resides, descends to the region of generation with the image [of the man] engraved in it, and it then firmly engraves his likeness in the matter that generates the fetus. But since such likeness is much better retained in the fantasies of women than of men, given that their animal spirit is stronger, that likeness—that is, the likeness of the man—is reproduced in the fetus. We are convinced that the likeness in the woman's imagination is much stronger [than that in a man's] by the frequency with which women look at themselves in the mirror; and for this reason, women, in their imagination, retain a stronger and clearer likeness than do men, who never look at themselves in the mirror.

This is why bastard children more often resemble their putative fathers than their real fathers: because of the retained image of the putative father in the woman's imagination, since women feel guilty when they are in the act of betraying their husbands and therefore recall the image of their husbands, fearing them. Similarly, this is why, as Aristotle reminds us, a white woman could give birth to a dark black child, having at the moment of conception recalled the image of a black man in a painting in her chamber.[17] And from this we can also deduce why young lovers, when they first become pregnant, give birth to children who resemble their beloved. For the same reason, those women who are ugly, if they desire to have beautiful offspring, should avoid looking at themselves in the mirror and instead recall a beautiful woman and reflect on her beauty when in the act of coitus. This will certainly help to produce beautiful offspring.

Furthermore, there are those who say regarding this matter that, assuming that menstrual blood contributes to generation, and that it has more affinity with the mother, then this menstrual blood, controlled and also aided by the generative power of the mother, will result in the birth of a son who resembles her. Even though the strength of the menses and the generative power of the maternal seed may have outweighed the father's formative power with regard to features, form, and heat, it has not, however, been able to prevail on the issue of sex, which is why it is a male child who is produced, who resembles the mother. And I hold this opinion supported by what has already been said, and as a response to this disputed question, because it would take too long to expound further these complex matters on which physicians disagree with philosophers.

17. This is a recurring tale, traditionally attributed to Aristotle. The narrative is somewhat confused, however: Heliodorus wrote in his *Aethiopica* that Persina, the queen of Ethiopia, conceived with King Hydustes, himself an Ethiopian, a daughter who was white, after focusing on a painting of Andromache. The anecdote of a black child born to white parents is attributed to Quintilian, and occasionally to Hippocrates and Aristotle.

And having already said so much about the age of the young man, we will now shift our attention to the age of the young woman, emphasizing as did Avicenna that before she is mature, her uterus is not well developed nor is it disposed to generation.[18] If she does become pregnant and give birth, her child will be weak, frail, and imperfect: it will be sickly and live only a short life. But it is certainly true that the level of maturity of the uterus varies according to the girl's constitution, since girls with different types of constitution have diverse life courses. For instance, those with a sanguine temperament live longer than melancholics, and mature later; wherefore, in women of sanguine complexion, maturity will be reached in the twentieth year, whereas in melancholic women, it will be in the sixteenth. But in conclusion, as it is written, we will say that a young woman's maturity is reached in her eighteenth year. As Aristotle maintains when he says: "because of which, it is appropriate for them to get married around the age of eighteen."[19]

And following this, he says of the man: "marriage will be suitable for those around the [age of] thirty-seven, in respect to the perfection of their bodies and in the convenient time in order to procreate children."[20] Aristotle's theory may seem extreme, in that it surpasses by so many years the maturity of the man; so we will say to satisfy readers that Aristotle did not maintain that thirty-seven years was the earliest a man should copulate with a woman. When both the man and the woman have reached their perfect maturity, and their members are well-developed to the point that nature is no longer engaged in their development, and their genitals are well-developed, it is at this point that they may appropriately engage in coitus: for from these perfect beginnings, we may expect a perfect result. A man may, therefore, fittingly engage in coitus with a woman at the age of twenty-one, when typically he has reached his maturity: I say typically, for as it is certain that Aristotle maintained that an eighteen-year-old woman could lie with a man, and a man of twenty-one with a woman, we may therefore understand Aristotle's words to mean that thirty-seven is the zenith of a man's perfection, which physicians term "full manhood."[21] We should also understand that the beginning of this cycle

---

18. See Avicenna, *Canon*, Lib. III, fen 21, tract. 1, c. 11 (p. 929).

19. In Latin in the text: *propter quod has quidem congruit circa etatem decem et octo annorum coniugari.* See Aristotle, *Politics*, trans. Benjamin Jowett, ed. W. C. Davis (Oxford: Clarendon Press, 1905), VII.16, 1335a28–29.

20. In Latin in the text: *hos autem circa triginta septem aut parum in tanto omni tempore perfectis corporibus [coniugatio erit et ad profectum puerorum procreationis convenient temporibus] oportune.* See Aristotle, *Politics*, VII.16, 1335a28–29. As noted by Belloni (*DRP*, 62), Savonarola's quotation of this passage from Aristotle's *Politics* seems to be corrupted; the words in square brackets are missing in the Vatican manuscript, and I corrected *perfectum* in *profectum* according to the standard Latin reading of Aristotle.

21. The expression *etas consistentie*, in Latin in the text, is frequently used, for example, by Avicenna to define the male age between thirty and forty.

for a man is at the beginning of his twenty-second year, if we were to describe the perfect age for man to generate and produce the most perfect, robust, and long-lived offspring. And perhaps Albert the Great had this in mind when he comments in Book V of *De animalibus*: "for the human male has perfectly mature seed at the age of thirty, and he is able to generate up to age eighty."[22] We will deal with this later. So then it seems that at the age it reaches potency, semen is more perfect than at any other moment, but it is much more perfect at the middle of this age range, that is, when a man is more or less thirty years old.

And for similar reasons, we maintain that when a woman reaches her age of perfection, she more easily gives birth to stronger, more robust children with more perfect parts, and she accomplishes this with less pain, all other things being equal. And for this reason we should acknowledge that when infants are born with better body parts, the soul then will be able to perform its function better: therefore, they will be stronger, wiser, and have better memories and the capacity to learn the arts and sciences. And given this, we can understand why a horse-keeper, in order to have more beautiful and vigorous colts, mates stallions with mares—I don't mean decrepit horses, but animals having reached the mature age of ten to twelve, an age at which they are considered old, but not too old, since a horse's life expectancy is from twenty to twenty-five years, even though some reach the age of forty—and on this account, they are careful not to allow colts to mate with fillies. This is why in Puglia when praising a horse they say it "must be the son of an old horse."

And returning to our subject, we must recall that Aristotle emphasizes that before men and women reach maturity, coitus should not be attempted, because in such coitus essential spirits and nourishment are consumed and wasted and these spirits and nourishment should be used to promote maturity. This is why the church, in order not to stunt a youth's growth, does not require a young person to fast. Albert the Great resolves the question in book V of his *De animalibus*, where he says, regarding the perfection of the sperm: "it is suitable and good when the third seven-year period has been completed," and he adds, "for then the seed is thicker and more clotted, and its heat is made hotter as its superfluous humidity dries out, on account of which it is more suitable for generation." And in Book IX he says that

> sperm that is suitable for generation is that which is sufficiently de-cocted, and this is distilled in the third seven-year period. Before this time, as is seen in many cases, the seed is not perfected, not having

22. In Latin in the text: *homo enim masculus triginta annos habens semen perfecte maturum, potest generare usque ad octuaginta annos.* See Albert the Great, *De animalibus*, vol. 1, Lib. V, tract. 2, c. 1 (p. 431). Stadler's edition of the *De animalibus* differs, giving the age span as from age twenty to age seventy. Savonarola will quote this passage again in the next pages, giving the age of seventy. See note 29.

the perfected power of generating anything of human form, for although those of lesser age can generate something from their seed, what they produce is weak and infirm, not completing the full circuit of human life.[23]

And from this we can easily establish the proper time for appropriate matrimonial union.

Now perhaps you will say that "the law permits women to marry at the age of twelve and men at the age of fourteen," and I will respond that this is true with regard to the age of consent and with regard to their ability to perform; however, the law neither wants nor commands that they should engage in coitus at such an early age. The lawmakers who wrote this legislation simply did not consider the purpose behind the act of reproduction. With all due deference, I surely will not remain silent but argue with these men that a legislator is in charge of governing the republic, and considering that wisdom and strength are two qualities by which the republic is defended, wisdom in times of peace, and strength in times of war, it should be in his best interest that his citizens be born strong and robust, in order better to defend the land in times of war, and wise so that they may better govern during both peace and war. But as for those born from parents who are past their prime, or for those born to parents who are too young, I would like legislators to establish that no one can marry before the appropriate age. And this I would like to see written and enforced.

Finally, I would like to remind young women whose body parts are not quite ready for generation—that is, the uterus is not prepared to carry the fetus properly, nor is the exit for the fetus wide enough or naturally dilated enough—that when they come to labor, they will experience great suffering and because of the narrowness of the passage, will find it very painful. And many young women find themselves close to death, or mortally sick, because they have become pregnant too young. Avicenna notes: "and when a girl becomes pregnant who has not yet completed fifteen years, her death should be feared on account of the smallness of her womb."[24]

---

23. In Latin in the text: *conveniens autem et bonum est in tertii septenarii complemento*, et subdit *tunc sperma spissius et glandulosius efficitur, et suus calor calidior efficitur in ipso superflua exsiccata humiditate: propter quod convenientius est ad generandum*. Et in VIIII inquit *sperma quod conveniens est ad generationem filiorum, est illud quod est sufficienter decoctum: et hoc est quod in tertio distillat septuanario: ante hoc tempus ut in pluribus non est sperma complete habens virtutem generandi perfectum aliquid in genere humano: quia quamvis in minori etate parentum generetur ex spermate eorum, tamen illud quod generatur, fit debile et infirmum, non complens periodum humane vite*. See Albert the Great, *De animalibus*, vol. 1, Lib. V, tract. 2, c. 1 (p. 427); and vol. 1, Lib. IX, tract. 1, c. 2 (p. 680) respectively.

24. In Latin in the text: *et cum impregnatur puella que nundum consecuta est annos XV, timetur ei mors propter parvitatem matricis*. See Avicenna, *Canon*, Lib. III, fen 21, tract. 1, c. 11 (p. 929).

This is why nature has made women wider at the bottom, and those who are narrow like men experience great pain and difficulty during labor. Just as man tends to be broad on top and narrow below, the opposite is true of woman. This is why the women of Bologna and Padua have an easier time giving birth than those of Ferrara. Also, this is why, my ladies, you should retain a good midwife and learn, you mothers and fathers who love your daughters dearly, to keep your daughters at home until the right age and not risk losing them, together with your daughter's dowry.

What I have said is generally true; but sometimes one finds young women who even before the age of maturity are well-endowed, wide in the hips, and robust with prominent breasts; they are not afraid of a heavy weight, but bear such weight with ease. These girls can marry younger; perhaps, between the ages of sixteen and eighteen. Aristotle says that in certain areas of Greece, there exist temples where prayers are offered for young women, so that God may mitigate the suffering of young parturients, and care for their health and their offspring.

Chapter Two
On the time when the husband and wife should engage in sexual intercourse in order to achieve pregnancy

Having already discussed at length the appropriate age for coitus in marriage, it is now time to discuss what moment is appropriate for such activity in order to achieve the most perfect possible offspring. We will therefore first discuss in general what this is, and later we will deal with the specifics needed in order to achieve pregnancy.

On this topic, we will say, following Aristotle, that cold weather is much more conducive to pregnancy than warm weather. Therefore, nuptials should be in cool weather, whereas Aristotle says "as to the proper times in respect of the season we may accept what is customary with most people, who have rightly decided even as it is to practice marital cohabitation in winter."[25] And the reason for this is that in cool weather, bodies tend to be warmer, more filled with spirit and—all other things being equal—stronger; as Hippocrates says, "our innards are naturally hottest in winter and spring."[26] In cold weather, the pores of the exterior body constrict themselves and close up, and this is what causes the consolidation of the natural heat that makes a pregnancy stronger, and consequently, more effective,

---

25. In Latin in the text: *his autem que circa tempore vietatem, temporibus oportet uti, quibus multi utuntur bene et nunc determinantes hyeme fieri commemorationem hanc.* See Aristotle, *Politics*, VII.14, 1335a36–38.

26. In Latin in the text: *ventres vero hieme et vere caldissimi sunt natura.* See Hippocrates, *Aphorisms*, in *Hippocrates*, trans. William H. S. Jones (Cambridge, MA: Harvard University Press, 1931), 4:97–222, at I.15 (p. 105).

so that children born in cool weather tend to be more robust and strong. This is why shepherds, who understand this theory, when they wish to breed their sheep, make them turn their backs towards the north wind. Therefore, *frontoso*, if you desire your children to be fit and robust, get started with that pregnancy in winter or spring; additionally, in those seasons your body will have fewer ailments. And remember the common proverb: "June, July, August, oh wife of mine, I don't know you." Because it is certain that, due to the great heat in the summer months, our vital spirits are transformed, and bodies and genital members that are closed and strong in the winter become weaker and wilt in the heat, as experience shows us.

Therefore, if you desire, *frontoso*, strong and robust offspring, do not impregnate *frontosa* in the heat, or when you are weakened by great fatigue or other difficulties, from abstinence, or for other reasons, as, for example, when a scholar finds his spirits diminished: and you should take note of this, doctor. This is why physicians recommend coitus when the northeast wind reigns, because then the air is cold, more than when the hot southern wind blows. Children engendered in hot seasons or by those whose spirits are weakened by exercise, or study, etc., are often wretched and weak. O *frontoso*, learned scholar, keep in mind that Aristotle says that children born to a studious man, that is, one engaged in literary pursuits, are often wretched, and sometimes crazy, and the animal vitality of the generative spirit is often weakened because of excessive study; for it is certain that Venus [the goddess of love] does not mix with Pallas [the goddess of wisdom]. And you, who are a bit long in the tooth, pay close attention to what we have said: this business is not for you. Therefore, my dear readers, you who wish to revel or carouse, keep your shields up and practice moderation.

I will also not ignore here what Avicenna says about lustful old men: that it is more dangerous for old men to break their lance on such a shield than if they were to spread their blood forty-six times.[27] Remember this saying, old lustful man. This is why Aristotle sets man's age limit for generation at seventy and woman's at the age of fifty: this is the average, even though some men and some women find themselves able to generate even after this age. He says "there is fixed end of generation, the highest number of years for men being seventy in most cases, but fifty for women."[28] On this topic, Albert the Great writes:

27. Avicenna, while generally advising men (young or old alike) not to lie with women who are too old, sick, menstruating, too young, or virgins, did not in fact state that it is more dangerous for old men to copulate with young women than to be phlebotomised forty-six times when writing *de nocumento coitus* (c. 11, p. 902), *de regimine eius quem laedit coitus* (c. 35, p. 912) or *de regimine eius, qui plurimum utitur coitu, et nocetur eo* [. . .] (c. 36, p. 912); nor he did mention anything similar in the whole fen 20, tract. 1 (*De membris virilibus et coitu*) of his *Canon*, Lib. III, fen 20, tract. 1, cc. 1–48 (pp. 899–915). Similarly, Avicenna—unlike Savonarola—does not use any sexual metaphor, such as that of the lance and the shield which represent here respectively the male and female sexual organs.

28. In Latin in the text: *quoniam autem est determinatus finis generationis, ut ad plurimum est dicere viris quidem numerus septuaginta annorum ultimus, quinquaginta autem mulieribus.* See Aristotle,

for the human male has perfectly mature seed at the age of thirty, and he is able to generate up to age seventy, and sometimes, in the very healthy, this power is extended up to the eightieth year; but thereafter, only labor and pain results, and there is no power to generate however much one has intercourse.[29]

And if you protest that "the previously mentioned Messer Niccolò Pallavicino generated when he was over the age of one hundred," I will respond that this was something out of the ordinary, and there can be no science of such things, as Aristotle says;[30] one swallow does not make a spring.[31] And consequently he says about women "for the woman conceives and bears up to age fifty, and this happens only rarely."[32] And it is true that some exceed such a limit. Therefore, as we stated in the preceding chapter, the statements of philosophers and physicians on this matter for the most part should be taken as truth.

And now, getting to specifics regarding the right moment for coition, we recommend that intercourse should not be engaged in on a full stomach. This is because intercourse debilitates the natural power of digestion, and those who do not digest their food properly, are subject to many grave illnesses: moreover, in such an act the stomach is agitated, and thus grows weak, because it cannot digest properly, causing great suffering. O *frontoso*, remember this when you go to bed and have sex with your wife at night: don't be surprised to wake up with the taste of rotten eggs in your mouth, a gaunt face, and bags under your eyes. Beware, beware, and even if great desire strikes you, remember to go to sleep.

For the same reason, neither should one have sex on an empty stomach, that is, hungry, because in such a state the stomach is greatly weakened, adding more weakness to the already diminished natural heat, as its strength wanes as the body loses weight. Therefore, so as to achieve the perfect pregnancy desired, it is best to wait for the appropriate moment to engage in intercourse.

Next, we recommend that after the emission of bodily fluids, such as intestinal dysentery, vomit, and similar things, which weaken the body, and after

---

Politics, VII.16, 1335a8–12.

29. In Latin in the text: *homo enim masculus circa triginta annos habens semen perfecte maturum potest generare usque ad septuaginta annos, et raro in valentibus protenditur hec virtus usque ad octuaginta; sed post hoc labor et dolor et non est aliqua virtus generationis quamvis coeat.* See Albert the Great, *De animalibus*, Lib. V, tract. 2, c. 1 (p. 431). Savonarola had previously cited the same passage somewhat differently; see note 22.

30. See Aristotle, *Metaphysics*, VI.2, 1027a19–26.

31. This famous proverb is also found in Aristotle, *Nicomachean Ethics*, ed. William D. Ross (Oxford: Clarendon Press, 1908), I.7, 1098a18.

32. In Latin in the text: *mulier autem concipit et parit usque ad etatem quinquaginta annorum: et hoc raro accidit.* See Aristotle, *Politics*, VII.16, 1335a8–12.

great pain such as that felt from kidney stones or gout, one should not engage in intercourse. And for the same reason, a man should beware when he is weakened from too much heat or too much cold, or when his power is diminished for other reasons, as when he has recently recovered from a fever or other malady, that is, when he is convalescent. For coitus for a man in this condition can easily cause him to relapse. O thoughtless beast, who having a fever, or having just recently recovered from such an ailment if you lie with *frontosa*, you are not taking care of yourself, and by doing so you will fall ill again: Avicenna says "the relapse [into sickness] is worse than its root,"[33] so that what follows next may be death, or a dangerous or prolonged malady. So take note, *frontoso*, you who spend your winters waiting for your nightingale in the cold air, and do so again in the great heat under the rays of the sun, and you who have walked four or five miles so as to sing together the sweet song taught by nature, you know what I mean!

And for the same reason, intercourse should not be engaged in either before or after bloodletting, nor in moments of great melancholy, as fools do who hope to drive away their melancholy by means of carnal pleasure. For in such a case, the melancholy does not go away but persists, and the person becomes even more dispirited, and is further weakened by the act. As Galen says, the strong accidents of the soul such as anger, fear, and melancholy diminish strength in such a way that after the act, the body is left prostrate and exhausted. This is why those hoping to be fathers who are not cautious, as Aristotle says, not only harm themselves, but also their future progeny. He also says that such a man, in the act of impregnating his wife, transmits this bad disposition to his offspring, which results in his children being born weak and melancholic, or wrathful or timid; a similar reasoning can explain [how a father with a good disposition can generate] a spiritual, wise and speculative fetus on the same account, introspective, reserved, and introverted.

Now understanding, *frontoso*, all we have said, you may ask, what is the proper moment for coitus? My response is that the appropriate moment is when food has left the stomach and when the second digestion is complete, which is typically six to seven hours after a meal, when the third phase of digestion takes place in the veins: I say typically, because such time may vary according to the strength of the stomach and of the organs and the heaviness or lightness of the food, and therefore, the appropriate moment may be earlier in some cases and later in others. Let us also remember that, if possible, it is always advantageous to sleep after coitus, so as to regain strength: and also I will remind you that it is very beneficial for achieving pregnancy for women to sleep after "the skirmish," as we will explain shortly. And in order to address some common mistakes that men make, it follows that they are doing harm to themselves and to their expected

33. In Latin in the text: *recidivatio peior est sua radice.* See Avicenna, *Canon,* Lib. IV, fen 2, tract. 1, c. 95 (p. 100).

offspring if they go straight to bed after eating and immediately frolic with their wives. And to specify the correct time for intercourse, it is at the [canonical] hour of matins, especially for those who dine at regular hours—in other words, it should be done at nighttime.

And if you ask whether the man or the woman receives more pleasure in the act, I respond that it is the common opinion of doctors that man receives an intense delight that lasts briefly, but a woman's delight lasts much longer.[34] This is because the neck of the uterus, upon which such a delicious sensation is experienced, is much longer and broader than the head, or extremity, of the man's penis, in which man feels intense pleasure; and this is why a man feels that sensation more sharply and more perfectly than the woman.

And now to continue about the appropriate time for the woman, I say that the suitable hour for the woman is when she is clean from her menstruation, because finding itself clear, the uterus receives the semen with more appetite and delight and retains it better, and thus is not impeded by superfluities, which might corrupt it. Now take note, *frontoso*, if man lies with a menstruating woman against God's commandment, and she gets pregnant, he risks generating a leper, or a child whose skin is mottled, or one with the ulcerous skin condition doctors call *saphati*.[35] Therefore, *frontoso* and *frontosa*, I pray that you refrain from intercourse when the Marquis is galloping through town.[36] Also, I will not withhold what pro-

34. In his *Pantegni*, Constantinus Africanus asserts that women enjoy intercourse more than men do because men receive pleasure only from expulsion of sperm, whereas women enjoy themselves doubly (*dupliciter delectantur*), in expelling their own sperm and in receiving that of the male. See *Pantechni decem libri theorices* [*Liber pantegni*], 6.17, in *Opera omnia Ysaac* (Lyon: Bartholomeus Trot in officina Johannis de Platea, 1515), fol. 28r: *Delectatio in coitu maior est in mulieribus quam in masculis, quia masculi delectantur tantum in expulsione superfluitatis. Mulieres dupliciter delectantur, et in suo spermate expellendo, et masculi recipiendo ex vulve ardentis desiderio.* This passage is also quoted in Mary F. Wack, "The Measure of Pleasure: Peter of Spain on Men, Women and Lovesickness," *Viator*, 17 (1986): 177. In his introduction to *The Prose Salernitan Questions*, Brian Lawn adduces parallels from the Pseudo-Aristotelian *Problems*, Adelard of Bath's *Quaestiones naturales*, and the *Anatomia Nicolai*; Brian Lawn, ed., *The Prose Salernitan Questions, Edited from a Bodleian Manuscript, Auct. F.3.10: An Anonymous Collection Dealing with Science and Medicine* (London: Oxford University Press for the British Academy, 1979), 4. For a similar discourse in Avicenna, see *Canon*, Lib. III, fen 21, tract. 1, c. 2 (p. 923).

35. After Avicenna and Rhazes, medieval doctors named *saphati* the appearance of small pustules on the face or head, involving crustaceous ulcerations. See Treatise Three, 192.

36. The "Marquis" is a euphemism (still in use today) for menstrual period. According to Tullio De Mauro, editor of GRADIT [*Grande dizionario italiano dell'uso*], 8 vols. (Turin: UTET, 1999–2007), this meaning is attested since the fifteenth century and possibly derives from the old French idiom "Marquis," from *marquer*, meaning "to sign" or "to mark"; it was used with the same association in France, as attested by the English lexicographer Randle Cotgrave in his 1611 *Dictionarie of the French and English Tongues* (reprinted Columbia: University of South Carolina Press, 1950). Salvatore Battaglia quotes this very passage from Savonarola as the first Italian occurrence of the term: Battaglia,

verbially is said that because of this prohibition, "men go crazy," since they do not care to observe rules or limits; but instead that wise men in such an act (the sexual act) pull on the reins of the horse so that they do not stumble. Having already said so much about the right moment, I believe that for the present this will suffice.

Chapter Three
On pregnancy, and the rules that should be observed in order to achieve pregnancy

Since we have already discussed the appropriate age and the correct moment when married partners should participate in coitus, we will now proceed to define pregnancy—for, as Aristotle maintains, knowledge of the name is the principle of all doctrine[37]—and later we will explain clearly what is achieved by coitus, and how, and also what rules should be observed in order to achieve this desired effect.

As it is my desire that my writing should give readers great pleasure, I suggest that we reflect upon the great power of God and the vileness of man, as well as the great benefits received from God, so that man will be humbled and cognizant of the gifts he receives. O vile man, formed of vile substance, you who are the most noble and beautiful and most perfect creature under the heavens created by God, ask yourself with great wonder, out of what substance were you first created. O great and admirable power of God, who created from mud and earth something so precious as man; even though, in nature, from weak beginnings vile effects naturally follow, nevertheless, the work of God omnipotent, to whom all created things are subjected, is able to ennoble what is vile and make what is noble base. O ungrateful and proud man, think and reflect upon Adam, our first father, who was formed from vile earth by the sacred hand of God omnipotent: *For he formed Adam from the clay of the earth*,[38] Genesis 2. Remember that you were formed from vile and fetid matter, from the superfluous waste from the food you eat, from an element viler still than the first element created by God—*In the*

---

ed., *Grande dizionario della lingua italiana*, 21 vols. (Turin: UTET, 1961–2009). The same use of *marchese* for menstrual flow appears in the first Dictionary of the Accademia della Crusca (1612), where a similar example by the Italian satirical poet Francesco Berni (1497–1535) is given. According to the *Dizionario dei sinonimi* of the Istituto dell'Enciclopedia Italiana (Treccani), at <https://www.treccani.it/vocabolario/marchese_%28Sinonimi-e-Contrari%29/>, "*marchese*" is a euphemistic replacement for "mese" (month), i.e. "period."

37. Savonarola is perhaps referring to the *Posterior Analytics*, where Aristotle states that our knowledge always originates from a previous understanding, and that this understanding is often the recognition of a given meaning for a word or a phrase. See Aristotle, *Posterior Analytics*, in *Prior and Posterior Analytics*, ed. William D. Ross (Oxford: Clarendon Press, 1949), I.1, 71a1–2.

38. Genesis 2:7: *formavit enim Adam de limo terre*. The Vulgate reads: *formavit igitur Dominus Deus hominem de limo terrae*. Here and henceforth, the Latin Vulgate version is provided alongside Savonarola's where it differs from his own quotation from Scripture.

beginning God created the heaven and the earth,[39] Genesis 1—earth being such a useful and fruitful element. Remember that you were not formed by God's sacred hand, but instead by two of the most vile organs of the human body, loathsome to the eyes, organs that you keep covered out of modesty. From where then comes all your pride? What is the origin of your ingratitude towards God? Recognize his great power, the benevolence that God shows towards you and give thanks to him for all the blessings he has bestowed upon you, you who were born of such vile matter, and yet have been so exalted, that, as David the psalmist says, God has *put all things under [your] feet, all sheep and oxen, and the beasts of the field, the birds of the sky, and the fish of the sea.*[40] O man, as God has created you, is he not your father? Therefore, why do you not honor him, respecting his comandments: *Honor your father and your mother, so that you may live long upon the earth?*[41] You should fear and honor him, and you should be grateful for his priceless gifts. Assuredly, your great vileness should be made manifest to you, as has been said, by the matter of which you are made and the great stink that you emit when the soul is separated from the body, for it is so, more than that of any other corpse. O great is the power of God, which has conceded such dignity to such a vile body. Man should always be grateful and cognizant of such gifts. He will gain great happiness when his soul is glorified.

And now to proceed to our proposed topic, explaining that in medicine, this word, that is pregnancy, has three senses: conception, generation, and pregnancy. Conception is the enveloping of the seed by the womb,[42] and this is the first act, before pregnancy. Generation is the making or production of the embryo,[43] and this is the second act. After these follows pregnancy, which means that, by the previous two acts, the belly of the woman is filled, so that we can also say impregnation is so called because there is a beginning of the child.[44] Therefore, a woman should not be called *pregnante* until the vital, natural, and animal force enters the body of the fetus, which until the moment of entry of the soul is called *embrio*—with an "e," which means "out," and "brios," which means "limbs"—which is simply a clump of sperm and blood formed in the uterus without any distinction

39. Genesis 1:1: *in principio enim creavit Deus celum et terram.* The Vulgate reads: *in principio creavit Deus caelum et terram.*

40. Psalm 8:6–8: *omnia subiecisti sub pedibus eius, oves et boves, universa pecora campi, volucres celi et pisces maris.* The Vulgate reads: *omnia subjecisti sub pedibus ejus, oves et boves universas, insuper et pecora campi, volucres caeli et pisces maris.*

41. Exodus 20:12: *honora patrem et matrem, ut sis longevus super terram.* The Vulgate reads: *Honora patrem tuum et matrem tuam, ut sis longaevus super terram, quam Dominus Deus tuus dabit tibi.*

42. In Latin in the text: *Conceptio est seminis a matrice comprehensio.*

43. In Latin in the text: *Generatio est embrionis factio sive productio.*

44. In Latin in the text: *impregnatio quia nati impressio.*

of body parts, as we will discuss.[45] After the limbs are distinct, and he is able to move them, he is called an infant, or *infante*, as noted by Hippocrates. But it is true that at both stages of pregnancy, at the time of the embryo and of the infant, the woman may be called gravid, or *gravida*, weighed down by the fetus.

And now let us move on to material that will give everyone much pleasure. It should be known, having satisfied the goals announced for Chapter Two and addressing those promised at the beginning of the present chapter, that such a pregnancy is achieved in this way: by the man emitting his sperm into the uterus, so that the woman may become pregnant, and she, receiving it with the greatest eagerness, then emitting her sperm, converging with her menstrual blood, to the place of generation, that is, in the cell of the right- or left-hand side of the uterus, or in both. From these three substances, the fetus is generated in the womb/uterus, that is, from foul-smelling sperm and stinking and fetid menstrual blood. And do not forget this, O powerful, proud man! When with great pleasure the uterus draws up and tightly squeezes the head of the man's penis such that, if the man and woman concentrate, they will feel a sensation, then they will know that she has become pregnant, as we will discuss in Chapter Four, *on the signs of pregnancy*.

After this moment the uterus tightens so tightly that, as Avicenna describes, it could barely be penetrated with the tip of a very fine stylus.[46] And it is said "in one cell or in more than one," which means that in the uterus there are seven places, called "cells" by doctors, and in all of these the generation of the fetus is possible: three are on the right-hand side, three on the left-hand side, and one in the middle. A fetus can be generated in any of these; therefore, a woman can bear up to seven children in one labor. [47]

But, before writing about this, I would like to respond to a question: "why is it that a woman does not always become pregnant when a man emits sperm inside her uterus?" My response is that just as soil that is not prepared does not produce fruit from the seeds planted in it, so likewise the uterus needs to be well-prepared if it is to produce fruit from the seed emitted inside of it. Both great appetite and pleasure are necessary in order to prepare the uterus to bear fruit, so that the woman will emit her sperm at the right moment, and her pleasurable sensations cause the uterus to tighten, drawing all the sperm out of the penis, as we have said

---

45. Savonarola's etymology for embryo is not correct. The correct one is *en* (into)—*brúō* (swell, grow).

46. See Avicenna, *Canon*, Lib. III, fen 21, tract. 1, c. 1 (p. 920).

47. Notwithstanding the exposition of the so-called seven-cell theory of the uterus, of late-ancient origins, Savonarola will later specify that he, as a physician, does not embrace this theory; see *MM*, 79. For the theory itself, see Fridolf Kudlein, "The Seven Cells of the Uterus: The Doctrine and its Roots," *Bulletin of the History of Medicine* 39 (1965): 415–23; Robert Reisert, *Die siebenkammerige Uterus: Studien zur mittelalterlichen Wirkungsgeschichte und Entfaltung eines embryologischen Gebärmuttermodells* (Pattensen, Germany: Horst Wellm, 1986).

before. Next, the presence of menstrual blood is necessary, as Avicenna notes in fen 3, particula 1:

> and therefore we say that two things were at the origin of the gen-
> eration of our bodies, one of which is the sperm of the man, whose
> essence more certainly holds the place of the active principle, and
> the other is the sperm of the woman and the menstrual blood, a sub-
> stance that most certainly has the function of material principle.[48]

And therefore if sperm is thrust into a woman who is not well-disposed, pregnancy does not always follow.

Now returning to the topic from which we have digressed. Man usually feels
his seed ejaculating in spurts into the uterus, and not all at once. When the seed
ejaculates in spurts in different places and in sufficient quantity to impregnate,
multiple fetuses may be conceived with a single emission of sperm: and even two,
three, or five fetuses can be generated, as I have seen in my day. And setting aside
here the opinion of Aristotle, stated in the tenth section of his *Problems*,[49] and
instead believing the doctors, who base their opinions on experience and reason,
who say there are no such cells, and also to render our writing more pleasurable
to our readers, I will suggest another cause of multiple fetuses in one pregnancy.
And it is this: that when the uterus has its mouth wide-open in order to receive all
the sperm, as is most often the case, and it finds itself with a quantity that would
be sufficient for the generation of two or three fetuses, nature, which always tries
to do its best, generates from this superfluity many fetuses.

O *frontosa*, I pray that you well consider how noble is your pregnancy: for
even though you have two breasts, with which you could potentially nourish two
fetuses, nevertheless nature usually causes you to be pregnant with one single
fetus at a time, because it often happens that—given the great worth of the infant,
for no animal is more worthy than man—both breasts are not sufficient to nourish him. Take note of what Aristotle says: that sows can nourish as many piglets,
and can become pregnant with as many as the number of nipples they possess.
Thus nature has provided for the human fetus, and for this, more than any other
creature, it has expressed great concern. So God created women with two breasts,
so that if one becomes diseased, the other can supply what is needful to its noble
fruit. It is also true that breasts beautify a woman and make her more exciting

---

48. In Latin in the text: *et dicemus quoniam propterea quod generationis nostrorum corporum prin-
cipium res due fuerunt, quarum una est sperma viri, cuius essentie certius est quod locum tenet factoris,
et altera est sperma mulieris et sanguis mestruus, rei cuius certius est quod locum tenet materiei.* See
Avicenna, *Canon*, Lib. I, fen 3, c. 1 (p. 162).

49. See Aristotle [pseud.], *Problems*, X.28, 894a7–11 (p. 305); and X.61, 898a9–19 (p. 335).

to man during the act of coitus. In Negroponte,[50] a place made corrupt by [the practice of male homosexuality,] that vice against nature, a counsel of wise men decreed that women should keep their breasts all (or mostly) uncovered, as do many public prostitutes in our times, so as to summon the male penis back to its rightful path. As a friend used to say, breasts are a stone on which men sharpen their blades: you know what I mean. For your health, and so that you may avoid being likened to a sow or beast, my *frontosa*, beware of superfetation.[51] In other words, you should not bear three or four children at once, as beasts do. I want you to know that, although it is said that in the hour of impregnation the uterus closes so that not even the tip of a stylus can penetrate it, its desire and delight to receive the sperm of the man is so great that in the act of coitus it always opens its mouth, and swallows the sperm as a stomach absorbs delightful wine, and later closes itself again. In this way, if the uterus is well-disposed, as I have described, a new fetus is generated. And in this same manner, even three or four fetuses can be generated in different moments, and can be born at different times, as has happened in my time.[52]

O superfetation, how worthy are you to be abhorred by a woman! Learn from wild animals, *frontosa*: for we see bitches and mares and similar beasts, when they are pregnant, do not allow themselves to be mounted, holding such a new union as abominable. Now perhaps you will say that they refuse such pleasure precisely because they are beasts. But I would respond that you are a worse beast than they are: because by such superfetation of another new fetus, the new one

50. Negroponte, nowadays Chalcis, is the ancient name of the chief town of the Greek island of Euboea (or Evia). The name itself derives from an Italian corruption of the medieval Greek name Egripon, and was used to refer to the entire island of Euboea as well.

51. According to ancient authors such as Hippocrates, Aristotle, and Galen, the birth of twins could be explained by superfetation—although rarely, because, according to the same authors, twins are generally produced from one act of intercourse, as a result of an overabundance of generative matter—that is, the phenomenon in which a woman conceives a second time while a previous pregnancy is ongoing. This explanation, although described as less common, was soon connected to the idea of adulterous relationships. Medieval authors added on these ancient medical explanations the motive of female sexual pleasure, which causes the womb to open up again after the first fecundation has already taken place. Savonarola uses here the Latin term *superimpregnatio*, the same used in his *Practica*, tract. VI, c. 21, rubr. 25 (fol. 268r). On views of the generation of twins in the Middle Ages, see Johannes M. Thijssen, "Twins as Monsters: Albertus Magnus's Theory of the Generation of Twins and Its Philosophical Context," *Bulletin of the History of Medicine* 61 (1987): 237–46; and Gabriella Zuccolin, *I gemelli nel Medioevo: Questioni filosofiche, mediche e teologiche* (Pavia: Ibis, 2019).

52. According to Avicenna and medieval medical theories, the time interval between the birth of twins would have been minimum if their conception was the result of a single act of coition; see, for example, Avicenna, *Canon*, Lib. III, fen 21, tract. 1, c. 17. In the rare event of superfetation resulting from separate acts of sexual intercourse, twins could instead be born a number of days apart, and sometimes even weeks or months apart, as attested by the medical literature (and by miracle accounts as well) of the time.

takes away the nourishment of the first, and could cause the death of the first, or at least his weakening, and he would be born weak and would die young; or the first, similarly, could do the same to the second. Therefore, *frontosa*, pleasure of this kind brings weeping and sorrow. Even if the fetuses live, they are likely to live a wretched life: and if there are three or four, it will be even worse. So take heed, O wretched lady, and do not ignore the danger of your own death from delivering so many offspring. Those deliveries will be increasingly painful and are far more dangerous than would be the delivery of a single infant, which already puts you at risk.

O ardent, abominable appetite! It is certainly understandable that many of you, in your condition (that is, being gravid) feel the desire for such a union, but keep in mind what Albert the Great says on this topic in book IX of *De animalibus*: "No female of other animals except for humans receives or submits to intercourse after impregnation. But a woman after impregnation not only submits to coitus, but even desires now to have intercourse more, and even more often than she did when she was not pregnant, especially if she is pregnant with a female."[53] Therefore watch yourself *frontosa* and leave *frontoso* alone: you know what I mean. And here I will remind you, *frontoso*, what Aristotle says about the mare: that the pregnant mare allows herself to be mounted by the horse,[54] and this happens especially when she is well-nourished with good fodder and excellent feed. Therefore, *frontoso*, you should not allow your pregnant wife to become too plump, and think twice before giving in to all her cravings. Aristotle discusses such superfetation after having seen a woman give birth to twelve fetuses one after the other.[55] I personally witnessed a case in Bassano, of a woman who gave birth to five: three died in the two days following their birth, the fourth lived more or less till his second month, and the fifth, a female infant, lived for about seven months. Aristotle discusses a similar case in the *De animalibus* (*On Animals*).[56] He tells us the story of a woman pregnant with twins, who after her third month, became pregnant with a third child, who then died: and Aristotle recounts many such cases. For the moment, it is enough to mention these cases, though I will add what the Conciliator[57] says, that in his days, in the town of Abano, he saw sixty

---

53. In Latin in the text: *Adhuc autem nulla omnino femina aliorum animalium ab homine recipit aut substinet coitum post impregnationem. Mulier autem post impregnationem non solum substinet coitum, sed etiam desiderat plus tunc coire et sepius quam ante fecerat quando non fuit impregnata, precipue si est impregnata de femina.* See Albert the Great, *De animalibus*, Lib. IX, tract. 1, c. 5 (p. 694).

54. See Aristotle, *On the Generation of Animals*, IV.5, 773b25–29.

55. See Aristotle, *History of Animals, VII–X,* ed. and trans. David M. Balme (Cambridge, MA: Harvard University Press, 1991), VII.4, 585a.

56. Aristotle, *History of Animals*, VII.4, 584b, asserts that five is the highest number of children that can be born at one time (and have a chance of survival).

57. Savonarola refers to the philosopher, astrologer, and physician Peter of Abano by recalling the title of his better-known work, the *Conciliator differentiarum, quae inter philosophos et medicos versantur*

fetuses come out from one uterus, all of which had the appearance and motions of human bodies.[58]

I will also remind these unfortunate ladies carrying multiple fetuses that such superimpregnations may cause the miscarriage of the first fetus: and by allowing this outcome, they become the murderers of their own children. And you, *frontosa*, who excuse yourself and say that your husband is to blame—I say to you that this happens to those who find pleasure in the game of sex. Therefore, you should take heed, poor ladies; and for the well-being of your own body and soul, you should loathe this fetid and dangerous superfetation: because if you abhor it, you will not generate multiple fetuses and not take pleasure in such a game, out of respect and fear for your lives; and recall often how beasts of burden hold this in abomination. *Frontosa*, just as when you receive food against your will, you do not swallow it with pleasure, nor do you relish it; in this way, the uterus, when it swallows semen against its will, will not bear fruit, knowing the grave danger it portends for your soul and body. And in order to give pleasure to our readers, I will add to our digression [about multiple births] what Augustine says in the *City of God*, of two twins that were so similar that it was impossible to distinguish one from the other, so great was their resemblance. When one was hungry, the other also wanted to eat; when one laughed or cried, the other did the same.[59] When asked about this, Posidonius, the great astrologer, responded that such a thing occurs because of the position of the stars. Indeed, *frontosa*, it is certain that the power of the heavens also affects your pregnancy. This is why Aristotle says "the Sun and man beget man";[60] and Quintilian and the Master of the Histories[61] [Peter Comestor] make similar statements. I do not wish at this time to pursue this debate, that is, whether it is possible for two beings to be identical in every aspect;

(*Conciliator of the Differences that Exist Between Philosophers and Physicians*), composed between 1303 and 1310.

58. Albert the Great, *De animalibus*, Lib. IX, tract. 1, c. 5 (p. 693), recalls the birth of sixty fetuses at one time. I have not been able to locate this information in the *Conciliator* by Peter of Abano. In his *Practica*, tract. VI, c. 21, rubr. 25 (fol. 268r), Savonarola refers to a similar anecdote recorded by Peter of Abano, but the twins he mentions are six, not sixty: *Unde Conciliator noster dixit in villa sua de Ebano sex embriones ab una muliere emissos, quorum quilibet motum habebat, res quippe stupenda multum* (And our Conciliator said that in his own city of Abano a woman aborted six embryos, and all of them had their own motion, which was indeed amazing).

59. Augustine of Hippo, *De civitate dei*, ed. Bernhard Dombart and Alfons Kalb, 2 vols. (Turnhout: Brepols, 1955), vol. 1, Book V, 129 (chapter 2, ll. 1–6) and 133 (chapter 5, ll. 55–64).

60. In Latin in the text: *sol et homo generant hominem*. See Aristotle, *Physics*, ed. William D. Ross (Oxford: Clarendon Press, 1955), II.2, 194b13. See also Jacqueline Hamesse, *Les "Auctoritates Aristotelis": Un florilège medieval: Étude historique et édition critique* (Louvain: Publications Universitaires; Paris: Béatrice Nauwelaerts, 1974), 145.

61. Savonarola is referring to Peter Comestor (also named Peter of Troyes, d. 1178), the well-known French theologian and author of the *Historia scholastica*.

for given the diversity that is found in nature and in the stars, such similarity is not possible.

Let us now return to where we left off [in our discussion of impregnation], saying that when these three moist substances find themselves together, the male and female sperms and the menstrual blood, and when the mouth of the uterus is closed, and these three substances are warmed up by the heat of the uterus—which originates from its many veins and arteries, and from its own particular heat that is the warm generative spirit—which heat is not able to cool because, with the closing of the mouth of the uterus, there is no outlet, and so this mixture necessarily boils, and by boiling, it spumifies like boiling water in a cauldron, and is transformed into foam. Thus the first step before impregnation is spumification, fueled by the informative power by means of the generative spirit, in which lies the power of the animal, natural, and vital spirits. The material composed of the three moist substances mentioned spumifies, and does so especially in those places in which the three principal members are generated: that is, the heart, liver, and brain. The informative power first directs the generative spirit to that part of the man's and woman's sperm that are predisposed to the generation of the heart, and arrange that part for the formation of the heart, isolating and coagulating it in the midst of chaos—and this can well be called chaos, as Ovid refers to the chaos that existed at the beginning of the world—those parts being all mixed up/confused together, parts from which many diverse members will then be generated; and take note, poet, of the allegory behind this story. And this spumification generates a cavity, which in itself receives that part of the sperm prepared for the formation of the heart, and from that the heart is formed.

After this cavity is formed, the informative powers create two other cavities near that one: one for the brain, the other for the liver. And these new cavities remain close to the first one formed, and they even appear to be ramifications of the first one, at least at the beginning; but when they begin to grow, they become distinct, as Galen describes in his short treatise *On Sperm*, which, according to the new translation,[62] says:

---

62. Savonarola's statement that he is quoting a work entitled *On Sperm* (*De Spermate*) "secundo la nova translatione" deserves an explanation. In fact the quotation is not taken from the Pseudo-Galenic *On Sperm*—a twelfth-century embryological-astrological text—but from the *De semine* (*On Semen*) written by Galen, first translated into Latin by Niccolò da Reggio in the first half of the fourteenth century, and therefore unknown to the Latins before then. Soon after the translation, the original *On Semen* became part of the medieval Latin collections of Galenic writings, but in many manuscripts, such as the one most likely consulted by Savonarola, it bears the title *On Sperm*. Immediately attributed to Galen, also the pseudo-epigraphic *On Sperm* (also known with the title *Microtegni*), entered the corpus of the original texts of the Greek physician, although doubts about its authenticity were already advanced by Peter of Abano at the beginning of the fourteenth century. This explains the possible confusion between the two titles. Finally, the fact that the treatise *On Semen* circulated very little at the time of Savonarola makes it likely that he could consider it a new translation of an existing work,

The formative and animal virtue is at work but this does not appear immediately because of the small dimensions. But when [the cavities] do first appear, they are pressed together next to each other, one nerve announcing where the brain will be placed on the higher side, below which lie the heart and the liver. As time proceeds, the cavities previously mentioned stand apart more from the whole, for the animal and the body are being shaped. And the cavity in the upper part is filled with blood tending toward whiteness, on account of which the brain is white in color.[63]

These cavities separate one from the other because of the impulse of the informative power: and one goes to the superior part, and there the brain is generated; the other goes to the right side, where the liver is generated. Surely, such a process is a divine thing! After this happens, in the middle of that chaos, beneath the heart and the liver, an orifice or hole is created where the umbilical cord is generated. And nature completes this part before others, because without the umbilical cord, other parts could not grow, nor could they become properly formed, and this is because all the parts of the fetus need to receive nourishment through the umbilical cord.

Later, from what remains of this chaos, nature generates a membrane called *secundines*, so named because the fetus is the first to exit the body and later, or secondly, this afterbirth comes out.

Nature generates yet another membrane that is attached to the navel, by which the urine expelled by the fetus is led outside of its body and stored. This is a large membrane that breaks during parturition, and when it breaks, fluid flows out and lubricates its passage, so that the fetus may more easily leave the body. So when women see this water, they should expect to see the fetus shortly afterwards. And this membrane, called *bilis* by doctors, is divided in its exit from the umbilical cord by a little skin, which separates the passage through which the urine comes out from the passage where the blood and air enter. And nature created this membrane so that the urine expelled by the fetus would not be retained and injure the fetus, or the uterus, since urine is corrosive, as it would if it had no separate place to go but was allowed to flow into the uterus.

---

which was actually a different work (the Pseudo-Galenic *On Sperm*). The confusion would therefore not only concern the titles but also the content of these two different texts (also considering that the "real" Pseudo-Galenic *On Sperm* is never mentioned by Savonarla in his works).

63. In Latin in the text: *Hoc utique in principio virtus plasmans animalis operatur, et non apparet a principio pre parvitate. Sed quando primo apparent, sunt comprehense ad invicem adiacentes et contigue, hoc quidem nervo uno fieri nuntiatur qua cerebrum altiori sede locatum, subiacet enim ei cor et epar. Tempore vero procedente predicta principia distant magis ad totum quod plasmatur animal et corpus. Et impletur vesica que est supra, sanguine ad albedinem declive, propter quod cerebrum est coloris albi.* See Galen, *De semine*, Lib. I, c. 8 (pp. 540–41).

Nature also generates a third membrane that doctors call *abgas* [amnion], more subtle and thinner than the one previously mentioned.[64] This membrane surrounds the fetus, and receives the secretions, which is why nature made it so thin, so that it is suited both to absorb perspiration and to expel it. Because the fetus nourishes itself with blood, and since perspiration is a liquid drawn from the blood, mixed with choleric humour, it is necessary, because of the great heat, for the fetus to perspire. Moreover, because the blood on which the fetus nourishes itself is very refined, not having any earthy or heavy parts that might be transformed into feces, a fourth membrane, forming a place to contain the feces, is not necessary, as, in contrast, it is for the urine.

Having given order to such chaos, and having discussed the place of the three principal organs, we will now further proceed to discuss the distinction and formation of the other body parts. After the development of the first three organs in the first six or so days, comes the generation of the thorax, which generates and provides blood to the other parts of the body, from the top of the head to the bottom of the feet, and on the sides to the arms and hands. It generates a stomach, bones, kidneys, arteries and veins, and other parts of the body, generating testicles as the principal organs for the conservation of the human species, and later it converts the blood that has been shed into flesh, which refills the empty spaces that are situated between the different parts of the body, as painters do who first trace the outline of a figure and later fill in the flesh. And with this explanation, we have completed the second part of the chapter, on the cause of impregnation, and the material from which it is created.

Since the body of the pregnant woman becomes bloated, I would like to offer our readers here a section that discusses such bloating. It is important to know that the uterus is located in a woman's body over her intestines (called *gentile* by common folk, by physicians *rectum*) as if it was over a mattress, and above it, as a blanket, lies the bladder. Therefore as it grows in volume, the uterus presses on the intestine from behind: and it blocks the intestine so that the feces cannot leave the body as freely as before. It also compresses the bladder in the front. This is the reason for a pregnant woman's increased need to urinate. It is because of this growth in volume that the pregnant woman becomes constipated and urinates more frequently. O, you who are so proud and powerful, you should meditate on how you were born, and be humble. For remember that you were created by God so that you should serve him. And consider that our omnipotent Lord has offered you so great an example of humility, by incarnating himself and being born, and that he chose such a vile and stinking place to be born, where one finds only feces,

---

64. For the unassimilated Arabic medical terms *abgas* and *bilis*, see Federico Corriente, *Dictionary of Arabic and Allied Loanwords: Spanish, Portuguese, Catalan, Galician and Kindred Dialects* (Leiden: Brill, 2008), 10; and Riccardo Gualdo, *Il lessico medico del "De regimine pregnantium" di Michele Savonarola* (Florence: Accademia della Crusca, 1996), 57.

urine, and stinking blood. O omnipotent God of great humility, you suffered be-ing born not in a luxurious bedchamber, but as an example to us of your great humility, you chose to be born in a stable between two animals: that is, an ox and a donkey. The ox is a symbol of great humility and guileless simplicity, as Ovid maintains: "what have the oxen done, an animal without fraudulent deceits?"[65] The donkey teaches us his great patience, because surely the ass is the most patient and hardworking of animals. This is so true that people call a simple man an ox, and a man who toils and suffers much, an ass.

Now, perhaps, *frontosa* will ask, concerned about her fetus, how it receives nourishment while in her body. And to such an honorable query, since it is per-tinent to our topic, and also for the pleasure of our readers, I will not fail to re-spond. Through the navel of the infant pass two veins, which originate from the liver (which was formed before these veins), and two arteries that descend from the heart—for the heart, being the first source of life, is the first of all body parts to be generated by the generative power, as Avicenna states, and "the truth is that the first member that is formed is the heart";[66] even though Plato did not agree with this theory, and like many other philosophers maintained that the first member generated was the brain. These veins and arteries converge in the formation of the navel, as Galen states in the third book of On the Usefulness of the Parts, and as these veins come out from the navel they end in the membrane called *secundines*, from which they extend out, like branches, and connect to the capillaries of the uterus from which the placenta is suspended, and they are connected to these by cotyledons.[67] Just as fruit is attached to a tree by cotyledons, or *pecullo*, in the same way the fetus is attached to the uterus. And just as when fruit is ripe, it separates itself from the tree, so does the fetus leave the uterus when it is well formed and perfect. So, *frontosa*, know that it is more painful to abort than to deliver the fetus at its due time.

Through these venal branches, the fetus receives nourishment. Blood enters into the branches of these veins through the branches of the veins of the uterus, and later it is transported to the liver, and distributed to all parts of the fetus, providing the fetus with nourishment. And similarly blood cools down the heart through these same arteries, which receive air through the arteries of the uterus; it is also true that, despite the fact that it is closed, the cervix is not so closed that air, which is such a penetrative substance, is not able to get through and reach the

---

65. In Latin in the text: *quid meruere boves, animal sine fraude dolisque.* Ovid, *Metamorphoses*, vol. 2: Books 9–15, trans. Frank J. Miller (Cambridge, MA: Harvard University Press, 1916), 15.120.

66. In Latin in the text: *et veritas quidem est, quod primum membrum quod formatur est cor.* See Avicenna, *Canon*, Lib. III, fen 21, tract. 1, c. 2 (p. 920).

67. Galen discusses fetal development in various parts of his work, especially in book 15 (not 3) of *De usu partium* (*On the Usefulness of the Parts*), in *De foetuum formatione* (*Of the Foetal Formation*), and in book 12 of *De anatomicis administrationibus* (*On Anatomical Procedures*).

fetus, which thereby receives necessary ventilation. In addition, the fetus receives fresh air due to the porous quality of the body and from orifices like the ears, nostrils, etc.

And keep in mind, *frontosa*, what we have said regarding the blood with which your fetus is nourished, that it is most pure, etc.: in the first days of pregnancy, the blood is almost imperceptible, since the fetus does not need much nourishment, but as it grows, it needs more and more. When the fetus has grown as much as it should, not being satisfied by the nourishment provided by the uterus, nor by the air supplied for its ventilation, the fetus begins to move, and tries to leave in order to find more fresh air and more food, and it kicks. Kicking, it breaks the ligaments and previously mentioned cotyledons and the two membranes, urinary and sudoral, whereby the urinary and sudoral moisture escapes, which are naturally reserved to lubricate the birth canal so that the fetus may be delivered with more ease.

Now, *frontosa*, I want you to know that the most common labor and the best is at nine months, even though at times children are born at months seven, ten, eleven, twelve and fourteen. As Avicenna wrote in his *De animalibus* (*On Animals*), a fourteen-month child was once born who had already sprouted two teeth.[68] Such a late birth does not occur in other animals, in the timing of whose births there is little diversity. In the fourth section of his *Problems*, Aristotle asks the reason for this, and he responds that it is due to the great differences in the complexions of humans and the great diversity of their wills.[69] Since other animals, imperfect in respect to humans, live in a perfectly natural state and do not err by will and appetite in the so-called non-naturals, that is, in eating, drinking, coitus, sleep, waking, etc.—for animals do these things as nature directs, and following nature, they do not spoil their complexions, from which derive similar effects, so that the ass always gives birth after one year of pregnancy, and likewise, the others in their time. It is because man spoils his complexion, ruining his semen and changing the times in which he engages in coitus, that there is such variety in the time of delivery: because ruined and debilitated semen, which otherwise would be able to complete fetal development in nine months, cannot do so in less than ten or eleven months. This is because everything comes from the informative power that is in the semen, and this may also be ruined and debilitated.

Now you may wonder, *frontosa*, because of your devotion to Our Lady, about her pregnancy. And to this inquiry, I would respond that Our Lady carried

68. Avicenna, *De animalibus*, in *Avicenne perhypatetici philosophi ac medicorum facile primi Opera in lucem redacta, ac nuper quantum ars niti potuit per canonicos emendata* (Venice: per Bonetum Locatellum mandato Octaviani Scoti, 1508; facsimile reprint, Frankfurt am Main: Minerva, 1961), Lib. IX (fol. 24v).

69. See also Aristotle [pseud.], *History of Animals*, VII.4, 584a35, 584b1. See also Pseudo-Aristotle, *Problems*, X.9 and 10, 891b25–38 (p. 289).

the Son of God. And turning to philosophy for the most clear and direct explanation, we also note that the child's body parts were formed from the purest blood, blood which philosophers maintain is the substance of the fetus—whereas the Holy Spirit acted on behalf of the natural informative power that is in the man's semen. And this is what the angel meant when he said *the Holy Spirit will come upon you*,[70] because in man's place, there appeared the Holy Spirit. And when Our Lady later responded to the angel, *Behold I am the servant of the Lord, let it be to me in peace according to your word*[71]—in that instant, the substance was prepared, which is her most precious blood, to receive the form of the human body, and in that instant the soul of the son of God was introduced within that fully formed body.[72]

But as we have said, it is certain that pregnancy depends greatly on the heavens. As Aristotle says, and as noted earlier: "the Sun and man beget man."[73] This is why Christians should especially invoke God, our Lord in heaven, with great reverence and eagerness of the heart, so that God may bestow his assistance upon the union of man and woman, without which pregnancy cannot occur, so that the expected and desired pregnancy may result. Indeed, we read about many parents whose wishes were granted by prayer. And to understand fully the whole theory of pregnancy, keep also in mind the motions of the heavens; we remind you what philosophers claim, especially Alexander of Aphrodisias, about the influence of the errant stars [i.e. the planets] on the formation of the fetus, and their action upon the fetus in each month of its formation. In the first month of the formation of the fetus, Saturn converges, and the reason is that such matter—that is, the sperm and menstrual blood—are fluid and need to be united and coagulated together. Saturn accomplishes this through its influence and with its frigidity; and because united, the generative spirit and the informative power find themselves strengthened and more able to accomplish their duty.

In the second month, Jupiter sends its power—that is, its heat and humidity—to this matter. By warming it and providing moisture, Jupiter makes the fetus dilate and grow and come to life, given that heat and humidity are the principles

---

70. Luke 1:35: *Spiritus Sanctus superveniet in te.*

71. Luke 1:38: *ecce ancilla Domini, fiat mihi secundum verbum tuum in pace.* The Vulgate reads, omitting "in pace": *ecce ancilla Domini: fiat mihi secundum verbum tuum.*

72. For medieval theologians, philosophers and physicians alike the Virginal Birth of Christ, also termed as "divine embryology," was a common theme. The roles of Mary and the Holy Spirit, the influence of the stars, the timing of the formation of the embryo and its ensoulment, and the source of material from which it was formed, were the four most discussed issues. Most scholastics described the conception, development in utero, and birth of Christ in the same terms as ordinary generation, but Christ is an exception in that the forming activity of the Holy Spirit enables the rational soul to inform the body immediately at the moment of conception. On these topics, see Van der Lugt, *Le ver, le démon et la Vierge*, 371–473.

73. In Latin in the text: *sol et homo generant hominem.* See Aristotle, *Physics*, II.2, 194b13.

of life. It also drives away that bad influence of Saturn, its opposite, if there is any left.

Third, Mars appears, since the fetus needs to harden its parts. Mars, through its great heat and dryness, makes the parts hard, just as mud is hardened during times of heat and drought, and through that heat and dryness, it melts away the superfluities produced and begins to give movement to the fetus and its parts, as we know by experience.

In the fourth month, the Sun—also known as the heart of the sky—is influential. The Sun with its great life-generating heat brings to life the embryo and completes it, that is, spreads the vital spirit that is in the heart among all the body parts giving them life. This is why Aristotle has said "the Sun and man beget man."[74]

In the fifth month, cold and humid Venus is influential. Through its frigidity and humidity it moderates the heat and dryness of Mars; and Venus also does the same with the heat impressed on the fetus by the Sun. Later it helps the generation of the flesh, making it grow, and beautifully forming its parts.

Later, in the sixth month, Mercury, with its benign temperament, contributes to the formation of the body parts, producing balance for them. This is why astrologers say that, because it prepares the body parts in a tempered, balanced way, to be suitable subjects for the rational soul, Mercury was named god of the sciences and arts.

Lastly the Moon appears, with its influence, which, through its humidity, increases the fetus's needed nutrimental moisture, given that the fetus, at this point rather large, is in greater need of sustenance. It also moistens the uterus, rendering it more lubricated; since in the seventh month the fetus is perfectly formed with regards to all its limbs, and in this month, being complete and grown, the fetus tries to come out and kicks a great deal; and if it comes out at this moment, having been weakened by this movement, when it comes into contact with the air, it usually dies.

If the fetus reaches the eighth month in such a debilitated state, and encounters Saturn, cold and dry, then it experiences two qualities contrary to the qualities of life (warmth and humidity); this is why the fetus born in the eighth month does not survive. But if the eight-month fetus remains in the body, it is then restored when benevolent Jupiter, the friend of life appears (in the ninth month), and the fetus usually lives. This is why they call Jupiter "father of the gods and of humans."[75]

---

74. In Latin in the text: *sol et homo generant hominem*. See Aristotle, *Physics*, II.2, 194b13.

75. In Latin in the text: *pater deorum et hominum*. On the origin of the theory of planetary influences over the stages of gestation, see note 82 in the Introduction to this volume (28); Burnett, "The Planets and the Development of the Embryo"; and Saif, "The Universe and the Womb."

And concluding this part, I will satisfy a question, the answer to which I feel *frontoso* and *frontosa* are very eager to learn. They ask me, after having well understood the manner in which the fetus is generated, "in what position does this fetus lie in the body of the mother?" To them I respond that the fetus rests with its neck and shoulders inclined towards the bottom of the uterus—because in such a position it better protects the heart—and has its hands over its knees and its nose between these, and its eyes above these: so that it is curved with its head in the front and with its feet at the base. Such a position is advantageous for exiting the womb, as when young children wish to dive from a high point into a body of water, extending their arms and their hands towards their knees and curving over with their heads close to the water in order to dive into it.

And now that we know how a pregnancy is made and from what material, we will proceed to the third part of this chapter—that is, to explain how the partners have to position themselves to attain such a pregnancy.

And because in such a narrative and instruction, it might seem to some that I speak about shameful matters, I ask for your forgiveness and that you please keep in mind that I only speak of these topics so that honorable and glorious ends may be reached. As Aristotle says, everything should be praised or censured according to its ends: therefore, stating and rehearsing the means by which one achieves pregnancy, that glorious thing which is so desired by all, I believe that I should not be chastised because I write of these things; but nevertheless, I will make every effort to keep this section as proper and decent as possible. Naturally, in order to discuss pregnancy, which is achieved with those parts of the body that are shameful, it will not be possible for me to avoid certain sordid words, as I am dealing with sordid topics. But I will turn to my women readers and ask of them that just as they should not feel shame in this act, especially when it is done in a proper and honorable place, they should also not be ashamed to read and listen about this topic in an honorable and appropriate manner.

Now, having asked for such forgiveness, I wish for you to know, *frontoso*, as we have previously stated, that a woman cannot become pregnant without receiving great pleasure in the act, emitting her sperm at the right moment, and compressing her uterus, as it is written. Now, given that these things need to concur in order for pregnancy to be achieved, it may be necessary for men to add some spice to intercourse with their wives: I say this especially for those wives who cannot become pregnant without such spice, as is the case with those who cannot swallow their food if it is not tasty. Such foreplay may help the woman to prepare herself so that she may emit her sperm more quickly at the moment of coitus, since, all things being equal, it takes longer for a woman to ejaculate her seed than it takes a man. However, such caresses are not necessary if and when the opposite is true.

Because following the theories of the authorities, we will say that, in order to achieve pregnancy properly, a man should lie with a woman in the aforementioned hour, that is after matins, when sperm is most powerful; and also at the appropriate moment—that is, after she is cleansed, as earlier stated. This is because at this moment the uterus is free of its superfluities, and then the sperm is not impeded in any way, and the uterus may better receive and contain the sperm so that it will best execute all of its functions. And this cleansing, or her moment, is on the eighth day after the completion of her menstrual cycle.

And before both parties come together for sex, they should each focus their thoughts and concentrate hard on pregnancy. They should both call to mind men who have impregnated their wives and wives who have become impregnated, because certainly such a strong mental image often causes the imagined effect, as was the case with the white woman who became gravid with a black child, as mentioned earlier. We have also heard the story of the man who, not imagining a fall, is perfectly able to walk over a long and narrow plank; whereas, when he fears falling and imagines falling, he falls, which is why it is said that imagination causes the fall: *imaginatio facit casum*.[76]

After this, the couple should touch one another, especially the man should touch the woman, touching her and rubbing her pudenda with his fingers: because this is the exterior place where a woman receives the most pleasure, because of its proximity to the neck of the uterus, where women achieve great pleasure; and as a result of this rubbing, women are more easily stimulated to spermatize. Afterwards, they should continue to delay intercourse, and he should touch with his hands her breasts and lightly rub her nipples, kissing her cheeks, mouth, and other parts, and he should touch her especially the area under her abdomen, while bringing closer his penis, but not penetrating her just yet, continuing to hold off. All of these things should be done to stimulate the woman to spermatize. But it is also true that there are some women who are more ready than others—that is, they are more or less warm: hence it is necessary for the man to undertake such caresses with prudence and measure. There are also some women who do not care about such caresses, and they are fruitful without them. If a man caresses a woman too much, as he would a woman who is cold, and she is already hot by nature, she may disperse her seed too early, thus wasting his effort. Now, if for writing about this I am called a pimp, I will bear this accusation in patience, because I have written this for a good cause.

O *frontoso*, note that when you desire to impregnate your wife, you do not have to engage in "such games" too often, since as was stated earlier, sperm grows cold and renders itself infertile; nor should you prolong intercourse too much, because in such a prolonging, its heat is weakened. Instead, you should find the right moment, so that such coitus should be done when the sperm mixture is good and useful for impregnating, and this moment must be some time between doing it too often and waiting too long to do it, considering that [the sperm] also

---

76. For the Avicennian origin of this example, see note 77 in the Introduction to this volume (27).

depends on the complexion and different strengths of the bodies. And to satisfy my readers as much as possible on this topic, I will list in the section that follows the signs of the cold uterus and the hot uterus.

But first, in order to complete what we have already said about coitus, I would like to add just a few words. When entering his wife, after so many caresses, a man should consider the sighs of his wife, who begins to gasp louder and louder and speak almost like a stutterer: this is when the penis should make its entrance. The man should force himself to send his semen down all at once and not in spurts, nor should he raise his tool or lower it, as is often done for pleasure; rather, he should hold it directly over the hole so that air will not enter and corrupt the semen. And before moving on, you should know, *frontoso*, that in writing this, I have often burst out laughing, because these things can certainly sound humorous. But on the other hand, I have thought about the glorious fruit born of this act, and this is why I have not refrained from writing about it, and I have felt comfortable proceeding with my writing, as I recall other rules that should be observed to facilitate attaining such a pregnancy.

We will say, therefore, following our warnings on how to achieve the desired pregnancy, that after the man has ejaculated his semen, his wife should raise her legs, and after the man pulls out, the wife should tighten her thighs, legs, and feet together. She should keep these elevated for a sixth of an hour, so that the sperm will descend better into her uterus and so that it be better retained, and also so that air does not get into her and spoil the semen. Later, in order to accomplish this even better, she should immediately smell cotton infused with musk or pomander, labdanum, or a similarly fragrant spice—this should only be done by those who do not abhor fragrant things. And in this position, she should try to sleep, so that by keeping the heat inside, the generative power grows, and the sperm becomes warmer and stronger for the task of impregnation.

These fragrant preparations are helpful to women when taken one hour before such coitus or before going to sleep. Prepared as suffumigations and suppositories, they act to soothe the uterus and lower it in the body, so that it more easily receives the sperm of the man; and they warm the uterus, and because of their dryness, they draw up and remove any superfluities that could impede impregnation. But in the application of these remedies, it is important to be aware of the complexion of the uterus, because, as Avicenna says, heat should not be applied to things that are already warm, nor moisture to things that are moist. Therefore, it is necessary to show moderation in the application of this type of remedy, and for this reason they should not be applied by women, but by expert physicians. Therefore, in what follows, as I promised, I will note the signs of the hot and cold uterus.

Suffumigation to impregnate: take arbotani, and calamint, one handful of each; rosemary, roses, one-half handful of each; make a decoction in river water. This suffumigation would be much more beneficial if it were delivered through a straw, with one extremity in the water, and the other placed inside the vagina—I leave this decision to the attendant, male or female, and it is good when the uterus is cold. But here we must note that any such fragrant suffumigation made to be taken from underneath would be harmful if it were received through the nostrils: therefore, it is necessary to be careful that such a suffumigation is not inhaled. And if it is possible that she has inhaled it, she should immediately inhale the fetid substances here indicated, such as galbanum, feathers of burned partridges, burned shoes or cloth, and similar things, such as an extinguished tallow candle. An excellent suppository: take labdanum, one ounce; form it into a suppository. Keep this in for an hour before going to the act of coitus. Any similar suppository may also be useful. Also good for getting pregnant is the dung of a young goat, placed inside the woman after the cleansing of her menses, mixed with *bdellium*[77] and *galia muscata*,[78] especially when the uterus is cold and filled with moisture.

For this reason it is necessary here to specify the signs by which we can recognize whether the uterus is hot or cold. Avicenna says that the most obvious signs of a hot uterus are these:[79] that the woman feels very warm, [the uterus] having passed such warmth to the other parts of her body; through its veins to the liver, from where they originate; similarly through its nerves to the brain, where they originate; and through its arteries to the heart, their source. And this is a sign "inferred by a change in quality."[80]

The second sign is the paucity of her menses, because heat weakens and desiccates the uterus. But such a paucity can also originate from other causes, such as obstruction. Accordingly, to verify such a sign, one should perform the following test: take white strips of cloth, and keep them for an entire night inside of the uterus during the woman's flow, and then, let them dry in the shade. Later, remove them, and afterwards, consider the color of the cloth. If it is red or yellowish, this will be a sign that her uterus is hot, but if the color verges on white or melancholic black, this will be a sign that her uterus is cold. If the uterus is cold,

---

77. Savonarola uses the term *bdelio*. This substance is a resin that comes from the bdellium tree, commonly used by doctors and pharmacists for emulsions and poultices. Uterine suffumigations and suppositories were considered useful in accordance with the ancient medical idea that the womb is naturally attracted by perfumes and avoids bad smells.

78. *Galia muscata* is a medicinal preparation containing musk, mastic, camphor, cinnamon, cloves, nutmeg and rose water.

79. See Avicenna, *Canon*, Lib. III, fen 21, tract. 1, c. 4 (p. 924).

80. With the technical expression *sumpto a qualitate mutata*, in Latin in the text, Savonarola refers to a general way of considering the symptoms and causes of a disease: the symptom derived from "a change in quality" (which therefore concerns the four qualities of hot, cold, wet and dry; in this case the increased heat of the uterus), is contrasted with the symptom derived from "a damaged action" (*actio lesa*), and—unlike this second type—it damages the affected organ if and as much as the changed quality increases and lasts over time.

the strip will not have a foul odor; but if the cloth strip is black and has a stench, which will come from dry heat, this will signify a hot uterus.

Another sign of uterine heat is that the woman often feels pain in the area of her liver or hypochondrium, or tears or other ulcerations may appear in her uterus. Another sign is when the lips of her vagina are very dry. Another sign is a excessive hairiness especially near her pubic region, because hairy women are more often hot, and such heat moves to the uterus. So, when there is significant hairiness near the pubic area, given that hair is generated by heat, this is a very strong indication that the woman's uterus is hot. The color of her urine should also be noted, which is affected by uterine heat, although it may also be affected by the heat of the kidneys, *frontoso*, so beware of how you judge this; this is why Hippocrates says "beware, lest you have encountered a disorder of the bladder or kidneys."[81] When the uterus is hot, moreover, since it is connected to the heart by its numerous arteries, its heat is communicated to the heart, causing a greater need for ventilation, which triggers the speeding up of the pulse.

And take note, *frontoso*, and not be fooled by these signs, that the heat of other parts of the body, if they are hot, could transfer their heat to the cold uterus, accidentally warming it up. In conclusion, I will add here a suffumigation that should be applied when the uterus is hot, like those recommended for when it is cold. Suffumigation: take equal parts petals of roses and of violets,[82] and one-fourth as much of lentils, and one half as much of bay leaves, and boil them in well water. We will elaborate more on this later.

After having discussed the signs of the hot uterus, we will now speak of the signs of a cold uterus. The first is paucity of menses, with which whiteness is associated. And to resolve a question that arises, I say that just as heat causes paucity, as has been said, so also may frigidity cause paucity, blocking the passages; and just as a small or moderate quantity of menses is associated with whiteness, indicating frigidity, whiteness also indicates frigidity when the menses are watery. Another sign of a cold uterus is menses that are very black, which results from a decrease in heat, as happens with coal, and is seen when warm blood, which is red, after an hour or two becomes black. Another sign is that the cold uterus prolongs its cleansing, doing so in two ways. First, whereas the hot uterus cleanses itself in four or five days, the cold uterus can take as long as seven or eight, because its frigidity obstructs the passages from which a woman's menses ought to descend.

---

81. In Latin in the text: *cave ne vesice vicio aut renum capiaris*. The exact Hippocratic quote has not been identified. The same sentence is in Michele Savonarola, *Practica canonica de febribus* (Venice: Giunta, 1552), c. 16, rubr. 1 (fol. 82v); cited in *Works by Michele Savonarola*, #2.

82. Savonarola uses the term *foglie*, which literally translates as "leaves"; however, it is clear from this context that he is referring to the petals of roses and violets. Petals and leaves were not terminologically distinguished from one another until the late sixteenth century. Fabio Colonna is believed to be the first author to have coined the term *petalo* for the colored floral leaves in his herbal *Phytobasanos* (1592).

Second, whereas the hot uterus cleans itself out every month, a cold one takes as long as two or three months. Another sign is inferred from the regimen—that is, from having eaten and taken foods that are fatty and cold, from drinking cold water, and from excessive coitus: because of these, the uterus becomes cold in nature and cold blood is produced. Another sign is that a cold uterus, feeling a numbness in its upper parts, transmits its frigidity to the nervous parts, paralyzing them. To these should be added the signs that are contrary to those of a warm uterus: that is, paucity of hair and pallor of the urine, which quickly becomes foul. And with this we complete the third chapter.

Chapter Four
On the signs of pregnancy

Having written so much on pregnancy, and given that women still have doubts about their pregnancies (and are often fooled), believing that they are pregnant when they are not, it seems to me that I should write about the signs of pregnancy, so that my writings may be useful to these women and entertaining to my readers.

Proceeding in this manner, I will remind you here of what was discussed in the previous chapter about the first sign: and that is that if, during coitus, the couple concentrates on the moment when the semen is sent into the uterus, the woman will feel a compression of the neck of the uterus, which has received the semen with great desire, and the man will feel similarly a contraction in his penis, which will remain dry, the cause of which has been explained already. Regarding this, Avicenna says that from that compression the woman feels a warmth—that is, a titillation all over her body—that she feels when she spermatizes together with the man—similar to, but much weaker than the sensation, or titillation, that the man also feels when he emits semen.[83]

The second sign of pregnancy is the retention of menses. When a woman misses her period for two or three months and does not see any menses, it is a sign that she has become pregnant, and nature is retaining this blood for its needs. Normally, this blood is superfluous, so its retention is a very revealing sign, but only when the woman is neither feverish nor otherwise in ill health, because her illness may cause an imbalance, and she may retain blood and become weak for that reason. When this retention is because of pregnancy, the closure of the neck of the uterus contributes to the retention of blood.

The third sign of pregnancy is that the neck of the uterus is closed very tightly, as previously discussed. This may be determined by a midwife inserting her middle finger into the vagina. Galen finds this to be the most reliable sign, writing in the second book of *De naturalibus facultatibus* (*On the Natural*

---

83. See Avicenna, *De animalibus*, Lib. XV (fol. 48r).

Faculties) and fifth book of the *Aphorisms* that such tightness "is a great and certain sign for knowing if women have conceived."[84]

The fourth sign of pregnancy is that as soon as the uterus has drawn the semen into itself, the lips of the vagina become dry. This is proof that not a single drop of semen has leaked out and moistened them, and that the uterus has drawn the whole of it, and that for this reason it is tightly closed. And by a similar cause the lips are thin, because if they were engorged, it would indicate that some moisture had leaked out, and consequently the neck of the uterus would not be closed; and at the same time, the woman feels the lips of the vagina pressed together and closed. And these are signs discussed by Albert the Great in chapter three of book IX of his *De animalibus*.[85]

The fifth sign of pregnancy is that the woman's breasts begin to enlarge. This is nature's way of storing blood in the woman's breasts, generating milk for the future nourishment of the fetus. Initially, however, her milk is thin and watery; later, when the fetus is grown larger and has feeling and movement, it will nourish itself from the mother's blood, taking it from the navel, as said.

The sixth sign of pregnancy is that the body becomes round because of the elevation of the uterus to the upper front part of the body. Also, the pregnant woman feels a small pain under her abdomen, and this is because the fetus begins to expand the uterus beyond its natural size, and this mostly happens to young women in their first pregnancy.

The seventh sign of pregnancy, especially at the beginning if the fetus is somewhat large, is that the woman urinates frequently and with difficulty. This is because the uterus, being dilated, and lying near the urethra, puts pressure on it, so that urine is not able to flow freely. Because of this compression, pregnant women urinate more often.

The eighth sign is that the pregnant woman, unlike in the past, abhors coitus. This is, first, because having retained her menses, bad vapors rise, which cause an imbalance. Second, her stomach wants to vomit, and she is nauseous, conditions that offend the brain and the heart, etc.; and because they are so out of balance, pregnant women no longer care about sex. But of course, I'm not sure what I am saying, given that there are many gravid women who still also enjoy hunting bumblebees. But what I have said applies to most women, because nature clearly teaches animals not to superimpregnate themselves, as we have said before.

---

84. In Latin in the text: *magnum signum et certum ad intelligendum si femine conceperint*. See Hippocrates, *Aphorisms*, V.51 (p. 170). Also see Galen, *On the Natural Faculties*, trans. Arthur J. Brock (Cambridge, MA: Harvard University Press, 1916), III.3 (p. 231). The same sign is also noted in other works by Galen, as in *De usu partium* (*On the Usefulness of the Parts of the Body*), 15.7, and *De anatomicis administrationibus* (*On Anatomical Procedures*), 12.3.

85. Albert the Great, *De animalibus*, Lib. IX, tract. 1, c. 3 (p. 684).

The ninth sign of pregnancy is that women are nauseated and sluggish, and feel heavy in the body and suffer from headaches. And the reason for this is that, as we have said, the disagreeable vapors from the retained menses rise to her head, heart, and stomach, which, perturbing the spirits, render them sluggish, and distress these principal organs, provoking nausea. And likewise, women experience disturbing thoughts, or fear, or other problems, depending on the influence of the vapors with their noxious qualities. And because they are carrying the fetus, they become heavier in their movements, and they feel a weight in their groin from the hanging of the fetus in the uterus. And because of these factors their stomachs are upset, their appetites are ruined, and they often crave strange things; and this happens especially in the first months of pregnancy; and this is what the corrupt vapors caused by her retained menstrual blood do to her. As a consequence of these vapors, women belch and suffer indigestion from acidity in their stomachs. And likewise, these vapors have an ill effect on the brain and eyes, so that at times pregnant women may feel dizzy. And likewise, they feel a tremor, a frequent pulsation, in their hearts, because these vapors have reached the heart.

Moreover, the whites of the eyes of pregnant women are yellow, because their choler is agitated and its vapors rise to the eyes, yellowing them. Oftentimes, the eyes of the pregnant woman may recede, which happens particularly when the fetus is four or five or six months old: this is because the uterus interacts closely with the eyes, and its vapors rise up to them, filling them up and shortening the nerves; and because of this shortening, the pregnant woman's eyes may retract. Some women's eyelids, additionally, become soft, also because of the rising of humid vapors, which relaxes the eyelids; and the pupils become small because of the damage the rising vapors cause to the ocular spirits, and those spirits diminish in response to the vapors. Also, the color of the face and of all the body changes in a pregnant woman, especially in a woman who is carrying a female child, because she who is carrying a male child generates more heat, which melts away the superfluities that cause the discoloration, and so women pregnant with male children have better color.

Note that there are also women who feel pain in their hips or in the area near their hips, and when they are gravid, they no longer feel these pains. The reason for this is that the heat of the uterus, the fetus, and the menstrual blood consumes the gases that caused this pain. Some women also become soft in the beginning because of the many retained fluids.

Having enumerated here the interior signs of pregnancy, we will now move onto the exterior signs by which one can tell whether or not a woman is pregnant. First, to determine if a woman is pregnant, we should give her, when she goes to sleep, two ounces of honey mixed with two ounces of rainwater. After this, if she feels torsion and a prickly feeling in her stomach, she must be gravid. This is why Hippocrates states, "if you wish to see if a woman has conceived, give her melicrat to drink":[86] and this is because the gassiness of this drink, called melicrat, cannot escape because of the tightness in the intestines caused by the fetus. This is especially clear in those women who typically do not feel pain when eating honey, whereas many women do.

Also, wrap musk in cotton cloth, or *galia muscata* or something similarly fragrant, and put it in the vagina as deep as it will go. If the woman can smell the scent of the fragrance, this means she is not gravid. But if she cannot smell it, it will be, like the other signs, a sign of pregnancy: for this means that the passage is blocked by the fetus. Similarly, you may perform this test with a head of garlic inserted as deeply as it will go into the neck of the uterus: and this alternative is for impoverished women who may not have access to precious and fragrant things. But a further note: on the day that they want to try this experiment, women must work hard all day and eat very little, so that the passages will be open and not blocked by foods or superfluous fluids. A similar test can be done by inserting the root of aristolochia with honey. If she tastes its sweet or sour flavor, this means she is not pregnant, for the aforementioned reason.

Next, pregnancy is revealed by the quality of the woman's urine, as well as by its substance and content. If she is pregnant, it will be yellowish, verging on white, because of the moderate temperature of her body, since if it were too hot it would not be fit for generation, and the urine would be a strong yellow. In the urine, a substance appears that resembles combed cotton, and because such matter is spermatic in nature, which the uterus does not accept after impregnation, and since the substance is not necessary, nature expels it through the urine. Also, the urine may appear cloudy, and some grainy particles may be seen circulating in it: this is a sign that some gas is retained in the urine, which makes these particles of matter ascend and descend. And these signs in the urine appear at the early stages of pregnancy, whereas in later stages, the urine may look reddish; this is because at the later stages of pregnancy the uterus, discomfited by bloody fluids, expels them, coloring the urine. At the end of the pregnancy, if shaken in the urine glass, the urine gets turbid; but at the early stages, this does not happen. This is because, at the end of pregnancy, the uterus expels superfluities which, mixing with the urine, make it turbid

And take note, O reader, that of all the signs of pregnancy there is none more reliable than the one Galen described, even though it seems shameful to

---

86. In Latin in the text: *mulierem si vis videre si conceperit, melicratum da ei bibere*. See Hippocrates, *Aphorisms*, V.41 (p. 168). *Melicrat* is a combination of honey and water. *Hydromel* is instead referred to as an alcoholic bevarage made with fermented honey and water, or with honey and wine. For a set of different—and often confusing—ideas concerning the preparation methods for melicrat and hydromel at a time closer to Savonarola's, see, for example, the commentary written by the sixteenth-century doctor and botanist Pietro Andrea Mattioli on Dioscorides's *De materia medica*.

observe.[87] And surely it is the case that the physician should not immediately choose by which one, or two, three, or four signs he should detect a pregnancy, especially when there are so many to choose from. But he may judge as he prefers among the several signs of pregnancy that he observes.

And I also want you to know, *frontoso*, that there is another condition in women similar to impregnation, called "mole," which has tricked many excellent and famous doctors into judging as gravid a woman who was carrying a mole. Even the famous Marsilio da Santa Sofia and Magister Pietro da Tossignano, both physicians of the duke of Milan Gian Galeazzo, were fooled in the cases of two female companions of the duchess. And therefore, so that the midwives of Ferrara are able to distinguish well between a mole and an impregnation, I will add to this chapter a discussion on the signs of moles, so that they be well recognized, since in Ferrara one finds moles in great abundance.

And before distinguishing between the signs of impregnation and of the mole, I will supply these tests, for the pleasure of my audience, that can determine whether the woman is apt to become pregnant and the man to impregnate. And the first of these is as follows. Dilute saffron with saliva and apply this mixture under each eye and in the corners of the eyes near the nose. If after some time the man and woman taste the flavor of the saffron, it is a sign that they are fertile, for it indicates that the passage is open from which descends that part of the [spermatic] matter that needs to be sent from the brain to the testicles for the generation of the sperm, and this is indeed its passage.[88] But if they do not taste anything, this is a sign that the passage is closed. Therefore whoever does not taste anything is not apt to procreate. The second test is to put garlic or some other odorous substance inside the woman's vagina. As before, if she smells its odor, it is a sign that the passages are open and that the woman is fertile.

And returning to the mole, I will cite Albert the Great, in book X of *De animalibus*. He writes that a woman, believing that she was gravid—for she had a large body, and milk, and her menses retained, and had lost her appetite, and displayed other signs of pregnancy—having reached the ninth month and even the tenth without giving birth, remained with her enlarged body for four years; after which came a great flowing of blood, and she gave birth to the mole. Albert adds that "in certain women this infirmity lasts a very long time and can extend up till

87. Savonarola is here referring to the third sign of his list (mentioned earlier), which is the womb's tight closing at pregnancy, generally recognized by all ancient authors, including Galen but also, among others, Hippocrates, Herophilus, and Soranus, and eventually mentioned by Savonarola as well in his *Practica*, tract. VI, c. 21, rubr. 22 (fol. 263r).

88. As previously at pages 63 and 66–67, Savonarola once again seems to refer to the Hippocratic and Galenic doctrine of the pangenetic origin of sperm, according to which it would not derive from blood, as for Aristotle (hematogenesis of semen) but from all the organs of the body, and in particular from the brain. According to this medical theory, which admits the existence of a female seed, both male and female sperm would have identical origin from the brain and all the organs.

death."[89] Where Avicenna says that sometimes moles remain with the woman up till the end of life and are never cured.[90] I would say this about our greengrocer from the piazza, who has had a mole for twelve years, with a very huge body: that whoever opened her up would find inside of her uterus a piece of hard flesh, not too heavy, that was originally very soft, like live flesh. This is why it is retained and not pushed out of her vagina, and it does not bother her, because it is like hard flesh situated in the uterus——flesh which is so hard, as experience has shown, that it would be difficult to cut even with a cleaver.

And I must certainly say that it is very difficult to distinguish between mole and impregnation, because with moles one finds many of the signs of pregnancy, which is why it is so important to recognize these signs. This is why, we will say first, that one can feel the mole's movement when one presses one's hand against the abdomen, but otherwise it does not move; in impregnation, in contrast, one can feel that the fetus moves often and when it wants, without any external pressure from the hand. Also, a mole moves as if it were a stone or a dead thing: so that when the woman turns to the right or left side, she feels like a heavy thing that moves on the right or left side, depending on where she moves, and afterwards, it stops moving. But if she is gravid, she feels a movement with a certain wiggle, like a living thing, and often she feels this from the right or from the left, depending on how she moves. Also, when she puts pressure on her abdomen with her hands, the fetus does not move like a mole, because it is connected to the uterus, as we have said. The other distinctive sign is that with a mole the body becomes much harder than with impregnation, because of the hard flesh lodged in the uterus.

Also, women prone to moles have soft hands and feet that are weak or exhausted. This condition occurs because the uterus is damaged, and communicates its pain to the liver, with which it is closely connected; thereupon the liver generates unhealthy, watery blood, which, since it is not useful, nature sends to the feet and the hands, that is, to the extremities, rendering them soft; and it also sends this fluid to the face, causing it to swell. But perhaps you will say, *frontoso*, "how can the extremities be weakened and the face swollen? Why don't the hands and feet swell too?" I respond that, even though the authorities say they are weakened, they also appear to be swollen and bloated like the face; and they are weakened essentially because they did not receive the necessary nourishment from the liver, because of its weakness. And this kind of swelling and weakness are not found in women who are really pregnant.

Another way to distinguish mole from pregnancy, which is reliable especially at the beginning, is that the lips of the vagina are always moist, because

---

89. In Latin in the text: *in quibusdam autem mulieribus durat valde diu hec infirmitas et protenditur usque ad mortem.* See Albert the Great, *De animalibus*, Lib. X, tract. 1, c. 4 (p. 743).

90. In Latin in the text: *et quandoque protenditur usque ad finem vite et non recipit curationem.* See Avicenna, *Canon*, Lib. III, fen 21, tract. 2, c. 18 (p. 939).

of the descent of moisture retained in the uterus towards the lips of the vagina. Another test you may attempt is to take your middle finger and check if the uterus is closed. As has been said, in the case of mole, the uterus does not close. Another is that in the sixth or seventh month of a pregnancy, the fetus increases its movements, because it is looking for a way out; [whereas in the case of a mole, there is no increase in movement in later stages of pregnancy]. Another is that the gravid woman is always in a better mood than a woman carrying a mole, and this is because pregnancy is a natural thing, whereas a mole is against nature.

Finally, I want you to know, my ladies, that I will not at present write about sterility, so as to not interrupt our writing as planned in the table of contents; but at the end of our little book, for your use and pleasure, I will attempt to instruct you well about this topic, leaving the completion of this discussion to practicing physicians—of whose resources I advise you make use, given that their resources are not at all sterile, especially if it is your intention, assisted by their knowledge, to get pregnant.

Chapter Five
On conceiving male and female infants, and the techniques to be followed so that one sex or the other is conceived, and on signs that reveal whether the fetus is male or female

Given that pregnancy is cherished by all fathers, especially when a male child, rather than a female, is expected, I would like to discuss the reasons for this—why it is that humans give birth to some boys and some girls—while hoping that my discussion of this topic will offer pleasure to our audience.

We will say, therefore, that the first and foremost cause for the generation of a boy is the heat of the man's sperm, generated in the warm testicles of a sanguine or a choleric man. In contrast, the sperm of a phlegmatic or a melancholic man will cause the generation of girls. And there must be a great quantity of sperm, because all things being equal, the man is bigger than the woman. But you may ask, *frontoso*, "teach me master, how does one make boys?" I respond, based on what has been said, that in essence, hot sperm generates boys.

Second, the sperm of the right testicle is warmer than that of the left testicle, because of its proximity to the right kidney, from which it receives its warmth, and the kidney receives its warmth from the liver, which, also being warm, makes the sperm of the right testicle better concocted and thicker. And it is also true that spermatic vessels descend from the veins of the liver, [which is on the right side of the body]. This is why cowherds, when they want their cows to generate males, bind the left testicle of the bull, and you should do the same thing.

Third, as the right-hand side of the uterus is warmer than the left, I conclude that if the sperm from the right testicle should fall in the right side of the uterus, it will receive much benefit, remaining much warmer than if it were to fall on the left side.

Fourth, the hour of coition also plays a role in getting the wife pregnant, because it is at the hour of the cleaning out of her past menses that her new menses are purer and warmer, helping the sperm with their warmth, which causes the conception of males; for we have assumed from the start that males are warmer than females, and therefore require more heat in their generation.[91]

Frontoso: this is why, if you want to conceive a male child, you must make certain that your sperm is warm. And you will assure yourself of this by eating good foods, foods that are easy to digest, and warm things, not foods with cold properties; and similarly, you must drink the right wines—good wines that are warm and easy to digest. And take note, O women and men of Ferrara, this is the reason your *corbino* wines made with *uva d'oro*,[92] and similar wines that are difficult to digest, will stand in the way of pregnancy with a male child, because of the indigestion it causes, rendering the sperm of both the woman and the man cold and useless: so the use of warm and good things and warm suffumigations are advantageous in this case. And likewise, the consumption of *aqua marelli*,[93] greens, fruit, fish, date mussels, and other cold and humid foods causes the conception of females. And take note, O citizens of Ferrara, who consume so much of these

91. Throughout the Middle Ages, as well as in antiquity, menstruation, this major physiological difference between men and women, was mainly understood to be the female body's method of shedding accumulated and unnecessary blood. It was thought to be due to the looser and spongier texture of women's flesh, which accumulated more fluid than men's from the consumption of food and drink, as well as to women's sedentary lifestyle. If menstruation did not occur regularly, the womb would become overrun with fluid and surplus blood that continue to build up in the body, eventually provoking serious diseases or even death. This theory was in turn based on Greek and Roman plethora theory, which held that once the quantity of blood in the womb reached a critical level, it is expelled spontaneously: this mechanism, known as "critical evacuation," also explained nosebleeds and other spontaneous emissions. But menstrual blood also contributed to the formation of the fetus during pregnancy, both by generating flesh and by nourishing the fetus, and was eventually turned into milk after birth. This explains why Savonarola thinks that "new," warmer and purer menses are important to achieve pregnancy, and possibly a male offspring. For an updated bibliography on such topics as chatarsis, plethora theory, menstruation, and evacuation—in both women and men—encompassing antiquity, the Middle Ages, and the early modern period in Europe, see Cathy McClive, *Menstruation and Procreation in Early Modern France* (Farnham, Surrey, UK; Burlington, VT: Ashgate, 2015).

92. The *corbino* wine is a popular red table wine, now known as Corbinello. The "corbine" grapes take their name from the dark colour of the grape skin. Likewise, we can retrace the history of the "Golden Grape" wine, today known as Fortana wine, and also called wine of the sands. The name does not refer to white grapes but to vineyards growing out of the sandy lands and dunes of the coastal Ferrara area and the Po river's delta.

93. This beverage and its origins have not been identified. Gualdo, *Il lessico medico del "De regimine pregnantium"*, 208, similarly writes: *vino o bevanda di identificazione dubbia* (wine or drink of uncertain identification).

things, do not be surprised, on this account, if your female offspring multiply greatly.

And now turning to more specific things, we will say that a woman who wishes to become pregnant with a male child must avoid the cold, especially in her feet. She should not eat fruit and similar cold things, nor should she drink water or watered-down wine. Also, she must avoid things that are constipating, like eating pasta, cheese, cakes, and fish. She should only use mild spices, but if she has a cold complexion, she may use strong spices. Afterwards, she should take one drachm, that is one eighth of an ounce, of mithridate,[94] with close to a fifth of a glass of fragrant wine, two hours before getting up; and if she can in this time interval, she should sleep. And this she should repeat after cleansing for eight days in a row. Also, in order to produce heat in her uterus, after her cleansing, she should prepare a fragrance with *galia muscata* or labdanum: she should insert one fragranced suppository in her vagina, and she should keep it in for the entire night, for perhaps five or six days after the cleansing. After eight days she should copulate with her husband. She should also avoid sitting on the floor, but should instead sit on a chair with a feather cushion, and also keep her back warm.

It is also necessary that copulation not be too delayed because, as we have said, the sperm spoils, and its power is weakened, if coitus is too delayed. Furthermore, you should make sure, when sending sperm to the uterus, that as it descends, it descends to the right side of the uterus. Therefore, turn *frontosa* on her right side, and have her remain in this position for an hour, and also as the sperm descends, have her raise her buttock as much as possible, so that the sperm can better reach the fundus. As soon as you pull out of her, she should keep her legs together and turn onto her side as we have said before. It would be best if you can have intercourse in this position, and you must strive for this to happen, either by propping up the left side of her body with pillows or other objects that may elevate her, so that she will be facing the right during the act. This is why Messer Pietro Contarini, the Venetian gentleman who had seven daughters, after having been instructed by a physician on this remedy, and always following it, from that moment on only had male children. And I also believe that it is very helpful to bind the left testicle with a string as well.

And the same thing we said for the woman is also valid for the man's regimen, which must tend towards warm things. But note that if the woman is warm in the kidneys, uterus, and complexion, as are so many in Ferrara, caresses may not be necessary. However, it is necessary to accompany your ship to port with prudence. Couples [hoping for male offspring] should keep under their members, or nearby, musk, *galia muscata*, labdanum, aloewood, and similar fragrant and

---

94. In medieval medical terms, the drachm is a unit of weight measure equal to an eighth of an ounce (circa 3.5 grams, from the name of the Greek coin that originally consisted of 3.5 grams of silver). Mithridate is an ancient antidote for poison.

warm things; and they should think only of males, always keeping in mind some famous man.

And note, *frontoso*, that he who generates male children is strong in the body and robust. He produces sperm that is thick and well-concocted, and has large testicles and veins that are large and wide; he is naturally disposed to copulate, and is not weakened by such copulation. All of these are signs of a man's great heat and well-concocted sperm. The largeness of these parts is a sign that the testicles will produce the great quantities of seed necessary for the generation of males. Thus it is easy to know whether or not you are generative of males. Moreover, a young man should understand that if his right testicle deflates before the left during coitus, a male will be generated, because it will be a sign that the the sperm was first released from the right testicle, and as was said earlier, the sperm sent from the right side generates males. Another sign that a male will be generated is when the seed comes out quickly, which indicates that the man's heat has stimulated the expulsive power.

Similar signs identify those females who conceive males. A woman who is prone to conceive males is of good color, from which it is clear that she is not cold, but instead of a warm or temperate complexion. She is also of a good shape, usually not soft, but firm, and not heavy set, but very agile. Her menses are light in texture, not thick, but of a good color, not black or burnt, because such burntness signifies excessive heat. It is a good sign when a woman has a good appetite and digests her food well, thus making good blood, of which the spirit and the sperm are composed; and she should not evacuate too much, because through such evacuation the natural heat of the sperm is weakened. Nor should she be too constipated, or the vapors of her feces will be harmful to her menstrual blood. Also these women are happy, and their veins are visible: all of these are signs of heat that is not excessive. And finally, you should know, *frontosa*, that those who begin to have their period at the right time, at around the age of fourteen, are prone to conceive males: since this is a sign of abundance of blood and heat, both of which are necessary in order to conceive males.

Many say that if the sperm of the male descends from his left side to the right side of the female, a virago will be born—that is, a masculine female; but if the sperm descends from the male's right side to the left side of the woman, the child will be a feminine male or an effeminate one.

And given that couples are eager to know, when the wife is gravid, if she is gravid with a male or female, we will describe for their pleasure, and to conclude our chapter, the signs of how to judge whether the fetus in her belly is male or female. Let us say, first, that a woman pregnant with a male has good color, much better than the color of women who are carrying females. This is because the male is generated with warmer sperm, and with warmer, purer blood than that of females. And therefore a woman [bearing a male fetus] is lighter and more agile in her bodily movements, cleaner and clearer in the face, with a much better appetite and with many fewer pains and difficulties than other pregnant women tend to have, of which we will speak later. Since the blood of the female is colder, discolored, and not as well concocted, [a female fetus will] generate [in the pregnant woman] bad color, slow movement, and poor appetite.

Another sign that a woman is gravid with a male child is that she feels the weight of the fetus on the right side, because it is usually generated in the right side from sperm sent there, and because this side is much more apt to receive sperm descended from the right testicle than from the left. And similarly, women feel a male fetus move much more on the right side, and almost continuously.

Another sign [that a male is conceived] is that the right breast begins to change in color near the nipple and it is a red color that tends towards a dark shade, and similarly, the right breast begins to enlarge before the left one. And the reason for this is that when a male child is generated, nature sends greater quantity of blood to the right side of the uterus for its nourishment, and consequently it also sends more blood to the right breast for the future nourishment of the fetus; for males need more nourishment than females, and this is why men generally eat much more than women, since they are of a warmer nature and more robust. And take note, *frontosa*: in giving your child to a wet nurse, you must seriously take this into account, because male infants need more milk than females. And because such blood is a bit concocted, the color of the nipple tends to look a bit darker; and for a similar reason, milk appears first in the right breast.

Moreover, the milk often appears viscous and not watery. When squirting such milk over a fingernail, it stays still and does not drip down the sides. And if you spray it on a mirror in the sun, it stays firm like a large pearl or like a drop of quicksilver and it does not flow. These effects all derive from good digestion and a body's moderate temperature, not excessively hot. But note that Avicenna, in his *De animalibus*, treatise XVIII, corrects this experiment, stating that it is true in the eighth and ninth month.[95] Another sign [that a woman is bearing a male child] is that the nipple of the right breast begins first to enlarge and becomes larger than the other, and tends towards red color, and the nearby veins enlarge. We have already stated the reason for this: because males need more blood and purer blood for their nourishment.

Another sign [that a woman is bearing a male child] is that her pulse on the right-hand side is more frequent, because the warmth of the fetus is transmitted to the right-hand side, and so requires increased ventilation. This is why the pulse meets that need by its frequency, which it cannot do by greater force.

---

95. Savonarola is possibly referring to the following statement of Avicenna in *De animalibus*, Lib. XVIII (fol. 53v): *Et apparet error Empedocles, quoniam credit quod lac generabatur in octavo et quarto* (And the error of Empedocles is evident, since he believes that milk is generated in the eighth and fourth month).

Another sign, which is common knowledge, is that when a woman is pregnant with a male she moves her right foot first when walking, and will also get up from a chair by first putting forth her right hand. This can be seen through experience, and Avicenna notes this sign, citing the authority of other philosophers.[96] But maybe you will say, *frontoso*, "how can this be true, because if the fetus is in the right-hand side, the woman should feel more weighed down on that side, and by consequence, shouldn't her right side move more slowly than her left?" My response is that this sign is generally true in most cases, like the other medical signs; as Albert says, man and lions, among other animals, first move their right foot, indicating that this type of movement is natural.[97] The woman first places her foot on the ground, in correspondence with the load, in order to ground her movement, so that she can more easily stand up, afterwards raising up the lighter part [of her body] that is not loaded down [with the weight of the fetus]; thus she acts like a mason, who first builds a heavy wall, and after that, on that foundation, lighter walls. And responding to this argument, I say that even though the right side may be heavier, nonetheless, since nature is eager for the fetus, it sends more heat, that is, blood and vital spirit, to the right side, making those parts warmer and more agile and more capable of motion. Thus nature teaches that these parts move first.

It is also said that a woman pregnant with a male child has eyes that are more mobile, and her right eye moves better than her left. The other sign is that the male child begins to move at the end of about three months, whereas a female child does not move until about the fourth month, or in some cases even at the end of the fourth month. The reason for this is that while in the belly, the male develops more quickly than the female, while outside of the belly, the female grows faster. This is a great riddle to be solved, which I leave to those who wish to speculate. Another sign [of the sex of the fetus] is put forth by those who wish to speak on the subject: the pregnant woman should take a root of *aristolochia longa*, crush it well, make it into a suppository, moisten it with honey, and wrap it up with uncombed wool that is not washed. In the morning while fasting, she should insert this into her vagina, and she should keep it in until midday, remaining on an empty stomach. If she tastes a sweet flavor in her mouth, this means that she is expecting a boy; if she tastes a bitter flavor, a girl; if she tastes neither sweet nor bitter, this is a sign that she is not gravid. Of course, interpreting these effects should not be left to someone who is ignorant. Even though bitterness tends to come from heat more than sweetness, which is why it should be one of the earliest signs of a male child, it is also true that sweetness is a sign of good digestion, and bitterness of poor digestion, and therefore bitterness more often signals a female fetus. Those who reflect on this matter say that these tests stem from the occult;

96. See Avicenna, *Canon*, Lib. III, fen 21, tract. 1, c. 13 (p. 929).

97. Albert the Great, *De animalibus*, Lib. II, tract. 1, c. 2 (p. 230).

that is, they can't offer any evident reason for it. Albert, in book X of *De animali-bus*, says of this "but I wonder if this is true, and it requires great consideration."[98]

Another sign is that a woman pregnant with a female child has ulcerations on her thighs, and spots on her feet, and some pustules that break out all over her body. And these effects tend to happen especially when the uterus is weak, and therefore producing some superfluities, which nature later sends to the extremities and to the exterior parts.

Let these signs of the conception of a male suffice for now, while for a female, one must look for the opposite signs. And I will also add to these a sign which I have seen with my own eyes: that when inside the lips of the vagina, and near them, there is a fiery red irritation accompanied by itching, this is sign of a male child, and the reason for this has already been explained.

Finally, I wish also to recall the nine signs of a dead fetus: 1. that the pregnant woman will feel in the cavity of her uterus something like a rock that moves from side to side, moving in this manner from one side to the other; 2. her abdomen under the navel, which was warm earlier, is now cold; 3. her breasts shrink; 4. the whites of her eyes become dark; 5. her ears and the tip of her nose become rigid and as red as her lips; 6. The pregnant woman's body deflates, especially under the navel; 7. her breath stinks; 8. she puts her hands in that place where she once felt the fetus, keeping her mouth and nose closed tightly for a while, and if it is alive, it will move, and if it is dead, it will not; 9. often when the fetus is dead, some virulent and fetid fluids appear, especially following an acute fever or other great illness.

Here ends the first book.

Treatise Two
Chapters of the second treatise of our volume

- Chapter One: Of the pregnant woman's regimen with regard to what the physicians call the six non-naturals: air, food and drink, exercise and rest, sleep and waking, evacuation and repletion, and the accidents of the soul
- Chapter Two: On the conditions or states common to pregnant women
- Chapter Three: On the regimen of the woman who has given birth

---

98. In Latin in the text: *sed ego miror si hoc est verum, et indiget consideratione magna.* See Albert the Great, *De animalibus*, Lib. X, tract. 2, c. 3 (p. 757).

Chapter One
On the regimen of pregnant women

Pregnant women have two responsibilities in their regimen: the first is towards themselves, and the second, towards the child they carry in their womb. Regarding nourishment and the other five non-naturals outlined by physicians—that is, exercise and rest, sleep and waking, repletion and evacuation, accidents of the soul, and air—it is necessary that women closely watch themselves. And regarding eating and drinking, the sixth non-natural, which here we make the first, we will say that it is important to consider both quality and quantity of nourishment, which is certainly the first and foremost foundation of both lives, especially the life of the child. As philosophers and doctors maintain, and experience shows, nourishment not only affects a body's complexion, but also its species; this is why when a grain of wheat is cast upon eroded soil, oats and barley, which are of a different complexion and species, sprout instead of wheat. As the great physician Galen says in book III of his *Art of Medicine* if for a prolonged period of time one observes a regimen contrary to these six things called non-naturals, especially with regard to food and drink, a person with a melancholic complexion may become sanguine.[99]

And for this reason, *frontosa*, if you desire to have a beautiful child, a child of good complexion and gifted by nature, you must eat wholesome, beneficial, and easy-to-digest foods, such as those that will be listed later, and drink good and honorable wine, whenever possible, and avoid the bad ones, of which we will speak, such as *aqua marelli*, heavy wines and those that are difficult to digest, like wines made from *uva d'oro*.[100] For understand that if it is possible to transform an adult melancholic into a person of sanguine complexion, as physicians maintain, so then it must be even simpler to achieve such a change at the beginning of life, when the melancholic complexion is not yet fixed and habituated. Therefore, melancholic and weak-limbed couples, if you desire to have children of a good and robust complexion, you must be careful to follow a superior regimen, eating good things and drinking even better things, to speak plainly.

Keep in mind, *frontoso*, and you, *frontosa*, that all aspects of a good regimen are ruled by Lady Moderation; and furthermore, you must regulate the quantity of nourishment and the schedule you keep. On quantity, I will say the following: that

99. Although clearly stating that the different balancing of six non-naturals (i.e. air; exercise; sleeping and waking; food and drink; excretion; and emotions) can cause a change in complexion, Galen does not mention the passage from melancholic to sanguine in book III of his *Art of Medicine*: see Galen, *On the Constitution of the Art of Medicine; The Art of Medicine; A Method of Medicine to Glaucon*, ed. and trans. Ian Johnston (Cambridge, MA: Harvard University Press, 2016), Book III, ch. 25 (pp. 257–59); =Kühn, 1:372–76.

100. In Treatise One, at 102, Savonarola also warns his readers to avoid these drinks because they are too cold and humid and may lead to the conception of females.

as a pregnant woman's fetus grows in her womb, so should the amount of food increase accordingly, so that she will generate more blood, which is necessary for the nourishment of the fetus. But first, one must also consider the strength of the stomach. If possible, *frontosa*, you should eat three meals a day, spacing your meals as evenly as possible. And how you do this remains at your discretion, depending on your appetite; one hour more or less does not make a difference. And it is also true that pregnant women who are sanguine can perhaps get by with a lesser quantity of food; I say perhaps, because even among such women you find many who digest very quickly and are in need of a large meal. But I mention this here mainly for the benefit of our audience, so that they may remember to eat and drink moderately. Furthermore, moderation should be observed also according to season: since, of course, in winter one can eat more than in the summer—I say more quantity at a time; this is because bodies, as it is maintained by the authority of Hippocrates, are warmer in winter. Among Christians, the time between meals is from eight to nine hours. Nonetheless Avicenna, the Arab, says that in forty-eight hours, one should not eat more than twice.

In line with this chapter's objective, we will specify the most beneficial and harmful foods as well as the most useful and unsafe drinks for pregnant women; and of the other five non-natural things, we will also make recommendations, having first established some general rules, especially regarding foods: since all pregnant women should avoid foods that are harsh, gassy, constipating, and things that provoke a reaction—in other words, purgative and diuretic foods, that are too acidic and corrosive, because all of these types of food can harm the fetus, causing the woman to abort, or causing great pain or other hardships for the pregnant woman, as we will later describe.

Beneficial foods for pregnant women are the following:

Starting with bread: it should be baked from refined wheat, if possible, because this generates good blood above all other grains. I say "if possible," because impoverished women do not have the same access to it as do the rich. When bread is baked with bran, it becomes very harsh and it is likely to cause miscarriage. This is why Avicenna says "and let their food be white bread,"[101] that is, cleaned of bran. O impoverished pregnant woman who is forced to eat bran bread, I do feel compassion for you, and I also remind you that it is dangerous to eat this when you are pregnant, so if you can, stay away from it as much as possible.

Now, if you ask about bread made from millet, panicum, or sorghum, I would say that these too are difficult to digest, especially by delicate stomachs accustomed to wheat breads. These grains are constipating, and because of this quality, they are harmful to the pregnant woman, who is already constipated because of her pregnancy. These grains may harm the fetus because of their frigidity, and they do not generate the best blood: instead, these grains have the tendency

---

101. Avicenna, *Canon*, Lib. III, fen 21, tract. 2, c. 2 (p. 932): *et sint cibi earum panis mundus.*

to generate blood that verges on the melancholic. It is true that peasant women are more accustomed to eating bread made from these types of grains, and that it is therefore less harmful to them than it is to city women; and they also benefit from the great exercise they get, which makes them more robust. But remember that spelt bread is laxative, and so it harms the stomach and induces a reaction. Therefore, pregnant women should avoid this type of bread. Of chestnut bread, I will say that like bread made of millet, panicum, or sorghum, it causes gassiness, which causes pregnant women great pain.

Now, I mention all of this here, not because I believe that it will be fully heeded, but simply to make our audience aware of these facts. If they choose to overlook these recommendations, they should not stray too far, especially in the quantity or in the use of these foods; meaning that, when the pregnant woman feels a strong craving for something contrary to her well-being, nature often corrects the bad qualities of the food. Therefore, as long as this desire is not excessive, she may eat these foods in small quantities. This is what Hippocrates means when he says "plainer food is to be preferred to finer food, because it enhances the appetite."[102] Having talked about bread, which is made of water, wheat, or the flour of other grains, we will now pass to other simple foodstuffs, and we will first discuss meats.

On meats of quadrupeds. We will begin with four-legged animals, affirming that veal, beef, kid, milk-fed lamb, young mutton, and similar meats are easy to digest and therefore advantageous. The meat of a young pig (more or less one year old) is also advantageous and nourishing. As Galen observes, "pork is the most nutritious of all foods,"[103] although it is true that it is a little difficult to digest. It is said that pork should not come from pigs exceeding the age of one because the meat of half-grown pigs generates bad humors, and the meat of older pigs is very difficult to digest and generates melancholic humors. Pregnant women should also take care not to eat too much salted meat, noting the quantity. The best meat is that of the wild boar, and the meat of roebuck is also advantageous, while the meat of old deer generates melancholic humors. Pregnant women may eat hare, even though it stimulates urination, as long as they eat very little; and it is best when roasted over an open fire. Venison is difficult to digest for pregnant women and generates melancholic blood, although they can eat a little, but in any case, venison provides bad nourishment. Therefore, *frontosa,* you should exercise moderation in eating such meats and other foods that we will discuss that provide poor nourishment, even though you can eat them in small quantities. Let my advice guide you if you want your child to be beautiful, strong, and well-nourished.

---

102. In Latin in the text: *parum deterior cibus melioribus quidem est apetendus, quia apetitui dandus.* See Hippocrates, *Aphorisms,* II.38 (pp. 117–18).

103. In Latin in the text: *nutribilissimum omnium que novimus est caro porcina.* See Galen, *On the Properties of Foodstuffs,* trans. Owen Powell (Cambridge: Cambridge University Press, 2003), Book III, ch. 1 (p. 115); =Kühn, 6:661.

On meats of bipeds. The meat of hens, capons, chickens, francolins, pheasants, partridges, and pigeons is advantageous. O *frontosa*, who would not want to get pregnant and be treated to such dishes? The meat of duck and goose may also be advantageous: that is, the pregnant woman may eat these if she has a strong stomach, since they are difficult to digest, especially the meat of older fowl. Crane meat offers poor nourishment, generates bad blood, and is difficult to digest. The meat of peacock is likewise bad. The meat of the grey partridge and of the Greek partridge are advantageous and they generate good blood. Therefore you, *frontosa*, who are rich and privileged, when you are pregnant, you should seek such meats and other foods that generate good blood. You may eat turtledove as long as it is young and succulent, and avoid those that are old and thin; and when you want to eat turtledove, make sure that it is tender, because if not, it can be difficult to digest. You may eat quail, but in small amounts and seldom. Quail meat is difficult to digest and it makes the pregnant woman susceptible to fever; rather, when you have some quail, repay your physician by sending him some as a gift. Skip over the little birds, for they are too scrawny. Instead, eat birds that live in bushes and trees such as skylarks, thrushes, and blackbirds. Leave aquatic birds to fly through the valleys, since they generate bad blood, giving bad nourishment, as do chickens from Bondeno and Finale.[104] Therefore, *frontosa*, when you desire the well-being of the child you carry in your womb, look for foods that are easy to digest, that have few superfluities, and that generate good blood; those I have recommended to you and will continue to recommend without adding others.

On fish. Fish always generates phlegmatic blood since it is cold and humid, and although pregnant women may eat fish, sanguine and choleric women are able to eat it with less harm than phlegmatics. If phlegmatic women eat fish, they should roast it, or cook it in wine, or season it with cinnamon or salt or the like, to counteract the coldness and humidity of the fish. Melancholic pregnant women should prepare fish the same way, focusing more on the removal of the coldness than on the removal of humidity. The best saltwater fish are flounder, sea bream, mackerel, bleak,[105] eel, and similar fish: these, pregnant women can eat. I also recommend freshwater fish such as gudgeon and other fish that love stony river beds—pike, small fish sturgeon, trout, umber, and similar fish—even though these types of fish are difficult to digest. Pregnant women may have salted fish in moderation. Tench, however, provides bad nourishment and is very glutinous. Of eels, which are abundant in Ferrara, I say like Oribasius, and with the authority of Dioscorides, that they are very nourishing and that they clear the windpipes, and so also the voice. Therefore, *frontosa*, if you enjoy singing, you may eat eels.

104. Bondeno and Finale are municipalities located in the region of Emilia-Romagna, respectively some 12 and 18 miles (20 and 30 km) west of Ferrara.

105. Although Savonarola classifies bleak (*alburnus*) as a "saltwater fish," it is technically a freshwater fish.

However, to correct their harmful qualities, you should first boil them in water and later cook them in good wine and fragrant spices. But be careful when eating eels from the month of May because they copulate with grass snakes; if they come from flowing water, they will be better.

And not turning away from fish and its uses, I will say that its milt is harmful to you, because it corrupts other foods. Second, beware, pregnant *frontosa*, of roasted fish that has cooled off and of fish that has been covered after being cooked; because it has not been able to respire, it retains vapors, and it is harmful like poison. Lastly for now, I advise that when you want to eat fish, wash it and clean it, and then salt it one hour in advance. Later cook it in water and make sure the water is boiling before adding the fish, then add the fish to the boiling water with some vinegar and good spices. I do believe that for you it is more beneficial to boil fish than to fry it, even though Galen explains in book III of *De alimentorum facultatibus* (*On the Properties of Foodstuffs*) that fried foods are better for the healthy, but that for the convalescent, boiled foods are better.[106] Indeed, I think that pregnant women should count themselves among the convalescent, insofar as pregnancy is like a slight malady, even though it is natural; that is, the pregnant woman can expect all these bothersome symptoms to resolve themselves and that her pristine health will be restored.

On prawns, oysters, clams, and shellfish. After discussing fish, we will talk of prawns, oysters, and clams. Regarding prawns, the pregnant woman may eat them: they are one of the foods that, according to some, retain the fetus in the uterus. Despite the fact that Galen claims that shrimp are harmful to the stomach, they may also be eaten. Clams and oysters are not only difficult to digest, they are also harmful to the stomach and they produce gases, which induce stomach cramps in the pregnant woman, whose intestines are so constricted by the fetus that is in the womb; and given that the gases can be strong and the escape narrow, these gases cause pain. Now, there are some idiots who like this type of seafood, especially oysters, claiming that they keep their cocks hard when they need to be. O stupid fools! Oysters may make your poles perk up, but they don't bring with them the flour to bake the bread. I will recall here what I said to Marquis Niccolò on this subject when he asked me about oysters, knowing well the reason for his question. I responded to him: "an oyster is a baker who orders others to bake bread, but if there is no flour, the order is placed in vain." You know what I mean, *frontoso.* And you, pregnant *frontosa*, take care not to eat too many oysters and clams, especially in the last three months of your pregnancy: the bigger your belly gets, the more oysters and clams are harmful to you and the baby.

On fruits. Fruits are generally cold, humid, and gassy, and they generate blood that is cold and humid, as well as gases. Because of these properties, fruits may not be well-tolerated by the fetus, and because of the excess gases they

---

106. See Galen, *On the Properties of Foodstuffs*, Book III, ch. 29 (p. 142); =Kühn, 6:725.

produce, they harm the pregnant woman, just as we have said about oysters and clams, and because of this they also harm the baby. Therefore, *frontosa*, try to eat as little fruit as possible and, as they say, "don't undress too far from the bath." Certainly, there are fruits that are warm, dry and astringent: warm like the almond, pine nut, date, walnut, hazelnut, and citron; and astringent like the medlar fruit, pomegranate, serviceberry, and quince. We will elaborate on these fruits noting that, even though the almond is fibrous and bloating, it is also nourishing, which is why Avicenna says that "eating sweet almonds makes one fat."[107] Therefore, considering that the almond's harmful qualities are minor and its benefits great, and hoping—having considered the great appetite for almonds of pregnant women—that nature will correct their bad qualities, as Hippocrates said, I would say that pregnant women may eat almonds. O *frontosa*, you may also eat fresh almonds in their skin when they are in season, since this is a food that pregnant women find delectable; but though they cleanse the stomach by their detergent qualities, they are also difficult to digest. Therefore be sure to show moderation, in this case as with others, as we have said before on several occasions, and take into account the condition of your own stomach.

The pine nut is very beneficial, especially in the first months of pregnancy and even later. The date is not advisable for women of a warm nature, because it often generates choleric blood. But if the pregnant woman is strong, and not of a warm nature, and she eats dates, they may in fact give her strength and benefit her. Of walnuts, let us say that pregnant women may eat them, especially in the first months, roasting them over a fire first; and later in the pregnancy, she may eat them raw, especially when the pregnant woman is not too hot by nature. Nonetheless, roasted walnuts are difficult to digest, and fresh ones are less harmful to her stomach. Hazelnuts, especially fresh ones, are difficult to digest, and they promote gassiness; furthermore, hazelnuts are more constipating than walnuts, on which account, as they cause flatulence and constipation, pregnant women should take care not to eat too many hazelnuts, especially from the third to the ninth month. Yet moderation is recommended: pregnant women should not completely refrain from eating hazelnuts, but should consume them moderately, and we have warned them here of the dangers of hazelnuts so that they may practice moderation.

The citron in itself has different complexions that correspond to its different parts. The pregnant woman can sometimes eat it with other foods, but rarely, and if she does, she should eat the flesh of the citron together with the peel, because, speaking as a physician, the properties of the two parts balance each other out. The peel is truly difficult to digest; for as Avicenna says, "the rind is

---

107. In Latin in the text: *et commedere dulces impinguat.* See Avicenna, *Canon*, Lib. II, tract. 2, c. 58 (p. 271).

not digested,"[108] and it generates gases and severe intestinal colic. Therefore, pregnant women should not eat too many citrons, but instead, save them for special occasions. Medlars may be eaten in moderation. Serviceberries, which are more like medicine than food, given their constipating qualities, should be avoided by pregnant women, because they can be very harmful. Of quinces, I advise that they may be eaten on some occasions, in small quantities and uncooked, but they are less harmful if they are cooked; even though by nature quinces are constipating, they are also laxative, and may relieve the intestines of foods consumed. Now, everything we have said on the harmful and helpful qualities of fruit, we have said to remind pregnant women of all these properties so that they will exercise moderation in eating fruit, since they often err in determining the appropriate amount of fruit to eat.

Also, Avicenna claims that olives are harmful to pregnant women.[109] I say that this is true in that they are laxative and are difficult to digest; but insofar as they are astringent and bring relief to the stomach and increase appetite, pregnant women may use them in moderation, like the other foods previously mentioned. Certainly a pregnant woman must be more attentive to what she eats and drinks and to her other actions than women who are not pregnant, lest she abort her fetus or give birth to a defective child. *Frontosa*, I know that you understand me. The pomegranate, Avicenna says, is laxative, especially sour pomegranates, and so a pregnant woman should avoid sour pomegranates because they are harmful to the stomach;[110] sweet pomegranates, however, as well as those that are neither sweet nor sour, may soothe the stomach. Avicenna also says that pomegranate wine or juice is good for a pregnant woman's appetite.[111] Apricots, or *crisoloma* as doctors call them, may be eaten, meaning that they are better for the stomach than peaches, which pregnant women should not eat, especially following other foods, because they corrupt the stomach; instead, peaches should only be eaten before other foods, and in moderation.

Prunes or plums are good for choleric pregnant women and those who produce choler in the stomach, because they repress choler. They are also soothing to the belly, which pregnant women find beneficial and not harmful, since these fruits are mild. Pistachios are also beneficial: they soothe the stomach of the pregnant woman and prevent nausea, the desire to vomit, and even prevent vomiting. Grapes, if eaten freshly picked, may cause bloating; therefore, *frontosa*, refrain from eating grapes for a whole day, and later eat them, and they will comfort and benefit you.

---

108. In Latin in the text: *cortex eius non digeritur.* See Avicenna, *Canon*, Lib. II, tract. 2, c. 119 (p. 286).

109. See Avicenna, *Canon*, Lib. III, fen 21, tract. 2, c. 2 (p. 932).

110. See Avicenna, *Canon*, Lib. II, tract. 2, c. 319 (pp. 328–29).

111. See Avicenna, *Canon*, Lib. II, tract. 2, c. 319 (p. 329); see also Lib. III, fen 21, tract. 2, c. 2 (p. 932).

Raisins are beneficial and good for you. Galen claims that fresh figs are bad for the stomach, but dried figs are not harmful and they are very nourishing.[112] Even though they are laxative, you may eat them. But beware of figs that are too moist, because they may cause bloating. Similarly, show moderation with cherries when they are too moist; and remember that the sweet ones are better for you than the sour ones, which cause gassiness.

Authorities say that melons cause heartburn; therefore, the pregnant woman should eat them in moderation. Doctors also advise that pumpkins cause heartburn; and they are harmful to the stomachs of children, and particularly harmful to pregnant women who are melancholic and phlegmatic, although they are agreeable to cholerics. The turnip is warm and moist; so that roasted, it becomes less harmful to pregnant women; even if it is laxative, they may eat turnips in moderation. The same may be said for rutabaga, although it is a little hotter in quality than the turnip. Of cucumbers, Avicenna says that they generate bad humors and decay easily;[113] however, if there is choler in the stomach of the pregnant woman, cucumbers will not harm her; but since cucumbers are also laxative, I cannot recommend them. We may say similar things about watermelon, which is even more prone to putrefaction than cucumbers.

In general, on fruits I would like to say that those that are apt to be cooked are better because it is less harmful to eat cooked fruits than raw fruits. And to recapitulate, pregnant *frontosa*, if you love the baby you carry in your womb, be careful when you eat fruit and keep your hands on the reins. Finally, I will remind you that it is inadvisable to eat green apples when they first appear, and they are not yet ripe, because sour apples are cold and humid, and cause gassiness and bloating, generating pains in your abdomen, while sweet, ripe apples are temperate, slightly tending toward the hot. Uncooked apples, according to Avicenna, generate fever because of the bad qualities of their humors.[114] Fresh peaches, Avicenna explains, easily putrefy, but they keep the abdomen well lubricated;[115] therefore, they can be eaten before other foods since they soothe the stomach of the pregnant woman by waking up her appetite; but keep in mind, *frontosa*: Lady Moderation.

The reason why, my *frontosa*, I remind you about these properties of fruits that you should not eat when you are pregnant is so that you can keep yourself in check. Let me remind you that the most noble and beautiful fruit in the world is the human creature, and as for these other fruits, which are vile, harmful, and ugly, you must resist the sin of gluttony, most worthy of censure, in order to protect that

112. See Galen, *On the Properties of Foodstuffs*, Book II, ch. 8 (pp. 76–77); =Kühn, 6:570–73.

113. See Avicenna, *Canon*, Lib. II, tract. 2, c. 179 (p. 303).

114. See Avicenna, *Canon*, Lib. II, tract. 2, c. 569 (pp. 378–79).

115. See Avicenna, *Canon*, Lib. II, tract. 2, c. 571 (pp. 379–80).

incomparable, excellent, and precious fruit that you carry inside yourself. We will further elaborate on this later in this chapter.

Root vegetables. To continue with our lists of foods, we will now discuss the common root vegetables, such as parsley root, radish, and carrot, which are very appetizing and stimulative. A pregnant woman, however, must beware in eating these, especially if she eats them often and in large quantities. Avicenna says that celery provokes urine and menses and is therefore dangerous for pregnant women.[116] The pregnant woman should also avoid eating too much parsley root, which is in the same category. Radishes are laxative, difficult to digest, and induce nausea and generate gases, but they also awake and stimulate the appetite. Even though she may gain some benefit from these, a pregnant woman should limit the quantity of radishes she eats. We say the same thing of carrots. Next, the elecampane root also stimulates menses and urine. As Avicenna states, the use of this root makes a person urinate continuously:[117] therefore, *frontosa*, beware of it.

Section on seeds. Let us now move onto the seeds of melon, squash, cucumber, fennel, anise, coriander, and mustard. They are all appetizing, but melon seeds are laxative. Therefore, pregnant women should be careful when adding melon seeds to their diets, especially when they are sick, as melon seeds are less appetizing than the seeds of cucumber and squash. And the seeds of fennel and anise provoke urine and menses. Therefore, *frontosa*, I remind you that you must moderate your intake of these for your own health and that of your fetus. Mustard seeds are preferable to fennel seeds and anise. You may also eat prepared and sugar-coated coriander.

On grains. Next we will speak of grains, such as favas, beans, chickpeas, red chickpeas, lentils, peas or green peas, and similar foods such as rice, spelt, and panicum. You may eat rice, even though it is a bit fibrous, and similarly, spelt and panicum. You may also try beans with or without the shells, keeping in mind that they are very gassy, but without the shell they produce fewer gases and are less bloating; and you may also boil them and cook them well. However, women of Ferrara, you must know that the lupin variety of the bean, which is so popular among you, provokes menstruation, so beware of these, pregnant woman. Doctors strictly forbid beans for pregnant women because they stimulate menses—especially red beans, as well as the decoction of red beans with oil. And similarly stimulative are red chickpeas, although the white ones are less harmful. Eating these can cause abortion, and this is why Avicenna says "and let their food be like white bread; and let them avoid everything sharp or bitter, like capers and unripe olives, and everything that provokes the menses, such as beans and

---

116. See Avicenna, *Canon,* Lib. II, tract. 2, c. 56 (p. 271).

117. See Avicenna, *Canon,* Lib. II, tract. 2, c. 239 (p. 313).

chickpeas and sesame."[118] You may eat lentils, especially when they are boiled and also cooked as beans are: because prepared in this way they lose their bloating property. Peas or green peas also cause bloating, but less so than beans, especially fresh peas; but dry peas lose much of this tendency, and are safer to eat. Again, *frontosa*, the reason I continue to discuss the dangers of certain foods is so that you may moderate your intake of them.

On herbs. Having discussed grains, we will now move onto herbs that are commonly used with victuals, like savoy cabbage, chard, lettuce, spinach, endive, rocket, thyme, and marjoram. Savoy cabbage provokes menstruation, so when you eat it, make sure it is prepared with fatty meat, especially hen. Beware not to drink a decoction of Savoy cabbage cooked with oil and salt, as many of you often do. Chard is harmful to the stomach, a bit less so if it is cooked twice, as said of beans: and prepared in this way, a pregnant woman may eat chard. I do not find lettuce to have any dangerous properties for a pregnant woman, and therefore I grant ample license to the pregnant woman to enjoy it, especially in a salad with vinegar, which stimulates appetite. However, if she does eat salad, she must not add too many capers, hop shoots, or even hops, which are often eaten with salad. The warning about capers comes from Avicenna.[119] However, she may add a bit of hops, as long as she does this with moderation, because they are also laxaative. And we say the same about asparagus.

Of local endive, we will say that most certainly the pregnant woman may use it, and also the same of radicchio, also known as wild endive. This type does no harm to the stomach, but instead it soothes it more than the local variety. But the root of endive is difficult to digest, and it should be well cooked, in which case it prevents obstruction of the liver and the veins and soothes the liver and promotes good color. However, I believe that the use of this radicchio in Ferrara is prescribed by physicians, who have aided the bilious citizens of Ferrara, where many, and in the past even more, find themselves in this condition: therefore, *frontosa*, arm yourselves with radicchio. Spinach remains your friend, as long as you do not have a cold stomach. Rocket causes headaches when eaten alone, but when mixed with lettuce, its harmful qualities are removed. Of thyme, which is used in sauces more than in victuals, I say that it provokes menstruation. Therefore its use is dangerous, especially in victuals; however, it is fine to use thyme in small quantities in sauces. The same goes for rue, marjoram, sage, and rosemary.

---

118. In Latin in the text: *et sint cibi earum sic panis mundus; et devitent omnem acutum, amarum, sicut capares et olive immature, et omne provocativum menstruorum, sicut sunt faxolli et cicer et sisamum.* See Avicenna, *Canon*, Lib. III, fen 21, tract. 2, c. 2 (p. 932).

119. See previous note. Avicenna states that capers induce menses also in the *Canon*, Lib. II, tract. 2, c. 141 (p. 293).

On acrid foods.[120] On acrid foods such as garlic, onions, leeks, and scallions. Garlic produces gases, especially when it is fresh; and dried garlic weakens gases and often disperses them. It also provokes menstruation: therefore, *frontosa*, keep your hands on the reins; and garlic also causes headaches. Onions soothe the stomach and stimulate appetite, but they also provoke menstruation and bring on bleeding hemorrhoids. Therefore, *frontosa*, take care to control your intake of onions; they are better roasted under a fire and less harmful when eaten with vinegar. Leeks also stimulate menstruation and upset the stomach. The scallion is like a smaller onion; therefore, it is not necessary for me to repeat what I have already said about onions. But take note, *frontosa*, that all things that stimulate menstruation will make you abort, so use these things in moderation, especially of quantity, and I remind you of this often, so that you do not put your baby or yourself in danger.

On milk and dairy products. On milk and dairy products, like cheese, ricotta, clotted cream, and butter. We hold that dairy products induce bloating and cause stomachaches—especially ricotta cheese, which can be harmful to pregnant women. But it is also true that if milk is carefully boiled until it loses its watery part, it does not induce diarrhea. Eating too much ricotta may produce kidney stones, as can clotted cream: so I recommend, *frontosa*, that you do not crave these excessively. And note that in Ferrara kidney stones are very common because of the popularity of ricotta and similar cheeses. On cheese, I say that it is better for you to eat cheese that is neither too fresh nor too aged, but just in the middle, which you can eat in moderation. Now, when you crave cheese, it is better if you eat fresh cheese, as we will later explain. Of butter, I say that it is harmful to the stomach and takes away the appetite of the pregnant woman, especially when it is not fresh; and also note, *frontosa*, that the use of butter often causes ulcers or milk crust in babies.

On oils and fats. Know that the most soothing to the stomach of a pregnant woman is fresh oil, made from unripe olives, called *onfacino*; but pregnant women may also use oil made from well-ripened olives and it will not harm them. A pregnant woman may also use the fat of a chicken and of fresh pork: however, not too much because these fats take away her appetite.

On honey and sugar. Beware of honey and things sweetened with honey, because these things are gassy and cause pains in the stomach of the pregnant woman. And note, pregnant woman, that your use of gassy foods increases the gases in the stomach of your fetus, and upon leaving the belly, the fetus makes you pay for it by crying all night long from the pain caused by such gases. You can eat sugar and foods sweetened with sugar, since they are not by nature harmful.

---

120. Savonarola uses the category *agrumi* to mean foods with an acrid, pungent taste such as onions and garlic.

On spices that people often use. Among spices, you may use cinnamon. You cannot use pepper with the same confidence. And along with these you may use cloves.

I now maintain that this is enough for you on foods. And if you wonder which is better for a pregnant woman, food roasted over an open fire or boiled foods, I would say that boiled foods are better, because of a woman's constipation, especially from the fourth to the ninth month of pregnancy; but from the first to the fourth month, she may eat both roasted and boiled foods as she pleases. Similarly, she should eat moist foods such as broths rather than dry foods in order to keep her abdomen light and lubricated: as Avicenna says, "their foods should be white bread with *alesfidabegi* and *alzerbeiet*, that is, with fatty broths."[121] By now, *frontosa*, you have well understood the dangers of certain simple foodstuff: and I believe I have clearly explained to you the dangers of compound foods, such as spicy foods, cakes, gelatins, and pastries. So, therefore, we will not continue to write about these, but instead recall what Rhazes says supporting our points: he says that a pregnant woman should beware of all sharp and acrid foods such as capers, lupins, unripe olives, and everything that provokes menstruation,[122] especially at the beginning and at the end of the pregnancy. All of these have been mentioned earlier.

On wines and drinks. Let us now leave behind foods and move onto drinks, holding with Avicenna that the wine that the pregnant woman drinks should be subtle, aromatic, and aged—that is, not young wine.[123] And if you say "such wines are laxative," I respond, first, like Rhazes, in his *Liber ad Almansorem*, that such wines should be mixed with water,[124] so that through water the penetrative power of the wine may be reduced. And this is true of white wine, like malmsey,

---

121. In Latin in the text: *sint cibi earum panis mundus cum alesfidabegi et alzerbeiet, idest cum brodiis pinguibus.* See Avicenna, *Canon*, Lib. III, fen 21, tract. 2, c. 2 (p. 932). *Alesfidabegi* is an Arabic "unassimilated technical term" to refer to a lamb stew with coriander. See Corriente, *Dictionary of Arabic and Allied Loanwords*, 54. *Alzerbeit* (from *zerbagi*) likewise is an unassimilated dietary term, and refers to a "fat soup made with vinegar, dried fruit, saffron and cumin." See María Concepción Vázquez de Benito and María Teresa Herrera, *Los arabismos de los textos médicos latinos y castellanos de la Edad Media y de la Modernidad* (Madrid: Consejo superior de investigaciones cientificas, 1989), 280.

122. See Rhazes, *Liber ad Almansorem*, in *Opera parva Abubetri filii Zachariae filii Arasi [Rasis] que in hoc parvo volumine continentur* (Lyon: Impressa per Gilbertum de Villiers, impensis Johannis de Ferrariis, alias de Jolitis, ac Vincentii de Prothonariis, 1511), tract. 4, c. 27 (fol. 75r): *Pregnans ab omnibus cibis in quibus est acuitas et amaritudo abstinere debet: ut sunt cappares et lupini atque olive immature et his similia. Omnia etiam que urinam et menstrua provocant.* For similar advice in Avicenna, see note 118.

123. See Avicenna, *Canon*, Lib. III, fen 21, tract. 2, c. 2 (p. 932): *Et vinum earum sit odoriferum, et subtile, antiquum.*

124. See Rhazes, *Liber ad Almansorem*, tract. 4, c. 27 (fol. 75r): *de vino etiam boni odoris parum bibat, quod temperate sit aquarum.*

Ribolla, Tyre wine,[125] and strong white wines. But second, we may reason like Hippocrates, that a pregnant woman's wines should be red and subtle,[126] for these are not as dangerously laxative as white wines, and they should not be watery, such as *marello*, nor heavy like many Ferrarese wines, which are often dark and heavy. Whereas Avicenna, citing Hippocrates, says "Hippocrates said that she should take dark wine to drink, and it seems that he wished us to understand by this 'subtle dark,' whose darkness is due to its strength, not because of dregs";[127] therefore, the wines she drinks should be very good, inclining towards the red and *goreto*.[128] And you should stay away as much as possible from white wine, even though you may think that white wine suits you more in the morning. I will add, however that in the ninth month, in my opinion, the use of white wine is good for you and beneficial, especially near the end of the pregnancy, in that it facilitates in childbirth.

You may use the wine of pomegranates that are neither sweet nor sour, as well as sweet ones, as I have already mentioned. Also, cooked, reduced wine may be used as a pleasant seasoning for your food. You may use sour wine and vinegar in flavoring food or with meat, and better yet, with fish. And note, *frontosa*, that although vinegar may soothe the stomach, especially when it is warm, and it may stimulate the appetite, it also hurts the pregnant woman by cooling off the uterus; and its continued use could cause a woman to become pregnant with a female infant and to become dropsical. So take note of this, *frontosa*, you who have strong cravings for vinegar.

Beware of drinking cold water: it is not good for the fetus and causes the generation of females, especially here in our region: so instead, take to drinking wine.

On motion and rest. Having discussed food and drink, let us now move onto the other five so-called non-naturals, proceeding to discuss movement or

---

125. Malvasia (malmsey) wine grapes historically grew in the Mediterranean regions, especially Greece and Italy. Ribolla is, still today, a white Italian wine grape grown most prominently in the Friuli Venezia Giulia region of northeast Italy. Wine of Tyre, already known to Greek and Romans, originated in Tyre, modern Lebanon.

126. See for example Hippocrates, *Diseases of Women*, 1–2, ed. and trans. Paul Potter (Cambridge MA: Harvard University Press, 2018), ch. 1, at 267.

127. In Latin in the text: *Et Hipocras quidem dixit quod sumat in potu vinum nigrum, et videtur quod voluit intelligi per illud subtile nigrum, et sit nigredo eius propter ipsius fortitudinem, non propter fecem.* See Avicenna, *Canon*, Lib. III, fen 21, tract. 2, c. 2 (p. 932).

128. The same, otherwise unknown, word *goreto* (the word does not appear in the TLIO) is used by Antonio Cermisone, one of Savonarola's masters, in his *Consilia medicinalia* (Frankfurt: ex Collegium Musarum Paltheniano, 1604), 56 and 72, to refer to a wine *mediocris vinositatis et saporis*, that is to say a light wine. In Treatise Three, chapter 2, at 185, Savonarola refers to the same wine as *gorreto* or *gauro*. Mount Gauro (nowadays Mount Barbaro, near Naples) was known for its vineyards since Roman times.

exercise, as well as rest or inactivity, that the pregnant woman should engage in so that she will not make mistakes and she will not miscarry. I say, therefore, along with our authorities, that pregnant women should have moderate and not excessive exercise, because too much exercise causes miscarriage, just as "sailing on the sea upsets the body,"[129] as Hippocrates says. Furthermore, a pregnant woman should walk at a moderate pace, that is, slowly, because moving with great exertion can cause miscarriage.

And the reason for this advice is, as we have said, that the fetus is connected to the uterus just as a blossom or fruit is connected to a tree; and excessive movement caused either by wind or other movements may cause the blossoms and fruits to be detached from the branches and fall from the tree. In the same way, if the fetus is agitated because of excessive movement, it separates from the branches of the veins of the uterus to which it was attached. For as it is enveloped in a membrane that hangs down heavily, being weighed down by retained blood, any agitation detaches and breaks the cotyledons, that is *peculli* or ligaments, by which it is attached to the uterus, and it descends like a weight towards the neck of the cervix, where nature, irritated, tries to abort it. And you, *frontosa*, take good notice that it is more dangerous to exercise excessively in the first and last few months of pregnancy: because in the first months, like a blossom, the fetus is delicately attached; and in the last, the fruit is ripe and ready to fall, so that even the smallest jolt will dislodge it. Wherefore Avicenna states: "it is necessary that they occupy themselves in mild exercises and light walking without any excess. For excesses cause miscarriage, and this is because they are loaded down as a result of the retention of the menses."[130] And since "deficiency and excess in amount lead to the same differences,"[131] we believe that excessive rest can also cause miscarriage, especially in women who are very humid by nature. This is because too little exercise increases the superfluous humors, which weakens the ligaments, and the slightest movement can cause miscarriage. Perhaps this is the reason that Madonna de Monferrato could not retain her fetus; although she was often gravid, she would miscarry in five or six months, because she had retained an excess of blood. And this was the case until a physician—considering her sanguine complexion and her retention of so much blood, which hurts the fetus because its great quantity causes it to weigh on the ligaments, already weakened and

129. In Latin in the text: *manifestat autem navigatio quoniam corpora perturbat.* See Hippocrates, *Aphorisms*, IV.14 (p. 137). Hippocrates refers to the seasickness experienced by those traveling on rough seas.

130. In Latin in the text: *Oportet ut occupentur exercitiis temperatis et deambulatione tenui absque superflua. Superflua enim abortare facit: et illud ideo, quoniam ipse replentur propter illud quod accidit eis de retentione menstruorum.* See Avicenna, *Canon*, Lib. III, fen 21, tract. 2, c. 2 (p. 932). On menstrual blood retention, see Treatise One, Chapter Four, 95.

131. In Latin in the text: *defectus et superhabundantia ad easdem ducunt differentias.* See Galen, *The Art of Medicine*, Book III, ch. 26 (p. 261); =Kühn, 1:376.

moistened by her humidity, and by her great inactivity—prescribed bloodletting every month until the sixth, little by little reducing the bloodletting; and thus she retained her fetus and she was able to bring her pregnancy to fruition.[132]

Therefore, the pregnant woman should exercise in moderation, so as to rid herself and the fetus of her superfluities. And because baths may be a form of exercise, we will speak of them. First, many recommend that pregnant women visit alum-rich drying baths to rid themselves of their superfluities. But I certainly do not rush to praise these alum baths, as many do, because it is a dangerous thing, and only an experienced physician should prescribe thermal waters.[133] But instead, as we will later see in discussing ways to facilitate labor, I suggest it would be more prudent that a pregnant woman, as she enters her ninth month, especially if she is young and this is her first pregnancy, should soak once a week in a warm tub filled with ordinary water. She should stay covered in the bath for a quarter of an hour or so, and then get out before the water becomes cold.

But Rhazes also says "when the hour of birth draws near, the parturient ought to be put in a bath, and let her sit each day in a sitzbath, anointing her belly and ribs with an unguent."[134] This is because such a bath dilates and lubricates the passages and facilitates the delivery of the fetus with less pain for the parturient. This is why Avicenna says "a bath is terrible for them, unless they are approaching birth,"[135] and in fen 21 of book III, Avicenna says "when the pregnant woman approaches birth, then it is necessary that she bathe regularly and employ the

---

132. The same anecdote is reported by Savonarola in the *Practica maior*, tract. VI, c. 21, rubr. 30 (fol. 270va), under the heading *De conservatione embrionis et cautela aborsus* (On embryo preservation and abortion prevention): *Et credo quod Domina Marchionissa de Monte ferrato ob hanc causam abortiebatur. Et quidam medicus cognoscens causam phlebotomavit et foetus ad lucem venit, ante autem semper faciebat mortuos, et sic filiis carebat* (And I believe the Marchioness of Monferrato used to miscarry for this reason. And a certain physician, knowing this reason, drew out her blood and she gave birth to a child, whereas before she always used to miscarry and had no children).

133. In his Latin editorial success *De balneis* (see *Works by Michele Savonarola*, #10), Savonarola strongly argues for the therapeutic role of hot spring waters. In the part dedicated to alum-rich waters, which have strong astringent and haemostatic properties, Savonarola correctly indicates their usefulness for those who have skin conditions, gum problems, wounds and genital ulcers. Since it "prohibits the flow of blood and superfluities, and their effusion," Savonarola also writes that, when drunk or used as a subfumigation, alum blocks the abundant menstrual flow and prevents impregnation. He writes nothing about the usefulness of these waters for pregnant women in the *De balneis*, but—by comparing the two works—one can easily understand the caution with which in the *MM* Savonarola advises against the use of such a powerful coagulant water for pregnant women. See Savonarola, *De balneis*, in *De balneis omnia quae extant*, fol. 12ra.

134. In Latin in the text: *cum hora partus apropinquat, parturiens in balneo mitti debet, et in tina singulis diebus sedere, ventrem et costas cum unguento ungere.* See Rhazes, *Liber ad Almansorem*, tract. 4, c. 28 (fol. 75v).

135. In Latin in the text: *balneum namque eis execrabile est, nisi apud propinquitatem.* See Avicenna, *Canon*, Lib. III, fen 21, tract. 2, c. 2 (p. 932).

sitzbath."[136] We will speak of this later in the chapter on facilitating parturition. Note that Rhazes also says "they should take care not to dally too long in the bath or the sun."[137]

On sleep and waking. On sleep and waking, we say that it is better for a pregnant woman to get plenty of sleep rather than not enough, because the fetus is better nourished when she sleeps. But both sleeping and waking should occur in moderation.

On evacuation and repletion. On repletion we say that she should beware of it because it hurts the fetus badly, constricting it from so much food, especially when it is gassy, which makes it even more harmful. For when it feels constricted, the fetus moves around excessively, and this type of motion can cause it to become detached from the uterus. Similarly, the fetus moves when it feels hunger, which also weakens it. This is why, *frontosa*, you who so devoutly bend down each day to sweep the church floor, beware of fasting too often when pregnant, and especially from the end of the third to the ninth month, because the more the fetus grows, the more it wants to eat; and let the friars say what they will, they who often preach without any discernment. Overeating is also dangerous in the first months, that is the second and third, because of the weakness of the ligaments, since the fetus is not strongly bound to them, which is why Avicenna says "and it is necessary to avoid overeating."[138] Also, repletion is harmful because it causes obstruction of the veins and the passage of the blood needed to nourish the fetus; and it may stimulate desire for coitus, whereas fasting limits it.

I also want to advise you on this: that you must especially beware of intercourse in the first and second months of pregnancy, because the fetus is weakly attached, and during coitus, the uterus moves. And you, *frontoso*, note that knocking on the door may cause the fetus to move inordinately. It is safer and more praiseworthy if you leave *frontosa* to lie undisturbed in the bed; and if you must have her, act with care, with smooth and few movements, so that when the *bricola* enters, no inordinate movement causes the lord of the manor to exit from his castle.[139] Similarly, in the ninth month, when the ligaments are mature and weak,

---

136. In Latin in the text: *cum pregnans apropinquat partui, tunc necessarium est ut assiduet balneationem et tinam.* See Avicenna, Lib. III, fen 21, tract. 2, c. 23 (p. 941).

137. In Latin in the text: *caveant sibi ne in balneo vel in sole longam faciant moram.* See Rhazes, *Liber ad Almansorem*, tract. 4, c. 27 (fol. 75v).

138. In Latin in the text: *et oportet ut devitet repletionem cibi.* See Avicenna, *Canon*, Lib. III, fen 21, tract. 2, c. 2 (p. 932).

139. The *bricola* (plural *bricole*) is the Venetian name given to those large wooden poles that (still today) can be seen in the lagoon of Venice . Positioned in the water in groups of three, they indicate the deepest canals, i.e. those navigable even at low tide. Savonarola uses the term *bricola* as a metaphor for the penis, which enters the manor (pregnant belly), and disturbs and endangers the lord of the manor (the fetus) with inordinate movement. Another metaphor, this time "oenological," immediately follows.

take care not to make the wine flow from the barrel before its time, causing great danger and potential harm. This is why Avicenna says, "and it is especially necessary to avoid intercourse."[140] Not eating excessively limits the need for evacuation by medicine, by mouth, by clyster [enema], or by bloodletting; and if any of these is necessary, it must be performed with great caution. First, laxative medicines are strong and at the same time dangerous, and even more in the first, second, third, seventh, eighth, and ninth month. This is why Hippocrates states: "it is suitable that pregnant women be purged between the fourth month and the seventh, but in the earlier months and the later ones it ought to be feared."[141] And the same is true of harsh enemas. Therefore, a pregnant woman's laxative medicines should be common and soothing substances, like cassia, manna, decoction of tamarind and of prunes, the fruit water described by Mesue,[142] and similar things. Avicenna says: "and it is necessary to employ soothing medicines of such a nature that their effects are always mild, such as fatty *alesfidabegi*, that is, fatty broths, and such as *siracost*, that is manna, and similar things."[143] Some doctors prescribe rhubarb, especially in the fourth, fifth, and sixth month, and others especially recommend that pregnant women take only aloe, which is certainly not without risks, especially because aloe might cause bleeding, even though Avicenna may say of this: "however, the virtue of pure aloe does not penetrate to those parts of the body which are far distant, least of all does it reach the liver."[144] But I recommend that the physician use aloe only sparingly, and only physicians experienced in its use should prescribe this medication.

---

140. In Latin in the text: *et oportet ut evitet coitum et proprie.* See Avicenna, *Canon*, Lib. III, fen 21, tract. 2, c. 2 (p. 932).

141. In Latin in the text: *pregnantes si purgare convenit a quarto usque ad septimum: iuniora autem et seniora vereri oportet.* See Hippocrates, *Aphorisms*, IV.1 (p. 135).

142. Johannes Mesuae Damascenus [pseud], *De re medica libri tres*, Iacobo Sylvio interprete [Jacques Dubois] (Lyon: apud Ioan Tornaesium & Gulielmum Gazeium, 1548), Lib. III.2 (p. 176), lists one *Syrupus acidus de succis fructuum* and one *Syrupus acidus de succis et aquis fructuum*. Both contain mainly pomegranate juice. This set of pharmacological books were most likely produced in thirteenth-century Bologna, compiled from unknown Arabic originals, by someone who adopted the name Mesuae to lend them authority. On the uncertain identification of the author and the mysterious origin of this important trilogy of works, whose composition in Arabic is "by no means certain," see Paula De Vos, "The 'Prince of Medicine': Yūḥannā ibn Māsawayh and the Foundations of the Western Pharmaceutical Tradition," *Isis* 104, no. 4 (December 2013): 682–85.

143. In Latin in the the text: *et oportet ut assiduent lenificationem suarum naturarum semper cum eis que leniunt cum equalitate, sicut sunt alesfidabegi pinguia, idest iura pinguia, et sicut siracost, idest mana, et similia.* See Avicenna, *Canon*, Lib. III, fen 21, tract. 2, c. 2 (p. 932). Synonyms for Arabic terms, preceded by "that is" (*idest* in the original), are not to be found in the *Canon* but are Savonarola's own additions.

144. In Latin in the text: *cum tamen virtus eius quod purum est, non penetret ad illa, que in corpore sunt longinqua, imo non pertranseat epar.* See Avicenna, *Canon*, Lib. II, tract. 2, c. 66 (p. 274).

I also say that soothing fatty clysters are not free of risks. Of bloodletting, I say that it can be done more safely in the first three months, but when the fetus is bigger, it is much more risky. This is because the pregnant woman is a fragile vessel; therefore, physician, do not perform this procedure too often, as Avicenna says: "and to the degree that the child is larger, to that same degree is phlebotomy more harmful to it."[145] And note, *frontosa*, when you are pregnant, do not allow the feces in your body to harden too much; because the retention of hardened feces will cause you much pain and much danger to your fetus, and you will risk abortion. *Frontosa*, I advise you to be aware that when large amounts of milk flow from your breasts, you risk miscarriage, and similarly when you have diarrhea, you risk abortion. These are the teachings of Hippocrates, that wise old sage.[146]

It is best if the pregnant woman stay clear from anger, deep sadness, fear, and similar emotions, especially in the first month, because the fetus can be debilitated through her weakened spirits caused by fear, anguish, or sadness, or a dangerous inflammation may be caused by her anger.

She should beware of air that is excessively hot or cold, because both hot and cold air, by extinction or intensification of the natural heat, debilitates the fetus and could possibly kill it. Thus great heat and great cold may have the same effect, even though they are opposites. But note, *frontosa*, you must avoid cold air, especially so as not to catch a cold that could bring on a cough: this could cause you to miscarry on account of all the inordinate shaking. Therefore, when you wash your hair, make sure to keep covered more than you are accustomed to do. Be very careful, because if the catarrh settles in the chest it brings on a cough, which if it persists, often causes miscarriage. Be especially careful not to let your feet get chilled and not to drink cold water, especially on an empty stomach.

This is why Avicenna says that in very cold regions, there is a greater number of abortions—that is, women often miscarry, because so much cold enters the uterus, extinguishing the natural heat of the fetus, as we see natural heat extinguished in those who travel through snow-topped mountains. However, we similarly see a great number of abortions, that is, miscarriages, in hot and humid southern regions, where the ligaments become moist, and so are weakened. In northern regions, in contrast, as in Germany, where it is not excessively hot, such miscarriages are not common, for the heat is retained inside the body and strengthened, but not extinguished. Which is as Avicenna says: "and in regions which are very cold, miscarriage is very common, and likewise in southern

---

145. In Latin in the text: *et quanto filius est maior, est nocumentum cum flebotomia in ipso plus.* See Avicenna, *Canon,* Lib. III, fen 21, tract. 2, c. 8 (p. 933).

146. See, for example, Hippocrates, *Aphorisms,* V.52, on milk flow in a woman with child (which indicates that the unborn child is sick), and V.34, on diarrhea during pregnancy as a sign of abortion risk (pp. 170–71 and 167 respectively).

climates; and this occurs less in more northern climates unless they are too cold, which is extremely harmful to the embryo."[147]

O *frontosa*, you who are pregnant in the winter and expect to give birth in the spring, note well what I tell you: if the winter is warm and humid, that is, not too cold, and the spring air is boreal, that is, cold, then you are at a greater risk for miscarriage. Therefore beware of dangerous activities such as excessive movement, lifting heavy weights, eating things that are gassy or very cold, overeating, and similar things that may induce abortion. And this advice is emphasized by Hippocrates, in the third section of the *Aphorisms*: "But if the winter prove southerly, etc."[148] And similarly, Avicenna says, "and when a warm southern winter comes, and a cold boreal spring follows it, then pregnant women who are due to give birth in the spring will miscarry from any sort of precipitating cause."[149]

We will leave the other reasons for miscarriage to the practicing physicians, having dealt with those that are of concern to us, and will close by saying that you should beware of the heat of the sun. O impoverished pregnant *frontosa*, who, in the country, must bear the sun and the summer heat, I have great compassion for you. I remind you of these things for your benefit, so that you may take care of yourself as best you can, because it is certainly a great sin to miscarry by your own negligence, and if this occurs, you may certainly expect punishment and retribution.

Chapter Two
On the conditions or states common to pregnant women

We will discuss common conditions and not the extraordinary ones whose care is left to the practicing physicians, because our intention is to only write of the regimen for pregnant women, and of the common conditions of their pregnancy, which indeed may be considered a natural infirmity. And so, in writing about those, we will say that the conditions or states that we wish to discuss are the following: first, the loss of appetite; second, gassiness, nausea, and vomit; third,

147. In Latin in the text: *et in regionibus quidem valde frigidis valde multiplicatur aborsus, et similiter in aeribus meridionalibus: et minoratur in septemtrionalibus, nisi sint frigidi, vehementer ledentes embrionem.* See Avicenna, *Canon*, Lib. III, fen 21, tract. 2, c. 8 (p. 934).

148. In Latin in the text: *si autem hiems austrina fuerit etc.* See Hippocrates, *Aphorisms*, III.12 (p. 125). The whole *Aphorism* would read in English: "But if the winter prove southerly, rainy and calm, and the spring dry and northerly, women whose confinement is due in the spring suffer abortion on the slightest provocation, or, if they do bear children, have weak and unhealthy offspring, so that they either die at once or live with puny and unhealthy bodies. Among the rest prevail dysentery and dry diseases of the eyes, and, in the case of the old, catarrhs that quickly prove fatal."

149. In Latin in the text: *et quando preterit hiems austrina calida, et sequitur illam ver boreale frigidum, abortiunt pregnantes, que pariture sunt vere, ex qualibet causa.* See Avicenna, *Canon*, Lib. III, fen 21, tract. 2, c. 8 (p. 934).

heart palpitations; fourth, menstrual discharge; fifth, miscarriage; sixth, constipation of the belly; seventh, suffocation; eighth, pain during labor; ninth, difficulty in labor; tenth, the birth of an improperly positioned fetus; eleventh, retention of the *secundines*; twelfth, excessive loss of blood after labor; thirteenth, retention of blood; fourteenth, fevers; fifteenth, dislocation of the sacrum.

First condition: cure for the loss of appetite of the pregnant woman. Most pregnant women, especially in the first few months, tend to have an unbalanced stomach. And this is why Avicenna, noting this, says, "a great diligence in the cure of their stomach is necessary, so let them be strengthened with things like geleniabin."[150] What Avicenna means is that a pregnant woman needs to have a healthy stomach and digest well, so that she may produce good chyle, from which good blood will then be made in the liver, which provides nourishment for the baby as well as herself. Therefore, *frontosa*, if you desire your child to be healthy and robust, take care to curb your appetite for the wrong foods, and make certain that you eat things that are apt for making good blood, as we have said. Also, use both internally and externally those things that soothe your stomach, such as things that benefit digestion, things that are fragrant, and not too hot or astringent.

For example, for rich women and those who can afford the expense: *Recipe* pearls not perforated, pellitory, one and one-half drachms of each; ginger, mastic, four drachms of each; zedoary, doronicum, wild celery, cassia, cardamom, nutmeg, mace, cinnamon, two drachms of each; red behen, pepper, and long pepper, three drachms of each; cinnamon, one drachm; very white sugar, an amount equal to all the other ingredients combined; and one spoonful of this should be taken by mouth every morning. This medication corrects the disposition of the uterus, from which originates the cause of this ailment, and settles the stomach. Whereas for impoverished women, we recommend the use of mastic, chewed in the mornings when they get up, as this is very beneficial to them. Or poor women may also chew cinnamon, that is *canella*;[151] they may chew two or three cloves one hour before meals in the morning and evening. Additionally, poor women should keep nutmeg in their mouths. The electuary *aromatico garifolato* described by Mesue[152] can also be useful, and the chewing of mint with some seeds of sweet, or neither sweet nor sour pomegranate can be beneficial as well.

---

150. In Latin in the text: *oportet ut vehemens studium sit in stomacis earum, quare confortentur cum eis, que sunt sicut geleniabin.* See Avicenna, *Canon*, Lib. III, fen 21, tract. 2, c. 2 (p. 932). The Arabic word *gele/iniabin, gelengibin* or *gelincabin* is an unassimilated pharmaceutical term. It means "confection of roses and honey." See Vázquez de Benito and Herrera, *Los arabismos*, 227, and Corriente, *Dictionary of Arabic and Allied Loanwords*, 316.

151. *Cannella* is Italian for cinnamon.

152. Mesuae, *De re medica*, Lib. III.5 (p. 235): *electuarium aromaticum caryophyllatum.* An "electuary" is a medication mixed with honey or other sweet substance. The base ingredients for this traditional

Externally, a woman should apply onto her stomach in the morning and evening, one half hour before meals, oil of mastic or wormwood, with clove powder, or she may apply the following stomach ointment: *Recipe* mint oil, absinthium oil, rose oil, one-half ounce of each; cloves, one-half drachm; myrtle berries, one drachm; cinnamon, one-half drachm; vinegar, two drachms; toasted breadcrumbs, and wax; and this should be applied as an ointment. Or take mint or wormwood and warm it up over a stone sprayed with dark wine and put it on the stomach; and when it begins to cool off, reheat it, and do this three times and afterwards reapply this ointment onto the stomach. Moreover, make a sachet with dried wormwood and place it on the stomach. Likewise, a woman can make a plaster out of the things mentioned, that is, mastic, clove, and nutmeg, and liquefy the mastic, and in this dilution add the ground clove, nutmeg and bog myrtle. After it is cooled off, this mixture should stay on her stomach like a poultice; and if preferred, a bit of resin may be added; and the use of sweet spices is also beneficial in this case.

Now if you ask the reason for such an imbalance, I respond to you with Avicenna, in the thirteenth fen of book III, on corruption of the appetite: "and sometimes corrupted appetite happens to pregnant women because of retention of the menses."[153] He says "sometimes," because numerous pregnant women do not feel an imbalance in appetite, desiring to eat one thing more than the other. Therefore, in these cases, as I have observed, the appetite does not diminish; neither is it corrupted, craving foods that are not customary, as many tend to do— not only strange things, but also more of one thing than the other. And it makes sense to speculate here why this disorder happens to some women more than others. As said, Avicenna maintains—and this has been established by other authorities as well—that such an imbalance comes from the retention of the menses, from which vapors and corrupt fumes rise, which offend the stomach, causing an imbalance in the appetite and in the digestion, such as is also experienced when feces are retained for too long; for these retentions cause harmful and bad humors to multiply in the stomach, which result in such cravings.

Now perhaps you will say, "why is it that this does not happen to those who are not gravid, but who retain their menses?" I respond to you that menstrual blood in pregnant women, from which such vapors rise, is much worse than the menstrual blood of non-pregnant women, because, as has been said, the blood of the pregnant woman is divided into four parts: one goes to the formation of the body parts; another nourishes the fetus; another converts itself into milk; and the

---

medication were cloves, nutmeg, zedoary, sandalwood, cinnamon wood, aloe wood, lavender, pepper, and cardamom.

153. In Latin in the text: *et quandoque accidit pregnantibus propter retentionem menstruorum apetitus corruptus.* See Avicenna, *Canon,* Lib. III, fen 13, tract. 2, c. 10 (p. 718).

fourth is foul and corrupt and remains so until the birth.[154] And this fourth part is by far the worst blood, the good blood being utilized by the pregnancy, which is not the case in women who are not pregnant; and as a result, its vapors ascend to the stomach and throw it off balance. But I will add that some women who are not pregnant find themselves with such cravings from the retention of their menses, but this is rare.

Next, to satisfy *frontosa*, I say that such vapors, which tend to be melancholic, originating in the blood made melancholic by its retention, as Galen explains, bring on unusual appetites for diverse foods.[155] This happens in the same way that melancholic vapors act on the imagination, bringing about many types of melancholic states. At times they may even cause a man to imagine that he is a goose—as happened in my time to Maestro Giovanni,[156] a surgeon of Verona, afterwards referred to as Maestro Giovanni Ocha [Goose]; or sometimes they may lead a man to believe he is a dog, and he will even bark and do similar things. Wherefore Avicenna notes: "and the kinds of melancholy are innumerable."[157] It is also impossible to define the causes of these different melancholic effects, for such effects come from the properties of these different types of melancholy.

And as Avicenna says, these effects of the corrupted appetite commonly appear in the first two months,[158] because in this period nature warms up the sperm, making it foam as previously discussed in the chapter on impregnation, and similarly, it shakes and warms up the menstrual blood so that it may form the parts of the fetus. Warmed up and shaken in this way, the blood spumifies more than in other months. In some women, these effects last longer, for up to five or

154. In Treatise One, Savonarola deals with the fivefold division of menstrual blood, as given in note 5 (62). Although he does not here mention the first type of blood ("the first and most pure, which tends to be white, generates together with spermatic material bones and nerves"), otherwise the classification is the same. For "spermatic" and "bloody parts" of the fetus, also see note 15 at page 65.

155. See, for instance, Galen, *On Diseases and Symptoms* (*On the Causes of Symptoms III*), ed. and trans. Ian Johnston (Cambridge: Cambridge University Press, 2006), ch. 11 (pp. 298–99); =Kühn, 7:264.

156. Since there are no records indicating that the famous Veronese physician and surgeon Giovanni Arcolano (1390/93–1458) ever suffered from mental instability, a search was made for this enigmatic character in the notarial archives of Verona. With regard to the fifteenth century, three surgeons named Giovanni appear, but none can be positively identified with Giovanni "da Oca/Ocha/ab Auca/Aucha": (1) Giovanni Bartolomei di Isolo superiore, active from 1414 to 1429; (2) Giovanni Becucii di S. Giorgio (da Sacco), active in 1418–1419, and again in San Zilio during 1422; (3) Giovanni Laurentii di Braida, active in 1440. Thanks to Dr. Claudio Bismara for his valuable help with archival sources.

157. In Latin in the text: *et indefinite sunt speties melenconie.* See Avicenna, *Canon*, Lib. III, fen 1, tract. 4, c. 19 (p. 489).

158. In Latin in the text: *deinde commoventur appetitus mali post mensem, aut duos menses.* See Avicenna, *Canon*, Lib. III, fen 21, tract. 1, c. 11 (p. 928). See also Lib. III, fen 13, tract. 2, c. 10 (p. 718): *et quandoque accidit pregnantibus propter retentionem menstruorum apetitus corruptus . . . et illud est usque prope duos menses aut tres.*

six months, while in others they continue until they are in labor; and this happens because the menstrual blood is more corrupted, or because of its greater quantity.

And in the same way that these vapors, and the humors they generate, cause unusual appetites, they may also cause the decrease or loss of appetite, and cause the pregnant woman to feel nauseous and vomit. Certainly from such weakness and discomfort of the stomach, the majority of pregnant women vomit and emit phlegm that is very bitter, with which they also emit some choler. Other women do not experience an imbalance of appetite, due to the good qualities of their blood; and often these women have better appetites than they did before pregnancy. This is because their organs are sucking blood through the veins for their nourishment as well as for those of the fetus, and in so doing, they deplete the liver, which in turn sucks blood from the stomach, resulting in an enhanced appetite.

As for the care of the pregnant woman and the fetus, we will first say that when the pregnant woman suffers loss of appetite so that she cannot eat, or eats without appetite, then she should avoid fatty broths and things that are too sweet, because such things fill up the stomach, relax it, and induce nausea. Instead, she should eat lighter foods that are easily digested, and foods more often roasted than boiled. She should begin her meal with things that stimulate the appetite like onions roasted under ashes, or raw onions with vinegar, but with moderation; for as Avicenna says, regarding onions, "it strengthens the weakened stomach and enhances appetite."[159] Likewise, she may eat garlic; vinegary foods; salted olives (in moderation); raw or cooked quinces; verjuice;[160] pomegranates, either those that are sweet or those neither sweet nor sour (but not vinegary); pickled radishes; salted and lightly salted meats; and similar things. At the beginning of meals, she should drink a bit of good fragrant wine, Trebbiano or malmsey, Tyre wine, Vernaccia, Ribolla, Romania, muscatel, and vino de la quaglia or just a good local wine.

Also, to reduce the bad humors present in her stomach, a pregnant woman should take the following drink: Recipe one-half mina of bran, well cleansed from its flour; put it on a cloth, then tie it, and let it soak in a pound of water for four hours; then press the water out, sweeten it with rose honey, then add a small quantity of vinegar, so that it acidulates a little, and then put it over a fire and with low heat bring it to a boil and then filter it. Take this drink for eight days in a row, warm, as needed, especially at the hour when you take the syrups.

Afterwards, the pregnant woman may evacuate with cassia, manna, or turpentine with which cinnamon is mixed. For example, for impoverished women and also for rich ones: Recipe turpentine, one ounce; cinnamon, one drachm;

---

159. In Latin in the text: confortat stomachum debilem et facit apetitum. See Avicenna, Canon, Lib. II, tract. 2, c. 122 (p. 287).

160. Verjuice, agresto in Italian, is a condiment made from the juice of sour and unripe grapes.

mix; take this with the *nevole*[161] in the morning three hours before eating. And regarding cassia, a woman may use it once a week, or in a month five or six times; and if she is constipated, she may take up to ten drachms, or up to one and one-half ounces without danger. Regarding manna and cassia, she may take from one ounce or more, depending on the constipation of her belly, the strength of her body, her age and habits, and as prescribed by her physician.

But perhaps you will wonder, *frontosa*, if "Avicenna maintains that in such cases pregnant women should use water, and says 'and drinking water is beneficial in moderation,'[162] how can this be, considering that water debilitates the digestive power of the stomach and produces raw phlegm, which also debilitates the appetite?" I respond that Avicenna's statement is especially valid when the stomach of the pregnant woman is warm, and the heat induces the fermentation of the humors that are inside it, converting them into phlegm, just as wine is converted to vinegar by fermentation. In this case, water is used to extinguish this heat; but even here, the use of water, as Avicenna states, should be in moderation.

And returning to the soothing of her stomach, we say that, besides the ointment described, the pregnant woman may also use a poultice of quinces and dates, with sweet flag and lavender, made with fragrant wine, taking equal parts of one as of the other.

And it is noteworthy that Avicenna recommends polypody in his discussion of the evacuation of humors of the pregnant woman, especially in those who crave coal, mud, ashes, or things like earth, stating: "and dried polypody is good for those craving to eat clay,"[163] and the reason is that it evacuates melancholic humors, from which the corruption of appetite originates. This polypody is a laxative grouped by Mesue among the powerful medicines called strong soluble laxatives.[164] However, considering the great risks for miscarriage, especially in the first months of pregnancy, it seems to me that it is better for the pregnant woman not to take polypody, but rather to give her dodder, a medicinal plant amongst the

161. In the Italian edition of this work, Belloni—following the Vatican manuscript—writes *novelle*, but he notes that the Venice manuscript has *nevole* instead. The third manuscript (Reggio Emilia, Biblioteca Panizzi, Codice Turri C 12), unknown to Belloni, also has *nevole*. Given that there is no antecedent for the plural adjective *novelle* (new) within the sentence, the second reading, the one discarded by Belloni, is preferred. Used in this specific context, a *nevola*, from Latin *nebula*, i.e. cloud, is an edible capsule or thin wafer (a combination of flour and water) shaped like a lens, containing a dose of medicine or powder, the equivalent of the French *cachet*. There is no mention of the word *nevola* in TLIO, but see its description in Costanzo Felici's sixteenth-century *Scritti naturalistici*, ed. Guido Arbizzoni (Urbino: Quattroventi, 1986), 116.

162. In Latin in the text: *et iuvatur in moderamine potus aque*. See Avicenna, *Canon*, Lib. III, fen 21, tract. 2, c. 4 (p. 932).

163. In Latin in the text: *et polipodium quidem exsicatum competit apetentibus lutum*. See Avicenna, *Canon*, Lib. III, fen 21, tract. 2, c. 4 (pp. 932–33).

164. See Mesuae, *De re medica*, Lib. II.2 (p. 88).

most highly recommended by Mesue[165]—that physician who was greatly reputed among physicians for his authority on these laxatives—and I recommend this especially since our human nature is so weakened now, as we will discuss. And also Avicenna himself agrees with me on this, when at the end of the chapter on polypody he says, "and in its place, dodder can be used."[166] And dodder should be used, therefore, as it has fewer risks than polypody.

Again, to evacuate melancholic humors, dodder is better, because, as Mesue says, dodder has greater properties than all laxatives for combating melancholic humors.[167] But because it is purgative and strong if there is a risk of miscarriage, it is good to mix dodder with some myrobalans [an East Indian fruit] and bring these to a boil in the water of a decoction of raisins or in whey, adding some salt. As the preparation of this medication is very risky for those who are not experienced in this art, it is not for the layman. This is why I feel that what has already been said about laxatives will suffice, and it is enough for the layman to use turpentine, cassia, and manna, and leave the decoction of myrabolans for the more experienced. After such laxatives, one should give the pregnant woman vinegary things and things with verjuice that soothe the stomach and also those that cleanse, such as honey water, water with sugar, and similar things, as we mentioned when dealing with rose honey. Avicenna recommends sharp-tasting foods such as mustard,[168] especially if flavored with honey, to restore the pregnant woman's appetite. Also beneficial is the use of salted capers with vinegar.

The last thing we will mention is that when the appetite of the pregnant woman turns to cheeses, it is preferable that she be given fresh cheese, since it is better for her, as mentioned earlier. And it should be somewhat heated, so that it better soothes her appetite with its moistness and very little dryness. Even though it is true that dry cheese has fewer superfluities, moist cheese better soothes her appetite.

Second condition: care for gassiness, nausea, and vomiting of the pregnant woman. Pregnant women, because of the increased presence of raw humors in their stomachs, tend to have gassiness, by which their stomachs feel pain or distress when they eat; and when the stomach feels these pains, it seeks to drive away the humors; and if it achieves its task, this evacuation is called vomit. Pregnant women commonly have the tendency to vomit; I say commonly, because some are not so afflicted.

---

165. See Mesuae, *De re medica*, Lib. II.1 (p. 72).

166. In Latin in the text: *et loco eius ponitur epithimum.* Avicenna, *Canon*, Lib. II, tract. 2, c. 542 (p. 373).

167. See Mesuae, *De re medica*, Lib. II.1 (pp. 72–73).

168. See, for instance, Avicenna, *Canon*, Lib. III, fen 21, tract. 2, c. 4 (p. 933): *et quandoque iuvantur ex acutis, sicut sinapi et similia* (and sometimes sharp-tasting foods, such as mustard and similar substances, are helpful).

Those afflicted by these symptoms have very different reactions depending on the variety and quantity of humors accumulated in their stomachs: some vomit often in the first two months of their pregnancy, while others continue to vomit until the sixth month, and many until their labor. To offer an example, my daughter-in-law in numerous pregnancies has been variously afflicted. In some pregnancies, she was vomiting until her second month, at times until her third month, at times until her last month, and in her last birth, even though she was carrying a boy, she was vomiting even on the day of her labor.

The cause of such vomiting is the presence in the stomach of phlegmatic humors brought about in by digestion, as has been said, and these humors cause gas and nausea.

On gassiness. To assist the pregnant woman with gassiness, we will list a series of helpful domestic remedies. First, when the pregnant woman feels discomfort from gassiness of the stomach, she should take cumin, first infused for eight hours in vinegar, and then roasted and crushed. She should take this powder with an equal amount of pulverized incense, so that all together it equals a drachm—that is, one eighth of an ounce—and in the morning, she should drink it with some warmed dark wine or with chicken or capon broth with a little red sugar over it. For impoverished ladies, I prescribe dry oregano powder.

Another beneficial remedy is the decoction of cumin made with water and drunk warm with red sugar. Rich women may take the electuary *aromatico rosato*, as described by Mesue,[169] in addition to the cumin confection made with the ingredients specified in the previous section. This may be taken internally and externally. However, if the gassiness increases, I recommend that they consult a physician, because they can become very ill. Be careful, *frontosa*, not to trigger these conditions yourself through your bad eating or drinking. Because it is the case that you women are quick to satisfy your appetites, following your whims and not regulating your desire with reason: this is why it is said that you always walk backwards.

On nausea. Having spoken about gassiness, we will now speak of nausea, which means an urge to vomit, even when vomiting does not follow. Nausea causes the retention of humors in the stomach, stressing the cardia, [the point where the esophagus enters the stomach]. Therefore, nausea, triggered by the presence of such humors, may be relieved if these humors are somehow removed or altered. For this reason, remedies prescribed for vomit will also offer relief from nausea. So we will proceed to discuss vomit and not speak more of nausea, mentioning only what Avicenna says regarding nausea: that Armenian bole is effective

---

169. See Mesuae, *De re medica*, Lib. III.5 (p. 234): *Electuarium aromaticum rosatum.* The base ingredients for this traditional electuary were red rose petals, liquorice root, aloe wood and sandalwood, cinnamon, nutmeg, cloves and cardamom.

in quenching the nausea of a pregnant woman.[170] This is especially true when putrid humors accumulate in her stomach, as this remedy works to rid the stomach of these humors, which is why it is also recommended against pestilence:[171] it actually possesses the qualities opposite those of putrefaction, that is frigidity and dryness, and it is placed among the cordial medicines. If you ask how it should be used, I respond to you that it should be taken with warmed water sweetened with honey; for example: warm honey water, 5 ounces; Armenian bole, 1–1 ½ drachms.

On vomit. Following with vomit, we will first recall what Hippocrates says for the preservation of a healthy body: he recommends provoking vomiting twice in one month, and it should be done two days in a row.[172] Avicenna writes:

> Hippocrates instructs that vomiting be provoked for two continuous days in any given month, so that on the second day is corrected what on the first day had been difficult to correct, and so that what had been disturbing the stomach is expelled. For Hippocrates swore by this as a way to preserve health.[173]

Here we need to discuss whether or not vomiting is beneficial for pregnant women. First we will demonstrate that it is not useful, citing Avicenna's text, fourth fen of book I, in the related chapter, he says: "more need not be done to make the pregnant woman vomit, because the superfluities of her body will not come out with it; and both vomiting and strain result in emaciation."[174] Further, because of the risks she might incur, such as suffocation or rupture of the ligaments, Avicenna advises that pregnant women not be made to vomit.[175] Moreover, we can confirm the harm that vomit induces, such as headaches, great pain in the

---

170. See Avicenna, *Canon*, Lib. III, fen 21, tract. 2, c. 4 (p. 933): *et bolum armenum est de eis, quae sedant earum nauseam* (and Armenian bole is one of the substances which mitigate their nausea). See also Lib. III, fen 13, tract. 2, c. 11 (pp. 718–19); and Lib. I, fen 4, doctr. 5, c. 15 (p. 217).

171. On Armenian bole used against pestilence, see Avicenna, *Canon*, Lib. II, tract. 2, c. 420 (p. 341).

172. See Hippocrates, *Regimen in Health*, in *Hippocrates*, 4:43–60, at 53: *He who is in the habit of taking an emetic twice a month will find it better to do so on two successive days than once every fortnight.*

173. In Latin in the text: *Hipocras precipit fieri vomitum in unoquoque mense duobus diebus continuis, ut in secundo emendetur illud, quod in primo die fuit difficile, et ut expellatur illud, quod advenit stomaco. Hipocras namque securitatem facit, quod cum eo conservatur sanitas.* See Avicenna, *Canon*, Lib. I, fen 4, doctr. 5, c. 13 (p. 216).

174. In Latin in the text: *amplius faciendum non est, ut pregnans vomat; quoniam superfluitates corporis ipsius cum eo non egredientur: et vomitus et labor eam ad extenuationem perducent.* See Avicenna, *Canon*, Lib. I, fen 4, doctr. 5, c. 11 (p. 216).

175. See also Avicenna, *Canon*, Lib. III, fen 21, tract. 2, c. 4 (pp. 932–33).

eyes, throat, teeth, chest, and other parts of the body related to the stomach, as Avicenna also explains.[176]

O *frontosa*, be careful; as I have warned, pregnant women often feel nauseous, and to almost all of them, vomiting seems to offer relief, especially when they feel heaviness and pain in the stomach. By vomiting, they find their discomfort is alleviated; and this alleviation is welcome, and they proceed to continue to vomit. Because of this, it is wise to understand some rules about vomiting. First, depending on the constitution of the pregnant woman; second, depending on the vomit, with regard to its gentleness and force, ease and difficulty; and third, with respect to the antidote, that is, the medicine that should be used to alleviate this condition.

Regarding the constitution of the pregnant woman, one must consider whether she has a narrow chest, so that frequent vomiting does not fracture her veins or cause her to become tubercular. Likewise, one must consider whether or not she has a weak throat. If this is the case, she may develop inflammation of the throat from vomiting, and consequently, frequent vomiting would be very harmful to her and would put her life at risk. This is why in such a case or in a similar one, it is much better for these women, when nausea arises, to be given the prescribed drinks, that is, warm sweetened water with a little vinegar or water and rose honey, etc., because taking these remedies will cause troublesome humors to be dismissed from below. Or these women can try to vomit by drinking a large carafe of sweet wine all at once—as prescribed by Giacomo da Forlì, my mentor, who reigns sovereign over the discipline of medicine.[177] However, this should only be done when it does not cause further difficulty. For if by her drinking this wine and other substances in order to vomit, the vomiting is made difficult, then I recommend that she should instead try to evacuate those matters and humors from below, always turning to the aforementioned remedies whenever such nausea arises. For those pregnant women who do not suffer from a weak throat and a narrow chest, I say that vomiting every day is beneficial. If the woman can't induce the vomit easily on her own, then she should make use of light emetics, such as the following: *Recipe* hot water, five ounces; vinegar, one-half ounce; comestible, sweet oil, one-quarter ounce; the emetic should be tepid; she should drink it in the morning when she feels nauseous. After one tenth of an hour, she should insert her hand or a greased feather into her mouth. Or she may take water or oximel: five ounces of water and one and one-half ounces of oximel.

---

176. See Avicenna, *Canon*, Lib. I, fen 4, doctr. 5, c. 14 (pp. 216–17).

177. Giacomo della Torre da Forlì (d. 1414) practiced medicine in Padua in the late fourteenth and early fifteenth centuries and was Savonarola's teacher and mentor. See "Della Torre, Giacomo," in *Dizionario biografico degli italiani [DBI]*, 37 (1989), online at <http://www.treccani.it/enciclopedia/giacomo-della-torre_%28Dizionario-Biografico%29/>.

Now, if you will advance the authority of Avicenna,[178] I will tell you how it should be intended: pregnant women should not be made to vomit with strong emetics, as with hellebore and similar things, because of the dangers that they could cause. Instead, they should focus on evacuation from underneath, as has been said, and take cassia, manna, or turpentine.

Therefore, moving on to the second point, a pregnant woman's vomiting should not be strong and difficult, but mild and easy, so that it is beneficial and helpful to them, because nature is attempting in this way to evacuate harmful humors. As Hippocrates says, "evacuate in the direction to which they tend, through the appropriate outlets."[179] And from this, it is clear what must be said with regard to the third point about the emetic that is to be given to pregnant women: that it should be mild and not strong. By saying this, we have answered the question about whether or not vomiting is good for pregnant women.

Because of the dangers that could occur, even to those who vomit gently, we will add what they should do after vomiting. First, since vomiting hurts the eyes, they should blindfold their eyes tightly. After vomiting, they should take off the blindfold and wash their foreheads and their eyes with vinegar. This should be done especially by those who have glaucus, or light-colored eyes, or for those who are otherwise weak from other conditions. Following this, pregnant women should eat something astringent that benefits digestion, like a piece of quince cooked with a little cinnamon, or pear or candied quince with spices, or mint with seeds of sweet or acidulous pomegranate, that is neither sweet not sour. Also, here I will remind you of clove powder, which may be taken with chicken broth; or for impoverished women, water from the decoction of cloves may be taken, for example six ounces of water with one eighth [of an ounce] of clove powder boiled together.

Here I also want to remind you of what is said about pregnancy: that it is a natural infirmity. Therefore, we must reason that its conditions are those of a natural malady. Therefore, when these conditions go beyond the natural, that is when they are not usual in nature, these conditions may become serious and require urgent care, and it will be necessary to consult a practicing physician, because this kind of treatment is no job for a woman or a layman.

Furthermore, it is important to know that after vomiting, pregnant *frontosa*, you should refrain from eating anything for an hour and a half to two. In this time, the relaxed stomach will settle and will gain strength against that part of the humors that has remained, restoring it to health, and healing it, and sending

---

178. See pages 134–35, notes 174–76.

179. In Latin in the text: <que ducere oportet> *undecunque natura repit, inde per convenientia loca ducere.* See Hippocrates, *Aphorisms,* I.21 (pp. 106–7). The text within angle brackets has been added for better understanding of the aphorism: "<what matters ought to be evacuated>, evacuate in the direction to which they tend, through the appropriate outlets."

it to the intestines so that you may evacuate from below. Therefore, to conclude on this topic, we will agree with Avicenna that, when a pregnant woman vomits after eating, she must eat as a second meal something aromatic and astringent, like cooked quince with cinnamon or pear or candied quince, as has been said.[180]

Later, she should apply to her stomach an ointment, plaster, or poultice as specified earlier. She should keep mint leaves, or pomegranate seeds in her mouth, and she should sip some quince syrup with some Armenian bole. And having spoken on vomit, we will now move onto the tremors of her heart.

Third condition: heart palpitations and rapid pulse. It sometimes happens that pregnant women can feel their hearts racing, or palpitating. And of this condition, Avicenna writes that it is most often caused by the humor that finds itself in the cardia and communicates with the heart, because of the proximity of the cardia and the heart and also because of the great connection between them.[181] So the expelling power of the heart moves the humor and in such a way as to drive away this threat.

This condition, Avicenna writes, is relieved with the sipping of warm water little by little,[182] because the water makes the humor descend to the bottom of the stomach from the mouth of the esophagus. It is also good to drink bran water, as mentioned earlier, and anything cleansing, as discussed in the preceding chapter. Afterwards, it is useful to move moderately, because such exercise fortifies the heart and increases its strength to weaken such a humor, or move it below.

Now we must note here, *frontosa*, that when this condition of rapid heartbeat grows and perseveres, it may cause faintness; and if it grows stronger, it may lead to death. This is why while they are intensifying, heart palpitations should be treated with more than just warm bran water. You should make sure that in this case, you immediately seek expert advice. But if the heart palipiations are not too severe, then you can treat them as we have said.

Moreover, if this condition comes from gassiness trapped in the panniculus of the cardia, then such remedies are useful. Heart palpitations originating from gassiness can be distinguished from those of other origins, because palpitations of the first kind quickly resolve themselves and pass; but those originating from the humor are more persistent. In this second case, together with the heart's tremor,

---

180. See Avicenna, *Canon*, Lib. III, fen 21, tract. 2, c. 4 (p. 933): *Ad vomitum vero earum fuper cibum, oportet ut dentur post cibum ea, in quibus sunt aromaticitas, et ponticitas, et stypticitas, ficut cydonia assata* (With regard to their vomiting after eating, it is then necessary that she is given foods with aromatic, astringent and constipating properties, like cooked quince).

181. See Avicenna, *Canon*, Lib. III, fen 21, tract. 2, c. 5 (p. 933): *illud quidem plurimum accidit ei propter communitatem oris stomachi, et causa humoris in eo* (and this often happens to her because of the proximity of the cardia, and due to the humor present in the stomach).

182. See Avicenna, *Canon*, Lib. III, fen 21, tract. 2, c. 5 (p. 933): *quoniam multotiens alleviat sorbere aquam calidam, et exercitium leve praecipitans illud quod est in ore stomachi* (since drinking warm water and moderate exercise, which makes what is in the mouth of the stomach descend, is relieving).

the pregnant woman may feel nausea, vomiting, and stinging; and when the stomach is empty, the tremor is relieved; and during digestion, it becomes stronger. For this there is one remedy for the pregnant woman: for her to vomit after eating. She should do this as long as there is no reason for her not to, as we discussed in the previous section. Also, she should drink warm water with oximel after vomiting, as this is very helpful in relieving the humoral residue from the top or from below. After vomiting, she should wait three to four hours before eating, depending on how much food she has disgorged.

However, if the pregnant woman's vomit comes from some other reason, she should consult a physician who is knowledgeable about this, and will treat the condition. But also, I will remind you here of a cure that is very beneficial in such a case: take half an *aureum*[183] of bugloss powder every night before going to bed, as Avicenna says, in the eleventh fen of book III: "and among those things that increase aid in heart tremor is to drink the weight of half *aureum* of bugloss at bedtime on subsequent nights."[184] And Avicenna adds that another excellent and effective remedy is for the pregnant woman to drink two ounces of sweet warm milk with half a drachm of cloves on an empty stomach, and continue to do this as she likes.[185] Impoverished women should take every morning half an *aureum* of marjoram powder, with cold water if they feel warmth in their stomachs; but if they feel cold, they should take the marjoram powder with warm wine. The pregnant woman may take this every morning, as much as she likes. And so what is needed has been said about heart tremors of pregnant women.

Fourth condition: menstrual flow of the pregnant woman. To speak in general of women's menstrual flow goes beyond the scope of this work and would be too lengthy a topic. Therefore, we will limit our discussion to the menstrual flow of pregnant women. During pregnancy sometimes menstrual blood may appear, indicating the pregnant woman is at risk for miscarriage. In order to remedy this, it is good to apply astringent remedies—astringents that are not fragrant, because those provoke miscarriage.

This is why experts recommend the taking of gall nuts, pomegranate rind, lentils, beans, pomegranate blossoms, acorns, oak leaves, leaves of walnut, and leaves of quince. Draw a bath in which these ingredients are dissolved and put the pregnant woman in it. This bath should not be too hot. In the summertime, it should be cool; in the wintertime, it should have lost its coldness; but first the water should be boiled and then it should be left to cool down. Or else take a great

---

183. The *aureus* is a unit of weight measure roughly corresponding to one and one-half drachms, and to one sixth of an ounce (circa 5 grams, from the name of the Roman coin *denarius aureus*).

184. In Latin in the text: *et ex eis, quorum iuvamentum magnificatur in tremore cordis, est potare pondus medii aurei de bugulosa in tempore sompni noctibus continuis.* See Avicenna, *Canon*, Lib. III, fen 11, tract. 2, c. 3 (p. 677).

185. See Avicenna, *Canon*, Lib. III, fen 11, tract. 2, c. 3 (p. 677).

big sponge, infuse it in the aforementioned decoction, and wring it out so that it does not drip. Afterwards, place it over the pregnant woman's pubic area, cold or tepid, depending on the temperature of the air. Or take some pomegranate blossoms, acorns, dry figs, bean or lentil flour, and mix these ingredients with water and strong vinegar to make a poultice. Place it on the pregnant woman's pubic spot, because that corresponds to the part where the uterus is located.

It is also helpful to place cupping glasses between the pregnant woman's buttocks and her lower back, after rubbing her arms, and these remedies should suffice for the exterior. By mouth, give her every day, if you can, yellow amber pills or sealed earth, two scruples in the morning,[186] either in powder form or pill form, with three ounces of plantain water and a little sugar. Afterwards, a very beneficial remedy is Fenonan triphera, recommended by Mesue in his book of antidotes.[187] This should suffice in cases where there is a small amount of menstrual flow. If the pregnant woman's menstrual flow continues to appear in great abundance, *frontosa*, you must call a practicing physician.

Fifth condition: How to care for the fetus so that it stays in the uterus and there is no abortion. A pregnant woman must be very cautious and take great diligence to maintain the health of the fetus that she has cared for with great joy and effort, so that she does not happen to lose it, since it is, as we have said, the most beautiful, most worthy, and most noble fruit on earth. Therefore, be very careful, *frontosa*, not to allow yourself to have a miscarriage through your carelessness. Because if this happens, then two souls die together, yours and that of your child, and God will ask you for an explanation on the day of judgment. If you are found guilty, you may then expect great punishment for your soul beyond anything you have received on earth. This is why, in the first chapter of this second treatise we have instructed you what things may cause miscarriage, so that you may remember them and observe them with care.

Leaving behind those non-naturals that concern you that have been discussed, we will now speak of medications, reminding you that above all else you should beware of strong laxatives, especially in the first months, that is, the first, second, and third, since in this period the fetus is weakly attached to the cotyledons of the uterus. Later, you should beware of strong laxatives from the seventh month onwards, that is, in the seventh, eighth, and ninth months, because at this stage, the fruit, being ripe, could be easily detached by a simple movement. This is why Hippocrates says "it is suitable that pregnant women be purged between

186. *Terra sigillata*, i.e., "sealed earth or clay," so-called because the pastilles prepared from these kinds of clay were marked with a seal. The best-known *terra sigillata* came from the island of Lemnos. The scruple (*scrupolo*) is a unit of weight measure roughly corresponding to one third of a drachm (i.e. a little more than one gram).

187. See Mesuae, *De re medica*, Lib. III.5 (pp. 244–45): *Tryphera antid. minor Phenonis*. Triphera was a powerful compound preparation made from several species of myrobalans, herbs and spices.

the fourth month and the seventh, but in the earlier months and the later ones it ought to be feared."[188] Any laxatives given in the first or last months pose a risk; and if they are administered, they should be given with great fear and caution. Laxatives used by pregnant woman should be mild, as discussed earlier, which is why their administration is not a job for the inexperienced.

This is why Avicenna says:

> a laxative drug is one of the principal causes [of miscarriage], for which reason it is necessary to take care in its use before the fourth month and after the seventh, as also in the interval between. Nevertheless, in the interval [between the fourth and seventh months] it is salubrious, and it should be used when necessary; and really there is no reason not to cleanse and purify her blood in these periods, so that the embryo is not corrupted by the foulness of her complexion: which is why it must be done with delicacy and skill.[189]

And note, *frontosa*, that sometimes you may become pregnant before being well-cleansed. If this occurs, and you are sanguine, any corrupt blood that has not evacuated may increase your retention of blood caused by your complexion. This blood firstly sickens the fetus, then weakens the ligaments in such a way that abortion may result. This is what happened to Madonna the marchioness of Monferrato, from whose children descends the present day Marquis of Monferrato.[190] And note, *frontosa*, when you feel that your uterus is moist, and that fluids descend from your vagina, and that the lips of your vagina are more moist than usual, and this continues for some time, beware of miscarriage.

In this case take the following remedy: galls, bone ash, mastic, bistort, one to two spoonfuls of each, and bring them to a boil in dark wine, and soak a piece of sponge in this mixture and then wring it out well, and afterwards put it in the vagina and keep it there for one sixth of an hour, and then repeat this two or three times. You should do this early in the morning and in the evening before supper, and also after supper if you feel it is necessary. And you should also take one eighth of [an ounce] of mithridate every other day in the morning one hour

---

188. In Latin in the text: *pregnantes purgare si convenit a quarto usque ad septimum: iuniora autem et seniora vereri oportet*. See Hippocrates, *Aphorisms*, IV.1 (p. 135). This aphorism has already been quoted at 124 [85] [p. 118].

189. In Latin in the text: *Et farmacum quidem solutivum est de summa illarum causarum, quare oportet, ut caveatur eius dispositio ante mensem quartum et post septimum, et in eo, quod est inter illa iterum. Verumtamen in illo, quod est inter illa, est salubrius; et ad ipsum pervenitur, cum necessarium est; et fortasse non erit excusatio in quibusdam harum horarum, quin solvatur, et mundificetur sanguis eius, ut non corrumpat embrionem propter malitiam complexionis: quare oportet ut fiat cum facilitate et subtilitate*. See Avicenna, *Canon*, Lib. III, fen 21, tract. 2, c. 10 (p. 934).

190. The Marchioness has already been encountered in Treatise Two, 121–22.

before daybreak. Do not exert yourself in this time period. Eat dry foods as much as possible, and above all avoid coitus. Act as if you were sick. Use turpentine or cassia as mentioned, at least once a day, or twice if you think of it, especially when your menstrual fluids are abundant.

Now I want you to know, *frontosa*, that such abortion may come from gassiness generated in the uterus, and you will recognize it from the escaping of wind from the front, or by the moving or burping sensation that you will feel. Also, such abortion may come from lesions or similar causes, the removal of which must be left to the practicing physician, because it is not the job of a layman. So that you may be more careful, and more knowledgeable of such miscarriage, I will state the many signs that pregnant women should recognize. The first is when her milk-hardened breasts soften and become smaller. The second is when milk begins to flow and leak out and her breasts become smaller: this is a sign of the weakness of the fetus, and abortion will follow. The third is when the pregnant woman feels great and continuous pain in the depths of her eyes: even though this sensation is strong, it is not in and of itself a reliable sign of miscarriage, but it may indicate that there is a problem.

Frontosa, know that violent and persistent coughing may cause miscarriage. For this reason, when you are gravid when the weather is cold, do not go out lightly dressed. Also, as we have warned before, be careful not to catch a chill when you wash your hair, as this could bring on catarrhal cough. Lastly, to keep your fetus, you should take cordials such as doronicum, zedoary, cardamom, and mithridate; and if you do not fear musk, the preparation of diamusk is good and beneficial for rich women, or nutmeg for the poor. Of remedies like zedoary and nutmeg, you must take two or three pieces the size of chickpea grains, and in the morning chew the first two one at a time and swallow, and keep the third in your mouth for two hours. Take of the preparation of diamusk a small dose in the morning, that is three-eighths of an ounce, and in the evening before supper the same; and you may also use ginger. Enough has been said in this section.

Sixth condition: constipation of the pregnant woman. Let us recall what we previously said of the position of the uterus: that it lies between the *rectum* (called the *gentile* intestine,[191] by which the feces descend to the anus) and the bladder. Therefore when the fetus becomes larger, the uterus also grows, and because of such a swelling, it presses against the intestine from behind, and in this way it obstructs the exit passage for the feces: this is why the pregnant woman becomes constipated. In the front, the fetus similarly presses against the bladder, which causes frequent urination in pregnant women, and this we have previously discussed.

Constipation is relieved by drinking the broth of chicken or well-salted, fatty veal, or by drinking broth cooked with salted meat a half hour before meals.

---

191. See the previous reference to the *gentile* intestine, Treatise One, 85.

Relief also comes from taking cassia, manna, or turpentine, as we have said in the first chapter of this second treatise. The pregnant woman will also benefit from enemas of broth, salt, and oil; likewise of oil and salt; likewise from the decoction of wallflower stems and chard and mallow, salt and oil; likewise from suppositories made with honey. Now, if you think these laxatives are too strong, I say that their laxative quality is actually quite gentle and their strength is also diluted by the water, so that the benefit is greater than the harm. Later the pregnant woman may also take chard, wallflowers, mallow, and fatty beef broth.

But note, *frontosa*, that in the first two months until the end of the third, the fetus is not very large, and the uterus does not swell very much, which means that the pregnant woman should not be very constipated, and therefore these enemas are not necessary as in the fourth, fifth, and sixth months. I also wish to say that given that in the first months the fetus is weakly attached, as we have said before, enemas may be risky, especially in weak women, those with weak backs, and in those who have the tendency to miscarry; therefore it is better to proceed with these clysters with great prudence. I say the same about laxatives, which are significantly riskier than enemas.

However, these treatments may be used in a safer way in the fourth, fifth, and sixth months. In the seventh, when the fetus is fully formed, such treatment should be done with caution, because the fetus moves around in this month searching for a route of exit, so that such agitation with a clyster or medicine could cause its premature exit. In the eighth month, however, it is safer to proceed with such treatments. But in the ninth I believe it is questionable to use a clyster, especially before the first half of the month—because the pregnant woman, surely, is like a fragile vessel and must be handled with care. However, in the last part of the month, I believe enemas to be very beneficial, as we will discuss in the chapter on facilitating parturition.

And on such caution with regard to constipation and bloodletting, Rhazes says:

that if it should happen that they become sick, it is necessary that they be treated without bloodletting or purging of the belly, but, if it is done, let it be done with great fear or with the highest diligence so that the fetus is maintained and the birth may be easy.[192]

Seventh condition: suffocation of the pregnant woman. The pregnant woman may fall into a fit and remain deprived of her senses. She may lose her sight and movement and lie like a corpse. This is from the ascent of perverse and corrupt

---

192. In Latin in the text: *quod si ipsas infirmari continga<n>t, oportet ut sine minutione et ventris solutione medicentur, sed cum maximo timore, vel maxima et multa diligentia fiat ad hoc, ut fetus remaneat et partus fiat facilis.* See Rhazes, *Liber ad Almansorem*, tract. 4, c. 27 (fol. 75v).

vapors rising from the uterus, and this also happens to non-gravid women when they retain their menses. These women are called "suffocated" by physicians.[193]

These pregnant women should avoid taking fragrant substances from underneath; and similarly, they should avoid all rerouting of the humoral flow from the buttocks down, such as the application of cupping glasses on the thighs, rubbing of the thighs and the legs, ligatures on the legs and on the feet. This is because all such remedies are stimulative and may cause miscarriage. Therefore the suffocated pregnant women differ from the suffocated non-pregnant women in [that they do not benefit from] these remedies, but they agree [among themselves] to benefit from remedies applied from the buttocks up.

First, in such a pregnant woman it is beneficial for a cupping glass to be applied between the buttocks and her lower back, where the uterus is connected to the back, and repeat. I once treated a woman who had hemicranea [persistent headache] because of the collection of vapors risen from the uterus to her head, which lasted from dawn to vespers. I placed a large cupping glass at the end of her tailbone or spinal cord, where the uterus is connected, and she was healed with the sole application of a cupping glass for one hour before her paroxysm. She applied it three days in a row, always at the same time of the day, and I prescribed her to keep it in place until after vespers. I have related this episode to emphasize the importance of the use of cuppling glasses to reroute of humoral flow. And these cupping glasses may be safely used on a suffocated pregnant woman.

Also take three tallow candles and burn them; after they are partially burnt, extinguish them; and put those fumes under the pregnant woman's nose, and such a suffumigation should be repeated. Likewise, the fumes of a burned shoe or cloth and the fumes of galbanum are useful. The fumes of partridge feathers also have beneficial properties. Take a small band of partridge feathers tied together, light them on fire, and afterwards extinguish the fire, make the feathers smoke, and repeat. Likewise, you may use the sole of a dirty shoe roasted over a fire and later greased with lavender oil and wrapped up in a strip of cloth. Also, the following

---

193. In ancient and Hippocratic medicine, suffocation is a symptom which can derive "from the womb," and is thus *hysterikos* (from the Greek *hystera*, or womb), reflecting the idea that the womb physically moved to cause a wide range of symptoms. Nonetheless, the belief in the so-called "wandering womb" (i.e. the belief that a displaced uterus could cause many related pathologies) is only partially related to uterine suffocation, because such ancient physicians as Galen and Soranus of Ephesus, in describing suffocation, strongly oppose the view of the womb as an irrational, roaming animal, and both insist that the uterus is stationary and that its symptoms are due to substances being retained inside it (menses or female seed). Hysteria as we now understand it was not an ancient medical category and was not so named by the Greeks: hysterical suffocation derived from a physical cause rather than a psychological one. See Sabine Arnaud, *On Hysteria: The Invention of a Medical Category between 1670 and 1820* (Chicago: University of Chicago Press, 2015), and Helen King, "Once upon a Text: Hysteria from Hippocrates," in *Hysteria Beyond Freud*, ed. Sander L. Gilman (Berkeley: University of California Press, 1993), 3–90.

plaster is beneficial: take galbanum, sagapen, castoreum in equal measure, which should be placed on a piece of leather five fingers in width and seven fingers in length, which, fairly hot, should be placed upon the pregnant woman's stomach. But first you should begin with the candles; later try the partridge feathers, the burned cloth, and the soles of shoes; and lastly, try this plaster, when the other things did not work. Likewise, the pregnant woman's arms should be tied, and her hair pulled back, and she should be calmed and not agitated, as is the case with the non-pregnant suffocated woman, always remembering that a pregnant woman is like a barrel surrounded by rotten hoops; if you are not careful when you knock the hoops into position, the barrel could break into pieces.

Eighth condition: pains felt by the pregnant woman when she is about to go into labor. When the pregnant woman feels a weight in the bottom of her abdomen, under her navel, and pressure, along with pains, in her back near the sacrum in the lumbar region, and when she also feels pain in her groin, then she is close to delivering her fetus. This is how the fetus descends in order to come out: it becomes heavy and breaks the ties with which it was attached to the uterus, causing pain when it is separated from the uterus, which, because it is connected to the back and the groin, causes pain in these places.

From the movement of the fetus and the warm fluid retained in the uterus, which must also come out with the fetus, the pregnant woman's belly feels much warmer than usual. She also feels great swelling in the orifice of the uterus, because of the humors retained, since at this moment they are filled with gas. She also feels great moisture in the neck of her uterus, which comes from the urine and perspiration retained by the fetus. These watery substances have been retained until this time so as to lubricate the passage for the fetus, as we have said, and to facilitate the labor. For this reason, the rupture of these membranes is a sign that the fetus is on its way out. When the pregnant woman feels that loosening and her groin is enlarged, she should expect the fetus within a short time, because that bloating comes from the descent of the fetus.

And because, *frontosa,* in such a moment you feel this pain and these symptoms, you should be treated as a sick woman with an acute illness, at the beginning of which doctors prescribe little food. This is because if the woman eats too much food, her strength will be diverted from her task and will render her weak; and for this reason, doctors recommend that a sick woman should be given little food. This is why Hippocrates says: "where the disease is very acute, not only is the pain extreme, but also it is essential to employ a regimen of extreme strictness."[194] And again, he says "it is when the disease is at its height that is is necessary to use the most restricted regimen."[195]

---

194. In Latin in the text: *ubi ergo secundum acumen egritudo fuerit, continuos et ultimos habet labores, ultima et tenuissima dieta necessarium est uti.* See Hippocrates, *Aphorisms*, I.7 (p. 103).

195. In Latin in the text: *quando egritudo erit in statu, tunc tenuissima dieta necessarium est uti.* See Hippocrates, *Aphorisms*, I.8 (p. 103).

Clearly, when the pregnant woman is in this condition, the pregnancy is ready to progress to the next stage, which is the exit of the fetus: "the culmination comes when the symptoms reach their peak."[196] This is because, as we know, pregnancy is a natural malady, as has been said, which has a beginning, development, culmination, and an end. This culmination is at the hour of labor, when the symptoms of her condition are at their most powerful.

Now, *frontosa* may complain about the prescription of a strict regime by saying: "This is not good advice for parturient women, who expect for their suffering great mouthfuls of plump chickens, capons, eggs, candies, and drink without restrictions, or excellent wines like malmsey, Tyre wine, Trebbiano and others mentioned earlier. Certainly, if Hippocrates and other physicians had ever given birth, I am confident that they would not have imposed such strict rules about eating and drinking." I respond to you that Hippocrates speaks soundly, and that you should pay attention, for when dealing with labor, the condition of the parturient, her strength and weakness, the intensity and weakness of the pain, the ease and difficulty of the process must be considered, and it is necessary that the parturient be supervised according to her overall condition.

For example, if the parturient is a weak woman, and her symptoms and pains are strong, and the labor is difficult, then she should immediately be provided with good food that is easy to digest—like fresh eggs, consommé, ground capons or hens, and other invigorating foods, which we will mention later in the section *On the Regimen of the Woman who has Given Birth*, and similar things—and excellent wines to restore her strength and weakened spirits. This is also the opinion of physicians with experience in labor, whereas Galen writes that "food ought to be given immediately when the symptoms exhaust the strength."[197] But these foods should be divided into many parts, given to her a little at a time, that is, every four to five hours, depending on the quantity and quality of the food taken. This regimen is up to the wisdom of the women caregivers.

Now I wanted to emphasize this point, not because I do not want the parturient to be fed, but because it is important to not overfeed her. You understand me, *frontosa*. And if it is the case that the parturient is strong, in good condition, the delivery very easy, then hold her hands and make her adhere to a light diet until after she has given birth, and do not stuff her, as is done with geese. After

196. In Latin in the text: *nam status est cum accidentia ultimantur.* See Galen, *De crisibus,* Book I, ch. 10, in Kühn, 9:385.

197. In Latin in the text: *accidentibus prosternentibus virtutem illico dandus est cibus.* See Galen, *Commentarii in Hippocratis Aphorismos,* in Kühn, 17.2:380. Savonarola is here quoting a sentence taken from Galen's commentary on the Hippocratic aphorisms, thus approving the exception that Galen seems to suggest with respect to the Hippocratic rule of restriction of the dietary regime. See Hippocrates, *Aphorisms,* I.9 (p. 103): "Take the patient too into account and decide whether he will stand the regimen at the height of the disease; whether his strength will give out first and he will not stand the regimen, or whether the disease will give way first and abate its severity."

the labor, you will care for her as we direct. Having completed the section on how the pregnant woman should be fed, we will now move on to the section on how to facilitate parturition.

Ninth condition: preparation of the pregnant woman to ensure that labor be fast and easy. It seems to me, *frontosa*, that you must be very eager to learn about this, and that you are desirous to be instructed on these things more than others, for these are the most important things for a pregnant woman to know, that is, all the things that will relieve her anxiety and bring her ease. This is why I want to make sure that I am clear and thorough in this chapter above all others, and I hope also to include advice here for pregnant women that is very useful and agreeable and likely to bring them great satisfaction. I will therefore attempt, with the help of our omnipotent Lord, master of everything, by the great grace he bestows because of the prayers of pregnant women, especially my Ferrarese ladies, who I am sure, given that I have put forth such an effort for them, will not be ungrateful for the benefits received, for women are rarely ungrateful.

Here we go, *frontosa*. Pay close attention, and understand that difficulty in labor may come from eight causes: first, labor may be difficult because of the pregnant woman; second, because of the fetus; third, because of the uterus; fourth, because of the afterbirth; fifth, because of the organs near the uterus; sixth, because of the improper hour; seventh, because of the fault of the midwife, that is, the birth attendant; and eighth, from any other exterior cause, such as, for example because of the cold or something similar.[198]

Now following this order, we will first speak of the pregnant woman. If she is too young, her passage is too narrow. If she is weak and sickly, her expelling power is weakened. If it is her first birth, or if she is frightened and has lost her vigor and courage, her expelling power may also be weakened. This is why the women by her side should comfort her and give her courage. Also in the case of a first labor, the ligaments have not yet been broken, and as well, the passage has never been used and these body parts have never been dilated, so these women will feel greater pain and their parturition will be more difficult.

Another reason her expelling power may be weakened is because of the cold, which prevents the dilation of the muscles of the abdomen. This is why in such a case, hot compresses should be continuously applied to the parturient, and if possible, she should be kept near a fire. Also, the movement of the pregnant woman from place to place—made because she does not want to endure pain—adds much difficulty to her labor. This is why the high-backed chair or birthing chair (which we will discuss here) should be used to facilitate labor. In fact, when sitting on this chair and not moving from there, the pains continue and become

---

198. In Belloni's Italian edition of the *DRP* the numbering of these eight causes of difficult labor is incorrect (because both the Venice and Vatican manuscrips report an incorrect lesson). The third manuscript of the work (Reggio Emilia, Biblioteca Panizzi, Codice Turri C 12), unknown to Belloni, contains instead the correct list.

more intense, because nature, afflicted by these great pains, thus uses all its force to bring the fetus to the front in order to expel it. And in this way, the fetus will come out more easily, as we will later explain.

With respect to the fetus: there are multiple factors that can complicate its birth or delivery. Given that the fetus must change position on its own in order to be born, it may happen that the delivery of the fetus could be difficult: and such changes we will also address here, recalling several unnatural positions that the baby may take in exiting from the belly of the mother. However, first we will name the natural position and how the fetus should naturally exit head first, with its face turned towards the backside of the mother. Therefore, the first altar the baby kisses when he arrives in this world is his mother's ass, which will grant it pardon for any sins committed in her womb. Take note, O proud reader, how in this decrepit old age of mine I have come to understand what was said to me by children in school, wanting to insult me, who cried out "ass kisser"—which is exactly what we have all done.

We have already recalled the correct position of the baby in the belly of the mother, that is with his head between his knees and his hands extended over his knees. When it comes time for his delivery, he extends his arms and hands beside his thighs, as children do when they go swimming and want to dip into the water, extending their hands along their thighs, and with heads first they dive in: and this is what the fetus does naturally in order to exit easily. This is therefore the natural position for the exit of the fetus, and any other position we may call unnatural. And nature has done this, so that the head of the fetus can break the urinary and sudoral membranes, from which fluids come out that moisten and lubricate the passage, preparing it for an easy exit in labor. Nature also sends the fetus out head first, since at this point the fetus is large and lacks sufficient air to cool off his heart, so that he can cool off by breathing through his mouth and nose. For these reasons, this is the position in which the fetus usually comes out.

In addition to this position, there is another similar one, and that is when the fetus is positioned feet first, also with his hands extended over its legs. In this case, the midwife should gently pull the baby out by his feet; because just as in the normal position, his head breaks the urinary and sudoral membranes, in this position he breaks those membranes with his feet; and we will speak more of this later. It also happens that the fetus, because he is wrongly positioned in the uterus, may be ready to come out in many other positions, as with his arm first, or with his head and feet at the same time, etc., as will later be explained. All of these positions are wrong, and they are dangerous: sometimes the fetus dies, sometimes the mother dies, and sometimes both die. So take note of what we have said: a nine-month fetus who is not able to receive sufficient oxygenation from the artery in the womb, will suffocate if his exit is too delayed and if he does not exit with his his head first.

Continuing with our discussion of parturition, we will say that labor can become more difficult depending on the sex of the baby, as the delivery of a male is much easier, because the movement of the male child is stronger, and he helps himself more in his exit. Likewise, a large head or body makes labor more difficult, as does a small fetus, whose strength is diminished. Also, at times a fetus may have two heads, as I myself have encountered,[199] and as Augustine describes,[200] two twins who had two heads and one body, as also happened in Padua in 1320.[201] In these cases, labor became very difficult.

Also, labor becomes difficult when there are many fetuses, which, constricting the belly, push one another to exit, as happens with twins, or with quintuplets, as I have seen, and septuplets, as occurred in my time in Padua, and more powerfully if they are noticeably big. I say "noticeably," because if they are extremely small they are unable to push one another, as was the case recounted by the Conciliator, which I will also recall here.[202] He relates that in Abano, a village near Padua, there once was a pregnant woman who had sixty fetuses, and they all had movement and human form; which I believe, because he was a man worthy of much authority. Confirming this possibility, Avicenna says: "and sometimes there is a very large number [of fetuses] in one cell [of the womb]."[203] To return to causes of difficult delivery, when the fetus is dead in the uterus, labor becomes difficult: this is because the fetus has no movement and so cannot help himself get out.

O coddled pregnant *frontosa*, you who believe that you are so much more than a woman, just as the ass believes he is more than a beast—and I am not referring, of course, to my noble ladies of Ferrara, beware and believe me that when you go into labor and you throw yourself carelessly here and there on the bed or birthing chair, first stretching out, then curling as though you are especially delicate, by these erratic motions you may cause difficulty and greatly harm your fetus, shifting the fetus into an unnatural position, and this may cause your own death as well as that of your fetus. You should be obedient and stay still and patiently tolerate your pain, which we will now discuss. This is what Avicenna

---

199. Savonarola does not mention this specific case in his *Practica maior*, although reporting some other "monstruos births" his father personally witnessed. See Ynez V. O'Neill, "Michele Savonarola and the *fera* or Blighted Twin Phenomenon," *Medical History* 18 (1974): 222–39.

200. Augustine, *De civitate dei*, vol. 2, Book XVI, ch. 8 (p. 509, ll. 53–57), and ch. 5 (p. 133, ll. 55–64).

201. Chronicler Giovanni Villani reports the birth of a two-headed infant near Florence in 1317, but no similar birth is noted in Padua in 1320. See the cases included in Lorraine J. Daston and Katharine Park, eds., *Wonders and the Order of Nature, 1150–1750* (New York: Zone Books, 1998). On two-headed twins in particular, and other cases of conjoined twins in the Middle Ages, see Zuccolin, *I gemelli nel Medioevo*, chapters 4 and 5, at 125–93.

202. On the same anecdote, see Treatise One, note 58.

203. In Latin in the text: *et quandoque est numeratio plurima valde in kisti una*. See Avicenna, *Canon*, Lib. III, fen 21, tract. 2, c. 21 (p. 940).

meant when he said "or on account of the great restlessness of the parturient."[204] Wherefore you should know, *frontosa*, that when your breathing becomes regular, and you feel the pains cease in the fundus, and the fetus stops kicking, then you can be sure that the labor will be safe: since these are certain signs that the fetus will exit easily and properly, especially if your breathing is regular.

With respect to the uterus: labor may become difficult when the uterus is small, narrow by nature, and too closed, or if it is full of ulcers or scars, or if there is an abscess in it, or lesions or hemorrhoids, or other such causes that impede the exit of the fetus. Now you, *frontosa*, who suffer from hemorrhoids of the uterus, know that if you become gravid, your labor will be very difficult and painful.

With respect to the afterbirth: labor becomes difficult when the afterbirth is so massive that it cannot be easily separated from the fetus.

With respect to other organs close by that can complicate the birth: one of them is the bladder, especially when it has lesions or when it is harmed by the retention of urine; similarly the intestine, when there is a lesion in it and a mass of hardened feces. But note, *frontosa*, that hemorrhoids of the intestine also make delivery difficult, as Avicenna says: "either hemorrhoids or sores of the anus."[205] Surely I feel great compassion for the many Ferrarese women afflicted with these maladies; and I also feel for those who are too narrow—that is, in the loins—because such narrowness causes tightness in the passage through which the fetus must travel.

With respect to the time of birth: delivery becomes difficult when the fetus attempts to leave before its time and so is not assisted by nature as it would otherwise be. And premature delivery may be attributed to some exterior cause—fatigue, for example, from lifting heavy weight—and similar things.

With respect to the exterior causes of difficult delivery: delivery becomes more difficult if it is very cold, which constrains the exit passage; this is why, *frontosa* midwife, you must always make sure to have warm blankets available to protect the parturient from the cold. And because of the harmful effect of the cold, deliveries in the northern regions are both more difficult and more dangerous, as are those occurring in the winter rather than in the summer. But when there is a great heat spell, delivery is also difficult, since heat, sapping the strength of the parturient, weakens her. Therefore, moderate temperatures, tending more to warm than to cold, are more advantageous to deliveries than any other. *Frontosa* pregnant woman, know also that melancholy makes your labor more difficult,

204. In Latin in the text: *aut propter multitudinem inquietudinis parturientis*. See Avicenna, *Canon*, Lib. III, fen 21, tract. 2, c. 21 (p. 940). The beginning of the sentence, configured as a list of causes for difficult births, reads: *Et quandoque fit difficultas propter* . . . (and sometimes there is difficulty [in labor] because of . . .).

205. In Latin in the text: *aut emoroidis aut ragadie ani*. See Avicenna, *Canon*, Lib. III, fen 21, tract. 2, c. 2 (p. 940).

weakening the spirits. This is why those who spin crooked spindles,[206] because they must conceal their illicit labor, will suffer greatly for their sins. Melancholy also causes miscarriage, as we have said. O rich and refined *frontosa*, know that the use of fragrant things by mouth makes your delivery difficult, because the womb[207] is naturally attracted to good odors, and draws itself upwards when these are used.

With respect to the birth assistant or midwife: I will now offer clear instruction for all women who are midwives and assistants, so that they may learn the rules that must be observed in the parturition of the fetus; for surely, due to the ignorance of these midwives, many children and their mothers either die or endure hardship. I will also explain various modes of assisting with the many unnatural positions in which fetuses often present themselves upon reaching the exit of the uterus.

And to start at the beginning, we must first discuss how to facilitate the labor, which, because of its difficulty, often leads the pregnant woman down the wrong path, so that she ruptures a vein in her chest which makes her consumptive, or she suffers swelling or spasms, leading to her death and that of the fetus, as has been said. *Frontosa*, know that, when you feel pains in your front, and they descend near your pubic area, then get ready to give birth soon, because these pains travel to that place where your fetus will exit. And similarly, if those pains remain after the fetus has exited, know that the afterbirth with all its encumbrances will soon present itself. But when the pains start at the back, this is a sign that labor will be difficult, for the opposite reason, as they will not be located near the point from which the fetus will exit; similarly, an easy labor will follow if circumstances are the opposite of those mentioned here that cause a difficult labor.

But perhaps you will ask, *frontosa*, "tell me now, why has nature given so much pleasure to the man in impregnating and conceiving, and so much pain to the woman in giving birth? Just as coitus is necessary for generation and the conservation of the living species, so is childbirth, because without childbirth individuals could not multiply." And holding the opinion that man experiences greater pleasure in generation than woman, because he does not feel any of the pain that she feels during delivery whereas only by experiencing some pain he would have greater certainty of his actual paternity—I leave that question unanswered, so that the audience may have reason to dispute among themselves. Yet it seems that God has punished women much more than men, for God said to Eve *you will bear your children in pain*[208]—but since God created woman more fragile

206. This metaphoric expression, indicating deceit and betrayal, is documented in the Italian language since at least the thirteenth century (see TLIO, *sub vocem* fuso, i.e. spindle). The same expression exists in English, where it means "to make her husband cuckold; said of a women"; see Thomas Wright, *Dictionary of Obsolete and Provincial English* (London: H. G. Bohn, 1857), 2:895.

207. Savonarola uses the term *madre* (instead of *matrice*) here to mean uterus or womb.

208. Genesis 3:16: *in dolore paries filios tuos*. The Vulgate reads: *Multiplicabo aerumnas tuas, et conceptus tuos: in dolore paries filios*.

than man, sin should not be imputed less to man than to woman. And take note of this, you poor souls, who have taken a sinful woman as your wife.

O *frontosa*, I have great compassion for you and for all pregnant women. So that I may be praised by you and other women, and so that you will always pray to God for me, I will expound in the following section the many methods and rules that pregnant women should observe in order to have an easy delivery. And this is how I comfort all of you, by giving you these rules to learn and observe, if you want to easily empty your luggage. Don't object that these rules are novelties, because they are truly safe, authorized in writing, and have been successfully put into practice.

Following the logic of what we have thus far written, we should remember that there are two time periods in particular that we must focus on: the first is that time period that is near delivery, that is, ten to fifteen days before; the second is the moment when the pregnant woman actually feels labor pains. We must proceed in treating the pregnant woman as the physician does with the infirmities of the stomach or other parts, when it is filled with noisome and persistent humors. And for this condition, he prescribes medications that are digestive preparations for the humors, so that they are prepared to leave the stomach. Secondly, he prescribes medicine so that the humors prepared to leave the stomach may easily leave. Third, he offers relief through aromatic substances that are beneficial to digestion. In the same way, we may say that pregnancy is a natural sickness of the uterus, which nourishes the fetus within it, and within it also is retained blood, and so we must prepare the easy delivery of the fetus and of the retained blood, which would otherwise be injurious. Accordingly, digestives must first be given; secondly, the pregnant woman should be given medicines that facilitate the expulsion of the injurious substance; and third, the uterus that has suffered injury for so long should be comforted.

The first medication or treatment that every woman may undergo, fifteen to twenty days before giving birth, is to sit in a tub or vat filled with plain water that is not too hot, five or six times a day, and she should stay in this bath, if she can, for a quarter of an hour or more. This bath relaxes and softens the ligaments and the organs from which the fetus must come out. Wherefore Avicenna says "when the pregnant woman approaches birth, then it is necessary that she constantly employ bathing and the sitzbath";[209] so it seems that Avicenna maintains that this should be done every day, if the pregnant woman can tolerate it. But you will say, "Rhazes says the contrary in his fourth treatise: "they should take care not to dally too long in the bath or the sun."[210] I respond that he prescribes this only in the first months,

209. In Latin in the text: *cum pregnans apropinquat partui, tunc necessarium est ut assiduet balneum et tinam.* See Avicenna, *Canon*, Lib. III, fen 21, tract. 2, c. 23 (p. 941). This passage had already been quoted in note 136 (123).

210. In Latin in the text: *caveat ne in balneo aut in sole longam faciat moram.* See Rhazes, *Liber ad Almansorem*, tract. 4, c. 27 (fol. 75v). This source was previously quoted in note 137 (123).

but in the last months he recommends the bath, saying "when the hour of birth draws near, the parturient ought to be put in a bath, and let her sit in a sitzbath each day."[211] And if she would rather not enter the bath, it will be very beneficial to her every day to sit over pieces of cloth soaked in hot water for half an hour; even though a bath is much better, this treatment softens the abdomen and causes feces to exit the body, which often cause problems in labor, as we have said. And when you do this, *frontosa*, take care not to catch cold. This is one of the first treatments.

The second treatment is to spread an ointment on the orifice of the vagina and over the pubic and pudendal areas, and also on her limbs: and for this chamomile oil is best, or sweet almond oil, or also the oil of wallflowers. The pudendal area may also be anointed with chicken fat and with one of these oils and a little wax. If possible, she should do both of these things at the same time: that is, the bath, and anointing after getting out of the bath, twice a day for those fifteen to twenty days, while keeping continuously in the vagina a ball of washed uncombed wool soaked in one of the mentioned oils. It is especially important to do this at night, but she may also keep it in during the day.

The third treatment is a clyster made from fatty broth, or from pure olive oil, or from oil and broth together, or decoction of flax seed and oil. This type of clyster should be used by the pregnant woman on the third or fourth days in those fifteen to twenty days.

The fourth treatment is for the woman to continue drinking as much fatty broth sweetened with barley sugar as she can before meals, or eating as much fatty chicken meat, capon, and similar meats as she can. She should take the broth of spinach or of lettuce prepared with fatty meats, etc., and stay away from constipating foods.

Having prescribed these treatments, we now come to medications. For when the day of labor arrives, when the pregnant woman feels she is ready to give birth, then she should be assisted with medicines, some of which are external and others internal. We will begin first with the external medicines that facilitate the fetus in its exit from the mother's body. These medicines are methods and practices that have been proven effective in helping pregnant women, just as physicians have devised ways to administer noisome medicines by mixing them with sugar and fragrant things so that they may be taken more easily.

Therefore, we will say that when the pregnant woman feels the pains of labor, she should immediately sit down and prop up her legs, so that the contractions will move to her front part. And she should stay in this position for an hour, if she can. Afterwards, for the same reason, she should lie down on a bed with her body facing up; of course, this should be done only if she does not yet hear

---

211. In Latin in the text: *cum hora partus iam apropinquat, parturiens in balneo mitti debet, et in tina singulis diebus sedere.* See Rhazes, *Liber ad Almansorem,* tract. 4, c. 28 (fol. 75v). Previously quoted in note 134 (122).

the baby knocking on the door. After having tried this, she should immediately get up and climb on top of a crate or other tall piece of furniture and climb down, repeating this several times, strongly hitting the ground with her heel bone, as if she were descending stairs. And if perhaps such climbing is too tiring, she may attempt this method instead: take two crutches,[212] and by using them stand on the tips of her toes; afterwards, she should raise her legs in the air and move them down to the ground, landing on her heels. After this, she should take in as deep a breath as possible and then close her mouth and nose, and then hold her breath as long as she can in the lower parts of her abdomen. She should continue to practice this remedy even after the midwife has determined that the baby is at the door.

We should also note that when the pregnant woman is panting and out of breath, some stay in bed with pillows propped up behind them, and this is how they give birth; some get down on their knees; some stand; some sit on a chair with pillows behind them; and of all these positions, the worst is to stand. But in order to assist in that way in which I can best assist women, from whom I hope to receive many benefits for my efforts, I will design a birthing chair that is both comfortable and suitable for facilitating parturition; and it is this: this chair should be made of strong and solid wood, so that it is firm and it does not sway. In width, it should measure two "vescovato feet,"[213] and the height of the seat should be one and one half feet. It should be closed on the sides with boards; and the seat, that is its depth or width, should be one and one half feet; but it should be carved out in the front, carved in the shape of a curve, so that the child can easily descend, while the mother remains seated. Also, on both sides there should be arms, so that she can hold herself up with her hands as needed; and the back of it should be tall. So that this chair may be better understood, I will draw roughly what my birthing chair looks like in the margins.[214] In this way, *frontosa* should stay seated on this chair—since they well deserve such a throne, bringing such a noble fruit into this world with such difficulty—and behind the seat there should be a cushion, so that she does not feel pain from the hardness of the wood. When the pains come, she should extend her back to the apsis of the chair, so that she may push hard directly with her back and focus her strength towards her front, and this is how the chair facilitates in the delivery.

212. Savonarola uses the word *crozole* for crutches. See Charles Du Fresne Du Cange, *Glossarium mediae et infimae latinitatis*, ed. Léopold Favre (Niort: L. Favre, 1883–1887), *sub vocem* crozola, vol. 2, col. 628b: *Baculus superne rostratus vel in formam crucis efformatus*.

213. This unit of measurement cannot be identified.

214. The sketch of the chair is missing in all the three extant manuscript copies of the *De regimine praegnantium*, and its textual description does not coincide with the drawing of the primitive chair (or better, of the "Y" shaped birthing stool) printed in some editions of the *Practica maior* (see, for example, Figure 1, 154). It resembles most the kind of birthing chair printed and described in Rösslin's *Rosegarden* (see Figure 2, 154). Also see Introduction, note 104 (34).

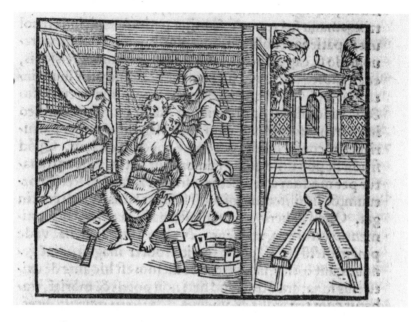

Figure 1. Illustration of birthing scene and "Y" shaped birthing stool – Michele Savonarola, *Practica maior* (Venice: Giunta, 1559), fol. 272rb.

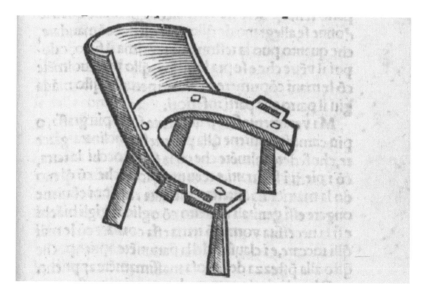

Figure 2. Image of birthing chair – Eucharius Rösslin, *Der swangern Frauwen und hebammen Rosegarten* (Strasburg: Martin Flach, 1513), without page number.

Therefore, as soon as the midwife perceives either with her eyes or with her hands the little head of the friar protrude, or the sack, if the water begins to come forth from the ruptured membrane, she needs immediately to make the pregnant woman expel as much air as possible. As said before, the parturient must then hold her breath and sneeze while holding her breath, covering her mouth and nose as much as possible: and she should continue with these two actions together as long as possible.

And if the water does not come, once the sack appears in the mouth of the womb, the midwife or birth attendant should pierce the water with her nail or with a thin needle, or with some round cutting instrument, such as this, in case she can't reach the place with her fingers or with a needle (see Figure 3). In doing this, she will encourage the fetus to come out more quickly. This is why every birth attendant should keep the nail of her index finger, that is, the one next to the thumb, long and sharp, like the finger of a harpist.

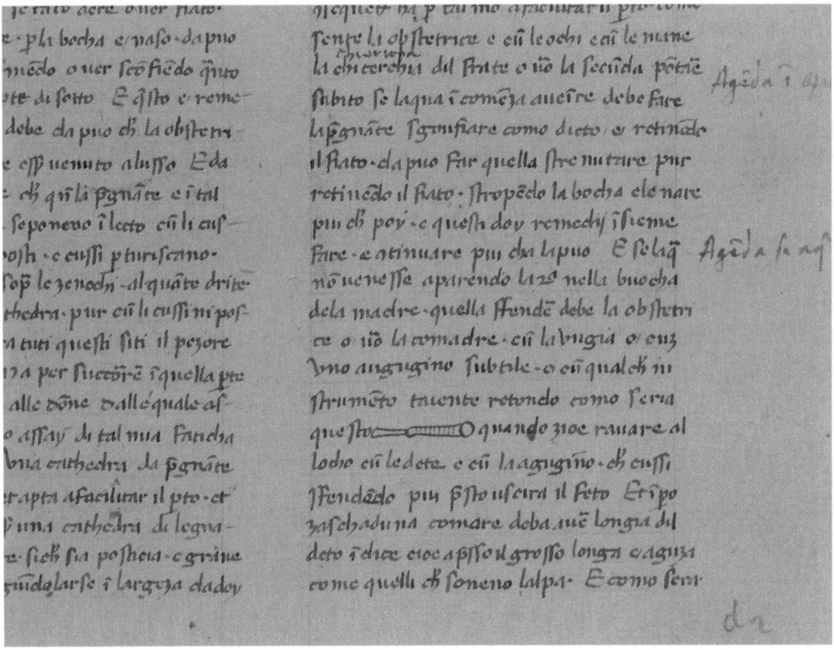

Figure 3. Image of page featuring small knife in red ink – Michele Savonarola, *De regimine praegnantium* (Biblioteca Panizzi, Reggio Emilia, Mss. Turri C 12, fol. d2r).

And when the water is broken, and even before, the midwife should apply fragrant perfume, that is, of *galia muscata* previously put on embers, so that the uterus will move downward. The assistant should spread or widen the legs of the pregnant woman, extending them as far apart as possible, to spread open the passage and to facilitate the delivery.

And know, *frontosa*, that screaming loudly in such a situation is very beneficial to you, which is why Avicenna says "do let her cry out";[215] and even if it does not hurt so much, I recommend that you scream loudly, so that your pain is believed, and your husband and family will feel compassion for you, lighting a great fire for you , and serving you capons, sweets, and excellent wines.

But note that while in labor, as we have said, your food must be small in quantity and highly nutritious, such as eggs, consommé and ground chicken, and excellent wine—not constipating dark wine, but light, white wine, as previously discussed.

Still, the best remedy is for the parturient to kneel down with her head on the floor, so that her knees squeeze against her abdomen, and she should keep herself in this position with her hands on the ground. Then the attendant should use her fingers to widen the vagina, after applying the previously mentioned ointments; in this way the delivery will be facilitated, especially for fat women. Therefore, *frontosa* midwife, when you see or feel the sack emerge, know that the birth is near, and therefore, make haste. If the water breaks on its own, this is good; but if it does not, you should break it with your finger nail or with one of the aforementioned instruments, because the flow of those fluids over the birth passage and pudenda will facilitate the delivery, just as water poured over river banks makes it easier for the barrels to roll down. And if, after all the fluid comes out, the fetus does not exit, beat an egg with the whites, chicken fat, and oil of dill, and spread this on the neck of the uterus and on the nearby area.

Even with all the aforementioned remedies, sometimes labor is difficult and the fetus does not come out. So in order to not fall short in my assistance to the women, for whom I have and will always feel compassion, after all we have said I will add some advice that I maintain is very useful, about which the authorities have written. Therefore, *frontosa* midwife or birth attendant, be careful, because when the baby does not come out because of the reasons previously mentioned, and the delivery goes on for a long time, you should make use of the advice that follows. Make sure that the parturient's mouth and nose are closed and have her blow as said before, and after this, the midwife should press into the belly with her hands.

If it still goes on for a long period of time, since the parturient has suffered pain and breathlessness for so many hours, it is necessary to keep up the strength of the mother: if she lacks her strength, the labor will be even more difficult. To

---

215. In Latin in the text: *et clamet*. See Avicenna, *Canon*, Lib. III, fen 21, tract. 2, c. 23 (p. 941).

help her regain her strength, she should be given fresh eggs that can be sipped, some consommé, ground chicken, or fragrant, excellent wine, and similar things. O impoverished *frontosa*, do as best you can: at least make sure you have eggs. If the parturient is debilitated for a long period of time, make her sniff fragrant wine, rose water, citron, violets, roses, and fragrant pomanders to enhance her vital strength. Even though fragrant things make the womb shift upward as said before, nonetheless, light fragrant things help to strengthen and comfort her more than they can harm her. However, if the parturient's powers are strong enough, such scents should not be used.

The second treatment should be a bath in tepid to hot water, in which calamint or rue or savin are first boiled. And in this tub the pregnant woman should stay up to her hypochondrium, that is, up to her waist, for half an hour. If the surrounding air is cold, light a fire, and if it is too hot, fan her lightly. Later, you may also spread chicken fat and chamomile oil on her pubic area and inside the vagina, as said before, as well as on the nearby areas. *Frontosa*, do not forget to breathe deeply and keep your nostrils blocked; this should be done continuously; and note that such remedies should be repeated.

After treatments such as digestives are administered, other medicinal remedies should also be given to her, and these are those things that enter the body either from underneath or from above: for example, suppositories and clysters, and simple or compound medicines taken by mouth. Among the beneficial suppositories is the myrrh suppository inserted into the vagina. Sowbread suppositories are also beneficial; they are made with aristolochia, or pulverized and mixed with opoponax as a treatment. Since this is a very strong remedy, first try the weaker treatments, such as inserting in her vagina uncombed wool soaked in the juice of rue or savin.

Of clysters, let us say that these may either be inserted from the front end or from behind. In the front, as the little head of the friar has not yet peeked out, you should inject the clyster into the uterus, with a cannula that is somewhat longer than the neck of the uterus (because it should be inserted deeply), and it should be long and thick as a thumb, and it should have only one opening in its extremity. Such a clyster should be made of lubricative things that are not harmful to the fetus, like a decoction of marsh mallow, flax seeds, fenugreek, with chamomile oil and similar things.

And since women often question and refuse such clysters, we turn to enemas applied from behind, such as an enema made from the decoction of red chickpeas, with fennel seed, rue, savin, annual mercury, garlic, sowbread, aristolochia: because all of these things make delivery easier. Wherefore the clyster for both poor and rich women may include red chickpeas, fennel seeds, annual mercury or rue or savin, flax seed or root of marsh mallow, butter, chamomile oil and salt, a bit of fatty broth or any other kind of broth: and all these things together tend to be very helpful in facilitating labor.

Having discussed clysters, let us now move on to things that should be taken by mouth to facilitate delivery. Let us say that all medicines that drive away worms make the fetus come out of the uterus; we will make this type of medication the focus of a section dealing with worms in Treatise Three.[216] But in order not to fall short of supplying aid that is needed so much, we recommend pulverized cinnamon drunk with celery water, or calamint, or maidenhair fern water. For example: take cinnamon, one eighth [of an ounce] and a half; celery water, or calamint water, or maidenhair fern water, three ounces. Heat these ingredients and add sugar. Afterwards, take water from the decoction of the leaves of marsh mallow with honey, taking five ounces at a time, also warm. These two waters facilitate labor and alleviate the pains of labor. Another excellent medicine: take myrrh, castoreum, storax, one drachm of each; cinnamon, savin, maidenhair fern, five drachms of each; form them into pills with honey; and let seven pills be given at a time with two ounces of maidenhair fern water sweetened with rose syrup. Also for the impoverished ladies, *somentina* pear may be given with honey, just as you would give children for worms.

The authorities say that holding a magnet tight in the left hand makes labor easier;[217] or you may also tie a string of corals to the right thigh. Both methods can be used by the poor as well as the rich. Having given this aid, in case the fetus is alive, I will add finally this poultice, which can be placed on the pubic area of the parturient if she wishes: take the pulp of bitter apple, rue—or even better, its juice—and myrrh, one-half ounce of each, savin and madder, two drachms of each, and once they are reduced to a powder, mix with honey and red chickpea flour to make a poultice.

Now, I have said "if the fetus is alive," because when it is dead, labor becomes even more difficult, wherefore it is necessary in this case that these medicines be repeated, especially those that are taken externally, because the parturient will be very weak and suffering great pains, and often a surgeon must pull out the fetus using cutting tools and hooks. The birthing attendant can at first be of great assistance, of course, keeping the parturient upright, with her pudenda raised and her head down, and having with her women who open the thighs of the parturient as much as possible, after which the attendant inserts her hands, well-lubricated with chamomile oil, inside the vagina, feeling the baby and attempting by her skill to give aid, continually greasing and smearing, as has been said. It is also beneficial in this situation to apply to the inside of the uterus a decoction of marsh mallow leaves and of flax seeds made with powder of dittany, which is an excellent remedy. The pregnant woman should force herself to keep the decoction inside her for at least one hour. Later, she should take white hellebore, sneeze as many

---

216. See Treatise Three, 206–209.
217. See, for example, Avicenna, *Canon*, Lib. III, fen 21, tract. 2, c. 31 (p. 943).

times as possible, and with her mouth closed and her nose blocked, she should release this decoction.

However, if the attendant's hands, and the lavage, and the greasing or the smearing, do not help, then it is necessary to turn to the practicing physician. If it seems that the pregnant woman remains strong and her labor still continues, the midwife should proceed with the prescribed treatments twice a day, early in the morning and in the evening. Then, if you give her the medicated water, she should wait at least four hours before having lunch, and the same is true for supper, and meanwhile she should also take preparations such as *diamargariton*[218] by mouth, taking them with some good wine. But if she is availaing herself of external remedies only, then she is allowed to have lunch and supper one hour from the administration of these remedies. And this should also be done when the fetus is alive and the parturient is suffering from a long labor. Be aware that these things depend greatly on the midwife or birthing attendant applying their wisdom to the task.

In conclusion, I also want to add the common practice, in the case of prolonged labor or labor with a dead fetus, of giving saffron with broth, sometimes with fragrant wine, more or less depending on the strength of the pregnant woman, but usually one eighth of an ounce. It is true that Serapion and Rhazes say that two eighths [of an ounce] of this mixture makes a woman give birth immediately.[219] But you must also consider the woman's complexion, fever, and strength, so that sometimes less should be given, and this is left to the prudence the midwife has gained from prior experience. Avicenna, in agreement with other physicians, is of the opinion that saffron should be used, tied and suspended over the vagina or to her right thigh, so as to speed the delivery of the fetus; and this works. It is also very useful to do suffumigations with just myrrh or with myrrh and galbanum.[220] And for the poor, the suffumigation of pigeon dung is useful.

Tenth condition: care in assisting labor when the fetus is improperly positioned for delivery. It happens sometimes that the fetus is not properly positioned for exit from the womb, and then labor becomes more difficult. Therefore, since I am eager to assist in this undesirable situation, I will describe some unnatural forms

---

218. A compound medicine made from pearls, or *margarite*.

219. See Serapion [Johannes Serapion the Younger], *Liber aggregatus in medicinis simplicibus* (Milan: Antonius Zarotus, 1473), tract. 6, s.n. (*sub vocem* Sulfur): *et quando mulier pregnans suffumigatur cum eo educit fetus* (and when the pregnant woman is suffumigated with it, the fetus comes out); and Rhazes, *Liber ad Almansorem*, tract. 4, c. 28 (fol. 76r).

220. See Avicenna, *Canon*, Lib. III, fen 21, tract. 2, c. 31 (p. 943): *Suffumiga eam cum myrrha quoniam est bona valde. Et iterum cum myrrha et galbano . . . aut sumantur sulphur citrinum* (Suffumigate her with myrrh because it is very effective. And the same is true for myrrh and galbanum . . . or take yellow sulphur). See also Lib. II, tract. 2, c. 59 (p. 272): *aquae sulphurae conferunt doloribus matricis* (sulphurous waters are good for uterine pains).

and positions of the fetus at the moment of birth, and explain how midwives should assist in those situations.

Although the fetus is supposed to come out head first, sometimes, as we have said, it comes out feet first instead. In this case, the attendant should lubricate her hands with chamomile oil and reinsert the feet, and lift them inside of the uterus, so that the head is pointed downwards, so that he is properly positioned for his descent. And if this is not possible, she should tie his legs with a good strong string, and pull the fetus out by force. And if this is not possible, iron tools may be used, a method that should be left to physicians, for this is not woman's work. Sometimes, as well, the fetus is doubled over inside the womb, in which case the best course, as in the previous case, is for the attendant to use her hands to gently stretch the fetus towards the upper part of the uterus, positioning it properly for delivery.

Sometimes, the fetus is so large that it cannot exit. In this case, he must be tied and pulled out by force, after the exit passage is generously anointed. And if this can't be done, and it appears that the fetus will die along with the mother, the authorities teach that we should treat it as if it were dead—that is, to cut it into pieces that can be removed from the womb. This decision I leave to others. And if the labor is complicated because of the death of the fetus, we have already discussed the steps that should be taken.

Wherefore, *frontosa*, I want you to know that the improper position of the fetus for delivery is often the cause of its death as well as that of the mother. Sometimes the mother dies and the fetus survives, and sometimes the opposite occurs, the fetus dies and the mother survives. Clearly, this is a situation of great danger. And this is why, *frontosa*, when you are gravid, take care not to tire yourself, stretch, bend, kneel down, or undertake similar acts, so that the fetus in your belly does not assume an improper position, and so that in delivery neither you nor your baby die.

Eleventh condition: care for the extraction of the afterbirth. Often it happens that the afterbirth does not descend from the uterus and instead is retained inside it, causing great pain in the head and in the stomach to the woman who has given birth. To avert this, we advise that when the afterbirth partially presents itself, it should be tied and carefully pulled out, the passage having first been lubricated and softened. At that moment, the parturient should sneeze, aided by the powder of white hellebore called *sternuto*,[221] and when sneezing, she should hold her nose and mouth, so that with the force of the sneeze the afterbirth comes out from below. If the afterbirth does not come out, tie a ligature to the thigh of the parturient or perhaps to both thighs, and take care not to break the placenta. For this reason, these measures should be performed with great gentleness, making the parturient sneeze often as has been advised, and treating her with perfumes, and with other

---

221. *Sternuto* (or *starnuto*) is Italian for sneeze.

things given to her by mouth, or with ointments or poultices, as has been said, to assist the delivery of the baby.

But if the afterbirth still does not come out, lubricate the passage with chamomile or wallflower oil and with chicken fat, and apply the perfumes mentioned earlier as well as galbanum, myrrh, and opoponax; then take a big ball of oakum to seal a wooden bowl upside down, over her navel, creating a vacuum. Then secure the bowl over her belly well with a cord, and then make the woman sneeze as said before. If the orifice of the uterus is too narrow, widen it with a hand lubricated with very hot chamomile oil or wallflower oil, called by physicians oil of *keiri*, or with strips of greased cotton or wool cloth, as it seems best to you. And have her lie down, if you think of it, because it is good for her; and also if necessary, apply a poultice on her in the front and behind, and pour the stimulative substances into her uterus, as we discussed in the ninth section on facilitating labor.

And certainly, because the afterbirth corrupts and putrefies and causes undesirable outcomes, we don't want to deny the parturient any type of assistance. Therefore, if necessary, put her in a tub filled with a decoction of leaves and stalks of celery, and also the leaves of marsh mallow and mugwart and the leaves of dwarf elder or leaves of laurel, wall pepper, which is one of the most recommended ingredients, and also the moss that grows on oak trees. These are all good for this purpose. Among suppositories, a suppository is recommended that is made with root of iris infused with honey and inserted into the vagina.

Several of the ancients have recommended that midwives learn to pull out the afterbirth with their hands, something which certainly causes great pain and damage. In contrast, Avicenna and the moderns dislike this practice.[222] Avicenna prefers using perfume made to enter the vagina by a tube while the pregnant woman rests on a fumigation stool for the duration of one to two hours; and this perfume should be made of strong things that impel the fetus: rue, horehound, southernwood, and others that were mentioned earlier.[223]

---

222. See Avicenna, *Canon*, Lib. III, fen 21, tract. 2, c. 16 (p. 938): *Et de antiquis fuerunt, qui praeceperunt obstetrici ut involveret manum suam in panno, et intromitteret eam et acciperet secundinam, sed haec cura est dolorosa: nam quum non egreditur secunda, tunc ipsa carminatur, et egreditur post dies* (And there were some ancients who prescribed that the midwife should wrap her hand with a cloth, insert it and take the afterbirth, but this cure is painful: therefore, when the placenta does not descend, it is necessary to purge it, and it will come out after a few days).

223. See Avicenna, *Canon*, Lib. III, fen 21, tract. 2, c. 16 (p. 938): *ut ponatur medicinae acutae, sicut ruta, et prassium, et abrotanum . . . et approxima ipsum scamno, super quod sedet mulier, et ponet cannam in vulvam eius ut non egrediatur vapor, et dimitte eam secundum hunc modum duabus horis, donec permutetur secundina* (use acute medicines, such as rue, and horehound, and southernwood . . . and take that chair, on which the woman sits, and insert a cannula into her vulva so that no vapour escapes, and leave the woman like this for two hours, until the afterbirth is detached).

Twelfth condition: on the treatment for excessive discharge of blood. After labor, many times the menstrual blood flows more than it should, that is, for a longer period of time and in greater quantity, and because of this, the puerpera—that is, the woman who has recently given birth—is weakened. Accordingly, she should be treated with medicines or procedures that redirect the humoral flow. First, the arms and the hands of the recent parturient should be tightly tied with a cord, and cupping glasses placed under the right hypochondrium. Afterwards, soak bandages in vinegar and place them, first, over her belly, and then on her backside as well, above the sacrum, near the lumbar region. Make constrictive suppositories by mixing balaustine powder, yellow amber roses, and incense with astringent dark wine, bringing these ingredients to a boil and soaking the bandages in the mixture of these ingredients; and when cold, insert these pieces, like a suppository, inside the vagina, and repeat often. There are many who claim that the best medicine is a suppository made with uncombed wool filled with pig's feces.

Thirteenth condition: on the retention of blood. Often after giving birth to the fetus, the recent parturient is not treated with warm compresses because of negligence of the midwife, and blood is retained, thickens, and does not flow, as happens to metal when it is being cast into bells. This often happens in the delivery of males, because the attendants are more solicitous of the male child than of the mother.

When this occurs, it should be corrected in this way: the retained blood should be warmed up, thinned, and encouraged to flow. You may come to the parturient's aid with an external liniment, laying over her belly bandages soaked in hot water and a decoction of savin, some rue, and similar stimulative substances previously cited. Some consider the remedy of water of cyclamen or sowbread—which is very potent, and held in high esteem by your apothecaries of Ferrara—a great medicinal secret. Also, make suffumigations of myrrh, galbanum, and similar things, as prescribed. Make her sneeze at this time, as we said for the facilitation of labor. Because, *frontosa*, that which is retained may cause a tumor in the uterus. And if such remedies do not suffice, it might be necessary to bleed her from the vein that is under her knee, on the right side as well as on the left. However, this should only be done with the advice of the physician.

Fourteenth condition: care of fevers. At times the parturient may come down with a fever. But if this is the case, her care should be left to a physician, especially when her fever lasts long or when it is high. In the first few days, it is sufficient for her to take barley water with sweet pomegranates. However, if her fever lasts longer than it should, be careful, *frontosa*, because more often than not this occurs from the retention of menstrual blood. And the cure is to bleed the woman from the large veins in her legs or from under her knees. Go to the physician for this treatment.

Fifteenth condition: treatment for the dislocation of the sacrum. Sometimes after labor a woman's sacrum [the bone at the base of her spine connecting to the pelvis] does not return completely to the joint, making her cry constantly. I was called to deal with such a case, and investigating the cause of the pain, I made the following correct judgment: I had the midwife relocate the bone using both her hands, and the pain ceased immediately.

Therefore, *frontosa* midwife, pay attention and learn about this kind of relocation, and make note of it. The way to relocate the sacrum is to make the woman cross her legs, and pull as hard as you think necessary, but always gently; and then, with your hands placed over the sacrum, relocate the bone.

Chapter Three
On the regimen of the woman who has given birth

Since the pregnant woman has suffered pain in her labor, and she has lost so much blood, it is reasonable that she feels drained and weak. Therefore, it is necessary to restore her strength, because as Galen says, "food ought to be given immediately when the symptoms exhaust the strength."[224] But since it is not possible to restore strength all at once, it is necessary that you do as did that man from Forlì who was dying of thirst. When he reached an inn, the Florentine host would put only small amounts of wine in his glass, because as soon as the host put wine on the table, the man from Forlì would immediately drink it; and as often as the innkeeper replenished the drink, the man from Forlì would take more. And the host asked him, "O my dear fellow, what are you doing?" And he replied, "you decide how little, and I decide how often."

In this way, my ladies, these women who have recently given birth should be fed often and in small quantities, and they should have light, easy-to-digest foods that are nutritious, such as fresh eggs, capons, chickens, and hens; and for the rich women, partridge, pheasant, francolins, and similar things, and good, fragrant wines, not astringent ones—ideally white wines, or perhaps lightly colored wines. It is right that the woman who has recently given birth should be well cared for in the first few days, because a bad beginning makes a bad end. I have seen poor care lead to a poor constitution, which persists for many years following. Therefore, those of you who have the means, make sure that you are well-cared for during your labor.

O midwives, take care of your puerperae, the women who have recently given birth. In the first days, do not provide them with a diet that is too heavy, as often is the case. Overstuffing the new mother may cause her to break out in a fever or overstimulate her production of milk so that her breasts become overfilled,

---

224. In Latin in the text: *accidentibus prosternentibus virtutem illico dandus est cibus.* See Galen, *Commentarii in Hippocratis Aphorismos,* in Kühn, 17.2:380. Previously quoted at 145.

causing her pain and possibly lesions. This is why Avicenna rightly advised: "and do not change her food suddenly to a heavy regimen because that gives her fevers and increases her thirst and perhaps causes dropsy: for, if her liver becomes hard with this regimen, there is no hope for her health."[225] Therefore, *frontosa* midwife, do not allow the woman who has recently given birth to overeat, so that she will not face risks that could lead to her death. And you *frontosa*, who do not want your breasts to become as big as barrels because of such overeating, take note of what we say.

Now perhaps you may ask, *frontosa* midwife, "Maestro, how should I take care of her?" I respond that you should first consider her age, strength, and habits, because young recent parturients need more food because of their age, and the same is true for strong and robust ones, as well as those who in good health are accustomed to eating very well. For all of these women, I would prescribe a balanced regimen. Therefore, the wisdom of the midwife should be helmsman of this vessel, at times raising and at times lowering the steering arm.

I say that for the first seven days the recent parturient should eat four meals. In the early morning, she should have two fresh eggs with a little marigold[226] and drink a glass of good wine, and afterwards she should sleep. Four hours later, she should eat chopped hen or capon or something similar with pulverized marigold in that mixture and drink good wine; and if she can chew, she should add some toasted bread to her broth with marigold dissolved in this, to regain her vital strength. Afterwards, she should wait for six hours and then make a light meal of an egg with marigold and drink a glass of good wine. Then she should wait four hours and dine as she has previously had lunch; and as mentioned, give her more or less according to age, strength, and custom, because there are some that cannot live with so little food.

After the seventh day, increase the amount of food you feed the recent parturient, giving her eggs in the morning, as prescribed, and also some meat that she chews herself, with the appropriate drink and prepared accordingly. If she is a woman of hot nature, choleric or sanguine, then you should add sandalwood and coral to the preparation in order to cool her down. Now, if you ask for foods that are good for her, I would say that we discussed this in detail in the first chapter of this book: refer therefore to that section, but remember that good food produces good milk. If *frontosa* is constipated, it is urgent that she address this

---

225. In Latin in the text: *et non permutetur cibus subito ad regimen grossum, quare faciat eam febrire, et multiplicetur sitis eius, et fortasse fiat idropica: quod si induretur cum hoc epar eius, non speratur eius sanatio.* See Avicenna, *Canon*, Lib. III, fen 21, tract. 2, c. 3 (p. 932).

226. *Margaritone*, i.e. *margheritona*. Marigold, or pot marigold (*calendula officinalis*) was commonly used to promote the healing of wounds and for pain relief. It was believed to have antiseptic and analgesic qualities which would greatly benefit the overall health of a woman whose body has recently endured the trauma of live birth.

through evacuation as previously stated, with suppositories, a clyster, cassia, or even stronger remedies, such as diafinicon, or diacatholicon,[227] keeping in mind the importance of her evacuation with respect to the strength in her body and to her habits and quantity of the food she eats. Clearly, her regimen for the most part depends on the prudence of the midwife.

Therefore, my ladies, keep in mind that you must watch what you eat: because certainly overeating will make you waddle like a duck. Anyhow it is also true that, more often than not, one errs by not eating enough rather than from eating too much, and it is easier to remove the harm that follows eating too much than that which follows not eating enough: this is why Hippocrates says "In a restricted regimen the patient makes more mistakes, and thereby suffers more."[228]

Treatise Three
On raising children

Having written in the opening section of this work that I would deal with the raising of children until the age of seven, I will divide this third treatise into five chapters. In the first four, I will discuss the raising of children and all that pertains to their health and the well-being of their bodies. In the fifth, we will speak about the things that pertain to their moral life and the well-being of their souls. We will now begin with those things that the midwife should do in caring for the newborn child, especially for the preservation of his health.

Chapter One
What the midwife should do with the newborn child

As soon as the child is born, the midwife should take him into her arms, holding him gently and tenderly, so that she does not hurt any of his limbs. Afterwards, she should tie that which women call *il maestreto*[229] near the navel, with a twisted and strong string. Now keep in mind that wool thread is much better than string

---

227. In modern usage, "diacatholicon" means a panacea, or all-purpose remedy. In earlier medicine, diacatholicon was the name of a specific laxative made of cassia, tamarind, rhubarb, violet, anice, polypodium, sugar and the seeds of cucumber, courgette, cantalope and watermelon. See, for example, the recipe given in Valerius Cordus, *Dispensatorioum pharmacorum omnium* (Nuremberg: Paulus Kaufmann, 1612; first edition 1546), *sub vocem* Diacatholicon Nicolai, at 92 (the name *Nicolai* testifies to the antiquity of the recipe, reportedly dating back to the ancient medical school of Salerno, where a *magister* Nicolaus is considered to be the author of a widely known *Antidotarium*). "Diafinicon" was an ointment or purgative electuary made of palm dates. See, for example, Mesuae, *De re medica*, Lib. III.5 (p. 235): *Electuarium diaphoenicum.*

228. In Latin in the text: *in tenuibus dietis magis peccant egrotantes, ideoque leduntur magis.* See Hippocrates, *Aphorisms*, I.5 (p. 101).

229. *maestreto*: the umbilical cord.

made of linen or cotton, because wool is soft and relieves pain. This binding of the cord must be performed gently and not made too tight, so that it does not cause the baby pain. For as we know, improper binding often causes children to scream with pain, and the mother and wet nurse do not realize why, and they often attribute it to other causes, such as cold drafts of air or a pain in their children's stomachs. For this reason midwives should always keep with them the right kind of string.

After performing this binding, the *maestreto* should be immediately cut with scissors or a razor, about four to six fingerbreadths from the abdomen. And after cutting it, the midwife should cover the navel with a linen cloth soaked in hot oil, to mitigate the pain and to soothe this area: and she should continue to apply this hot oily cloth until what remains of the umbilical cord falls off from the navel, which will happen within four to eight days at most. Applying this cloth will also help the stump of the cord to fall off more quickly and to mitigate the pain from the binding, if indeed there is any pain. Once the umbilical cord is detached, the common practice is to apply a bit of flour to the navel for a number of days. Some women use crushed coal; but myrrh is better, or dragon's blood with a bit of sarcocolla, or myrrh with a bit of cumin; the ashes of burnt clam shells are also good. And if the navel gets infected from the incision, take Celtic nard, turpentine, pine resin oil, and sesame oil, and mix them together to make a plaster and apply this to the navel. Also, the ashes of burnt clam shells are recommended for treating this type of incision.

After this incision, it is common practice to place the baby in a bath, washing and cleansing him, as well as shaping his head and limbs, as will be explained. However, before moving forward, trusting in my predecessors' patience, I will add my own opinion with regard to this common practice. Since the bath lessens the newborn's strength, both because of its real heat (indeed, Avicenna considers it equivalent to exercise)[230] and because the fetus is tired and drained from the effort and exertion of exiting the belly, it seems to me that after cutting the cord it is better to swaddle the child in a cloth or soft, warm, blanket, and to leave him to rest for a while, depending on his greater or lesser exertion from moving through the uterus. So let us say that he should rest for a minimum of one hour and a maximum of three before bathing. The midwife should always make sure that the baby does not catch cold.

And in the meantime, it is important to return to caring for the woman who has just given birth, and the cleansing of her uterus, and making sure that she does not catch cold, so that her menses are not retained.[231] And if they were retained, give her aid as is mentioned in the chapter regarding retained menses, adminis-

---

230. See Avicenna, *Canon*, Lib. I, fen 2, doctr. 2, c. 19 (pp. 119–20).

231. As noted earlier, Savonarola has no distinct word for the lochial flow: he believes that the woman's menstrual blood has been accumulating throughout the pregnancy.

tering substances that stimulate bleeding. Also, because she is so debilitated, assist her by giving her good food and restorative drink, as is mentioned at the end of the preceding treatise.

Now that the mother is being cared for, we should return to the child, who is all oily and dirty and tired, filled with gas acquired in the belly and outside from the coldness of the air to which he has suddenly come into contact. His skin is very thin and so delicate that the tiniest harshness does him great harm and causes him to cry. It is important to give him a good bath, which will cleanse him, soothing his weary limbs, relieve him of his gasses and of superfluous humors, and help him to harden his skin; especially the first but also the second bath.

It has been proven that a bath given with seawater or saltwater, with an abundance of sage leaves, is much better than a bath with plain water, as is usually given. Therefore, it is good to understand, *frontosa*, the reason why this salty or seawater bath is so recommended, as I too emphasize and write about this type of bath as authorized by Avicenna, who says "and one should hasten to salt its body with lightly salted brine, until its navel becomes hard and its skin firm."[232] Therefore a child's first bath should be lightly salted. So, I conclude that Venetian women and those who have access to seawater should bathe their children in saltwater. And they should especially do this for the child's first bath, and perhaps the second bath as well, since this type of bath will not cause any harm, but instead will be of great benefit to him. After this, bathe the child regularly in plain water. Water from a river is better for a child's bath than water from a well.

Before moving away from the bath, I say that in hot weather, the child's bath should be moderate in temperature, verging on the tepid, and in cold weather it should verge on the warm, but not too warm, as Avicenna notes: "furthermore, in the summer it ought to be bathed in mild and tepid water, while in the winter in water which tends to be warm, but not excessively."[233] Do be careful, *frontosa* with thick-skinned hands, that you are not fooled when you test the bath water. Have the attendant with thin-skinned hands test it too, because many children in my experience have been scalded. Next, as said before, if the baby is very dirty, bathe him in saltwater twice the day he is born. Afterwards, proceed to plain water, doing this twice a day and three times if necessary, if he is very dirty. And on the topic of the bath, we will discuss its timing and the length of time that the child should be kept in the bath, and also the form and manner in which the midwife should bathe him. He should be bathed after his long nap, according to Avicenna.

---

232. In Latin in the text: *et festinandum est ad corpus ipsius saliendum cum salamoria tenuis salis, quatenus eius umblicus indurescat et ipsius cutis dura fiat.* See Avicenna, *Canon,* Lib. I, fen 3, doctr. 1, c. 1 (p. 164).

233. In Latin in the text: *ipse preterea in estate aqua suavi equali balneandus erit, in hieme vero aqua, que ad caliditatem trahat non pungentem.* See Avicenna, *Canon,* Lib. I, fen 3, doctr. 1, c. 1 (p. 164).

The baby should stay in the water until his skin starts to turn red, and after this, he should be taken out.[234]

Now, according to the authorities, the nurse should bathe the child with one hand behind him and the other on his chest, not on his belly. And according to Avicenna, he should first be bathed with his belly down, and after he should be turned with his belly facing up.[235] This allows bending of his lower parts from the chest down so that they receive the benefit as do the other parts from the chest up; this action opens the kidneys and their passageways which had been constricted in the mother's belly. And for this reason, Avicenna adds that the baby's feet should be raised towards his mouth and bent back towards his genitals.[236] When the midwife places the child in the bath, she should always hold him with his head upright, so that water does not enter his ears; she should handle him with care and with her hands, softly rub him, focusing on his limbs, and in giving shape to them she must be very careful and precise.

And the nurse should especially take great care in the molding of the baby's head, which houses the brain, an organ so noble that it most assuredly deserves an appropriate home; and we know that a distorted head that is poorly formed will certainly cause damage to the brain. And if you say "I have seen many with distorted heads who are very learned and erudite," I say, "I believe you, but if their heads had been better formed, I tell you they would have been even more sharp and erudite." By the head, I mean the cranium or bone that contains the brain. For it makes sense that the better the worker's instruments, the better and more beautiful the works he creates: just as a carpenter using dull tools cracks and ruins wood, while the one using sharpened tools creates beautiful objects; and similarly, just as a barber whose razor is dull nicks the skin and does not shave well. Therefore, one must pay great attention to the formation of the head, because this is how the brain, well-functioning by nature, may be made better or worse. And such is the nobility of the brain that Plato maintained that it should be named the first and principal organ of the human body, even though Aristotle maintained that the principal organ was the heart.

---

234. See Avicenna, *Canon*, Lib. I, fen 3, doctr. 1, c. 1 (p. 164): *Hora vero ad ipsum lavandum, melior est post eius longum somnum. . . . In hyeme autem . . . ipse quoque non lavetur nisi usque quo eius corpus calefiat, et rubere incipiat: postea extrahatur* (The best time to wash him is after his long sleep. . . . In winter, then . . . bathe him until his body warms up and starts to turn red, then take him out).

235. See Avicenna, *Canon*, Lib. I, fen 3, doctr. 1, c. 1 (p. 164): *Deinde fiat ut in primis super ventrem sui iaceat, postea supra dorsum* (then make sure that first [the newborn] lies on his belly, and then on its back).

236. See Avicenna, *Canon*, Lib. I, fen 3, doctr. 1, c. 1 (p. 164): *Amplius in hora ablutionis ipsius studendum erit ut ipsius plantae ad dorsum eius eleventur et eius pedes ad caput eius subtiliter et suaviter perducantur* (Also, at bath time, make sure to turn the soles of his feet towards the back and then try to gently and lightly raise his feet towards the head).

But it only makes sense that the midwife wonders and asks: "Maestro, what can I do to improve the shape of the head? Teach me." I respond that you should first make sure that the head becomes as round as possible. Then, grasp it well from the sides, that is, at the temples, so that the back part remains wide and the front tends to be sharper. This is why Galen, addressing the correct formation of the head, said that it should be like a sphere of wax—that is, a round wax object, pressed on both sides.[237] Once the head is formed, the midwife needs to give shape to the nose, lengthening it and tightening it as she sees fit to give it a good and beautiful form, so that it is neither too wide, nor too narrow, nor short, nor long; she should pull on it, if it seems too short, always keeping in mind a beautiful shape. Next, the ears must be managed, and they should be pressed as much as possible towards the head.

Next the midwife must wipe the baby's eyes gently with a silk cloth, or with a very soft and worn linen cloth. Avicenna maintains that the eyes should be cleansed with oil, because oil is very cleansing and it does not irritate or cause harm: he says "and we should put a little oil in his eyes."[238] Similarly, she should swab the baby's nostrils with water and oil and brush his palate with honey. The palate should be spread with her little finger, whose nail must be trimmed as short as possible. This is why every midwife should keep the nail of her little finger trimmed, just as that of her index finger should be kept long, as noted previously.[239] Next, with this finger the nurse should also spread open the genitals: because I have certainly seen here in Ferrara a child born without an apparent sex, just as also I have known baby girls to have their sexes covered by a tissue with a little hole, which barely allows the passage of urine: therefore it is important that the nurse be made aware of this.[240] And these cleansings should always be done to the child when he is bathed—although when performing the saltwater bath, the midwife should not cleanse the baby's eyes.

Next, she should extend the child's arms and then cross them, since with this manipulation, the arms reach their natural potential, that is, their natural length, given that they were crossed for so long in the womb. She should also extend the baby's legs in the same way, gently, and also bend them, so that his

237. See Galen, *The Art of Medicine*, Book I, ch. 6 (pp. 178–79); =Kühn, 1:320.

238. In Latin in the text: *et in eius oculos parum olei iniciemus*. See Avicenna, *Canon*, Lib. I, fen 3, doctr. 1, c. 1 (p. 164).

239. See Treatise Two, 155.

240. It is interesting that this is the only point in the text where Savonarola raises the possibility of ambiguous genitalia. The biological phenomenon of intersex conditions was certainly known in medieval Europe and received attention in civil law and medicine as well as natural philosophy. See Monica H. Green, "Caring for Gendered Bodies," in *Oxford Handbook of Medieval Women and Gender*, ed. Judith M. Bennett and Ruth Mazo Karras (Oxford: Oxford University Press, 2013), 345–61; Eva Pibiri and Fanny Abbott, eds., *Féminité et masculinité altérées: Transgression et inversion des genres au Moyen Âge* (Florence: SISMEL, Edizioni del Galluzzo, 2017).

heels touch his buttocks, as a form of exercise. Next, the midwife should press on the baby's bladder so that the urine may flow out more easily. And if one of the baby's legs is longer than the other, the nurse should pull on the short one gently so as to lengthen it.

Now take note, *frontosa*, how much prudence and agility of hands the midwife or nurse must possess, and how strong she must be to handle the child. This means that when she is old and her hands tremble, she can no longer perform this job; however, she can still teach her job to others. But heaven help those of us who wind up in the hands of a nurse who is too old, who is often the cause of the death of our children or of their difficulties of body and soul. Since we surely want our children to be raised by the most expert nurses, every experienced midwife, as if she were a doctor, should mentor apprentice midwives and teach them all they know.

Now you may ask how often children should be bathed, and I would respond that there is no fixed number given by the authorities, but common practice is twice a day for the first month, and after the first month, once every eight to fifteen days. Many bathe their children every eight days, and many do not use water, but instead bathe their children in wine.

And so here the question arises: "Is it better to bathe the baby in water or wine?" To satisfy the reader, I will respond to this question respectfully following ancient authorities [*cum pace maiorum*]. We recommend a bath in water over a bath in wine, as do Avicenna,[241] Rhazes,[242] Galen,[243] and all the ancient authors, following common practice: because the wine bath is too warm and provokes too much of a change in the infant, which is not good for him. But many say, on the contrary, that with a bath of dark wine, the baby's body parts relax more and are comforted, and that the wine bath counterbalances the coldness of the air experienced by the child while exiting the womb. But I contend, with the ancient authors, that a bath with water is better: for the wine bath is too intense, and its strong vapors could seriously damage the baby's brain, and expose his brain to the dangers of the outside air; and it could impede his growth and ruin his constitution as we will later discuss.

Continuing with the bath, we will say that the child should be bathed as described and even much more: certainly until the age of five, children should be bathed at least three times a month, since this is very beneficial to their health and to their growth. Although this is not the common practice, it is to be recommended wherever possible, and especially for the impoverished; for the strength and beauty of the body is a great gift for the child, which is why the proverb says

---

241. As previously noted, see Avicenna, *Canon*, Lib. I, fen 3, doctr. 1, c. 1 (p. 164).

242. See Rhazes, *Liber ad Almansorem*, tract. 4, c. 29 (fol. 76v): *Postea vero in aqua calida balneetur* (Then bathe them in warm water).

243. See, for example, Galen, *De sanitate tuenda*, Book I, ch. 10–11, in Kühn, 6:47–59.

"he who is born beautiful, is not born poor."[244] And take note, *frontosa*, if you do not want your children to be puny, you should follow the advice of Galen[245] and Avicenna,[246] and bathe them often, even though it is not commonly done, and let those who disagree rail against you. And after having bathed and tended the infant, the nurse should wrap him in warm swaddling clothes, extending his hands and arms wide to reach toward the knees. She should extend them no further than four fingerbreadths: it is said that boys or girls who have arms and hands so long that they reach past their knees are kinfolk of the Virgin Mary—and I saw one in the city of Feltre. Therefore, *frontosa* midwife, you should extend the baby's limbs as stated and later swaddle him, covering his limbs in cloth that is soft, smooth, and plush, lacking any roughness.

Make sure to cover the baby's head gently with a moderately close-fitting hood, and tie it with a strip of cloth so that the natural shape of his head is not altered: Avicenna notes "and its head ought to be wrapped with a cloth strip, and a close-fitting cap should be put on it."[247] I am well aware, *frontosa*, that some people will object to my writing things that are against common practice; but I am guided by reason and moved to write as authorized by respected and honored philosophers. So be sure to wrap the child with the right kind of swaddling cloths, and be sure that you do this with great dexterity.

I also believe that due to the fault of a nurse unskilled in swaddling, many children are made imperfect and disabled. I have seen this happen in the Friuli region, where a great many are lame, especially among the peasants and country folk, for very few gentlemen of that region are lame. I hazard to say that this is because the gentlefolk give their children the best care. Moreover, the stars may have great influence, as in Apulia, where there have been reported cases of women

---

244. *Chi nasce bello non nasce povero.* This proverb is included in the *Raccolta di proverbi toscani* compiled by Lionardo Salviati in the sixteenth century. See Accademia della Crusca, Banca dati: Proverbi: <http://www.proverbi-italiani.org/index.asp?m=0>.

245. See Galen, *De sanitate tuenda*, Book I, ch. 10, in Kühn, 6:53: *Est ergo id ea ratione alendum, ut constitutionis suae integritatem perpetuo servet. Servabit autem si quidem annis solo lacte nutrias, ac balneo dulcis aquae et calentis utare; quo videlicet corpus ejus molle quam diutissime servatum ad plurimum augmenti perveniat* (He should therefore be fed in order to always preserve the integrity of his constitution. And this is possible if, for a few years, you feed him only with milk, and bathe him in warm, plain water, so that his soft body, preserved for the longest possible time, can grow).

246. See Avicenna, *Canon*, Lib. I, fen 3, doctr. 1, c. 1 (p. 164): *Et plerumque quidem est conveniens ut ipse bis in die lavetur, aut ter* (And in most cases it is convenient to bathe him twice or three times a day).

247. Avicenna, *Canon*, Lib. I, fen 3, doctr. 1, c. 1 (p. 164): *et ipsius caput instita ligetur, et pileus ei imponatur, qui super caput eius constringatur.* According to Du Cange, *Glossarium*, *sub vocem* instita 2, vol. 4, col. 383a, *instita* refers both to the sash on a woman's dress and to a baby's swaddling cloth: *Vitta seu latum cingulum, ut solet esse id quo parvi in cunis ligantur.*

who have given birth to monsters along with an infant child:[248] that is animals, like grass snakes, frogs, bats, hawks, and similar things; this is not the case in all parts of Apulia, but only in certain areas, which is why I say the stars may be to blame.

The child, thus well-swaddled, should be put in a warm place and covered well, so he does not catch cold. This place should be as dark as possible. As Avicenna notes, "in addition, put the child to sleep in a house of moderate temperature, and not cold; furthermore, the house should be shaded and somewhat dark, not brightly lit by the sun."[249] Thereupon he should be placed in bed with his head raised. And when he is moved, whoever moves him should do so with care; he should be lifted all at once and not in a lopsided manner, so as to not hurt any of his body parts; and when he is put to bed, he should also be put down all at once. And after eight days, once his limbs are formed and strengthened, he should be placed in a crib, covered with a sheet, and the crib should be rocked, and the child should be cared for according to the six non-naturals, as we will explain next.

And now, because it is the season of carnival and masks are everywhere, I will tell you the story of a young masked girl, who was pregnant and not a virgin but had come to give birth, whose kinfolk, not wanting her to be recognized because she was a noble lady, covered her face with a mask. Now as her labor pains mounted and she could no longer keep silent, she removed her mask saying, "I would rather live and be recognized than die." Therefore, my ladies, I don't know what I should say about a *frontosa* maiden, who has fallen in love, and who spins a crooked spindle in the dark,[250] yet cannot possibly survive without a nurse and the many other treatments that we have discussed in this book. I believe that she

248. The strange phenomenon reported by Savonarola—also in his *Practica maior*, tract. VI, c. 21, rubr. 23 (fol. 265rb)—in which along with a healthy baby a number of small lizards, frogs or snakes were born, is nowadays thought to be connected to the different gestational developments of twins and the death in utero of some of them at particularly early stages. See O'Neill, "Michele Savonarola and the *fera* or Blighted Twin Phenomenon"; Zuccolin, *I gemelli nel Medioevo*, at 47–54. Medieval Salernitan masters also discussed the phenomenon of the so-called *frater salernitanus* ("Salernitan brother"), variously known as *arpa*, *pecus*, *bufo* or *crapullus*—a kind of small monstrous animal who appeared to be born just before the delivery of a viable and fully formed fetus. The belief was that if the *frater* was allowed to touch the ground after birth, the mother would die. Ausécache explores the moral connotations that were attached to this condition, indicating that some medieval writers suggested that its root cause was immoral behavior; see Mireille Ausécache, "Une naissance monstrueuse au Moyen Age: Le 'frère de Salerne,'" *Gesnerus* 64 (2007): 5–23. Most medical writers, however, kept to naturalistic explanations (such as excessive sperm or menstrual blood). Later writers associated it with the uterine mole, a phenomenon recognized in antiquity and now understood to result when a fertilized egg undergoes abnormal genetic growth.

249. In Latin in the text: *in domo preterea temperati aeris, que non sit frigida, ad dormiendum ponatur; oportet autem ut domus umbre attineat et tenebrositati alinquantule, que a superante radio non illuminetur.* See Avicenna, *Canon*, Lib. I, fen 3, doctr. 1, c. 1 (p.164).

250. On this metaphoric expression, see Treatise Two, 150.

cannot do this without great danger to herself and her child. Scoundrels will say that there is not really such great pain and danger in childbirth—and this is why I, with you, pray to God that one day these men will be made to suffer the same pains that you endure.

Chapter Two
On the regimen of children regarding the six non-naturals

Physicians maintain that in the conservation and preservation of the human body, the first thing that should be considered is the regimen, which consists of six things called by physicians the non-naturals: they are as the air, eating and drinking, movement and rest, sleeping and waking, repletion and evacuation, and accidents of the soul. Of these we will write according to our knowledge, and the knowledge obtained from the authorities and from common practice. Later we will follow with the things that threaten the good health of babies and that endanger their well-being, placing each under its own heading, focusing on the care of the ailments of children. Now according to our purpose, we will begin by expanding on the child's regimen, and on the way these six non-naturals should be regulated in substance, quality, quantity, frequency, time, and order.

To begin, we will say that sudden drafts of air, especially cold ones, are a much greater enemy of children than heat; therefore, children should avoid cold drafts as much as possible. And although there are many that cannot avoid the cold, still, it is mentioned here, as are other details that we will discuss, so that fathers and mothers may have instruction on these topics, and so that they may better know how to deal with them. Parents should also keep their children from stormy weather, because the winds and humidity it causes often lead them to catch catarrhs, inducing coughing, upsetting the stomach, causing fevers, and increasing the phlegm that generates worms, as we will later discuss. And similarly, excessive heat is bad for children. It loosens the catarrh and makes it descend, as the cold does because of its compression. This is said especially in the case of children who spend great amounts of time outdoors, but also of those who mainly stay indoors and are well-clothed: they too should beware. So, in conclusion, we will say that all children should be kept from the cold, because it is the cause of multiple ailments, including pains, worms, cough, diarrhea, fever, and others.

Now, washing of the head falls under this first section. We will recall also that when washing the baby's head, you should first be very careful that the soap you use is not too strong, especially when washing those at a very tender age, but as they grow in strength, you may gradually increase the dosage and strength of the soap. Now here I wish to blame those ignorant mothers, who immediately after washing their children's hair, tie kerchiefs on their heads and allow them to play outdoors; and in so doing, as the hair dries, the dampness descends to their eyes and to their chests and to other places, causing an imbalance. Similarly, I warn about drying the head at the fire or while standing in the sun: instead, the head should be dried with a heated towel if the weather is cold, and in the warm weather with tepid or cold cloths.

After discussing the air, we will now proceed to the child's eating and drinking, speaking first about the food's substance, then about its quality and quantity, frequency, time, and order. The first food that the child should take is milk, which I want to discuss thoroughly as to its substance, quality, quantity, and the frequency of feedings. First, I will say that the best milk for the child, which is most beneficial for his health, is that of the mother, when it is good and not spoiled. This is because it is similar to the nourishment he was receiving inside the womb, that is, menstrual blood, from which milk is made, as we have already said.[251] And I say "if it is not spoiled" because if the mother were for any reason in poor health, then it would be better for the child to take the milk of another healthy woman who possesses the traits of a good wet nurse that we will describe.

The first requirement of a good wet nurse is that she should be young, between the ages of thirty-two and thirty-four, and no older than thirty-five. This is because at this age, a woman is strong and she has developed to her full potential. The milk of a young girl is neither as good nor as perfect, not having reached perfection with age. When you cannot find a wet nurse of this age, you should try to have one who is close to this age. So, we will conclude, that the closer she is to such an age, the more suited she is nourish children than at any other age, and using the distance from this ideal age as a sure measure, you will know whether her milk is good or less than good. Similarly, we may also suggest that the milk of these girls who have had their first baby around the age of twenty is worse than that of those who did so in their thirties, although this advice is contrary to the common opinion of women. But what about the milk in wet nurses over the age of thirty-five? I say that until the age of forty it is fine; but after this, lacking youth and blood, the wet nurse will not be as bountiful as a younger woman. It is also true young women between the ages of twenty and twenty-five have a greater quantity of milk than those thirty to thirty-five years old, but this milk is not better because it is more watery.

The second requirement is that the wet nurse should have good color, since good color comes from good blood, and from good blood comes good milk. The third requirement is that she should have a sturdy neck and wide chest, which signifies strength and robustness, signs that she is in good health and consequently will provide the baby with good and healthy milk. Fourth, the wet nurse should be strong, practice healthy habits, and be neither too thin nor too fat: this will signal the abundance of the nourishment she can provide. Fifth, she should possess good and praiseworthy manners; she should not be choleric—that is, she should not be

---

251. On the identity of menstrual blood (one part of it) and milk, see Treatise One, 62 and 96, and Treatise Two, 128–29.

quick to anger, so that she does not spoil the blood; and she should also not be very melancholic or capricious, for if she were, the wet nurse might decide, either because of the baby's crying or for other reasons, to withhold milk from him, not being his mother, or not to soothe him or to ease his discomfort. O *frontosa* mother, fierce harridan, moderate, moderate your anger and disdain for your reasonless baby, and make sure to soothe your baby as much as your duty calls you to do.

The sixth requirement is that the wet nurse should have moderately large breasts but not unusually large ones, and her breasts should be firm and not too soft, which is a sign of watery blood. The seventh is that her milk should not be too old; instead, it should be fresh, that is between one and one half to two months from her parturition. The eighth requirement, which ensures the good quality of her milk, is that she has given birth to a male child, since this is a sign that her menstrual blood is purer, warmer, and better than if she had given birth to a female child. The ninth is that she should not be pregnant, should not have recently miscarried, and should not have the tendency to miscarry; for these would all mean that the nourishment she can offer your child is faulty. The tenth requirement: the wet nurse should nourish herself well in order to make good milk, and not choleric, salty, or scorched milk, which would give the baby milk crust and other ailments. But perhaps you will say, "such a woman is a white crow, impossible to be found." My response is that the woman fulfilling all of these conditions should be regarded as ideal, and the greater the number of these qualities she possesses, the better.

Oh gentle and delicate *frontosa*, who possesses so many of these qualities, how can you not want to breastfeed your child, taking into consideration the quality of his care, his good health and well-being, and even your own health and longevity? By not breastfeeding, you will get pregnant again very quickly, and then for most of a year you will have a disordered appetite, stomachache, backache, and similar ailments, and the number of your childbirths will multiply. And remember that every birth is a great blow to your own life, shortening it, and often causing poor health, and since your life is affected in this way, you often die younger because of frequent pregnancies. *Frontosa*, I have known many who have not wanted to breastfeed in order to conserve the beauty of their breasts and to be able to show them off in public, like those women who keep their breasts beautiful so as to display them to admirers. I want to remind you that your own milk is best for your child, especially as you would give it to him with greater care than does a hired wet nurse: and consider how much more you would love the child you have breastfed compared to the one you have not breastfed, and also, accordingly, how much more you will be loved by the child you have breastfed. Consider all the difficulties the child might experience because of the wet nurse; for if her milk is inferior because of her bad diet, your baby will cry more often, he will not sleep, and, as you can imagine, he will spend more time in soiled clothes; while with you, he would not face these difficulties.

I would also like to remind you that God gave you breasts like other animals so that you might nourish your children.[252] And as we will later explain, bad nourishment spoils the baby's constitution. *Frontosa*, you should always keep before your eyes the humble virgin mother of the son of God, who breastfed her own son and took such great care of him. If you are able, you should breastfeed your child, for his well-being and for your own good as well. And always remember what is said about the nipple of one's own mother. O wretched woman, who has bestowed more love on her lovers than on her own children, I can say with certainty that you have given the devil much pleasure, and also, that your failure to breastfeed is frowned upon by medicine. If you are rich and noble, keep a maid with you to help you with the tasks you fear you cannot manage if you are breastfeeding your child.

Now, after so many digressions made about the wet nurse, let us return to the nourishment that she must give the baby, that is, to milk, the desirable qualities of which we will discuss. And take note, *frontosa*, that even though all these qualities cannot be found in one type of milk, we still feel that the best milk contains the greater number of these qualities, while the milk that lacks many of these qualities is inferior. We say then that good milk should be in substance halfway between thick and thin, equally viscous and fluid, so that it does not dribble out from too much thinness and fluidity, nor should it be too strong and therefore not flow because of its viscosity and thickness.

And this can be determined by squeezing a little milk on a fingernail: if the woman bends her finger and it flows quickly from her fingernail, then it is too thin and watery; but if, on the other hand, she bends her finger and the milk remains clumped, and doesn't flow, it is too heavy and thick. The substance of good milk will lie between these two extremes. To test milk for its wateriness, the following experiment may be conducted on milk poured into a glass: throw into it a pinch of pulverized myrrh, then with a finger mix it, and the watery part should separate from the casein; and if it is good, then these two parts will be equal or close to equal; but if it is not good, you will know this because it will either be too watery

---

252. The recourse to wet nursing was the norm for medieval elites. Savonarola's invocation of maternal breastfeeding (just as happens in contemporary discussions on the same subject) is based on partly medical and partly moral, socio-cultural and even religious reasons. Medieval preachers and confessors openly condemned mothers who do not breastfeed their children, accusing them of knowingly circumventing the ecclesiastical ban on having sex during breastfeeding in this way. The medical stance adds physiological reasons to this perspective, such as the continuity between gestation and breastfeeding (since milk was considered, as previously noted, a refinement of the same blood that had first formed and then fed the fetus in utero), and the Aristotelian idea that nature does nothing in vain. Since women are provided with breasts, as is the case with other animals, breastfeeding inscribes itself into the order of nature. Savonarola already explained this in Treatise One, at 79. For an in-depth examination of this topic, see Van der Lugt, "Nature as Norm in Medieval Medical Discussions of Breastfeeding and Wet-Nursing," 563–88. See also in this volume the Introduction, 39–42.

or have too much casein. Now believe me, *frontosa*, it is rare for this perfect balance to occur; but we have brought it up here as a sign, or measure, in order to better understand different components of milk, etc.

Milk should not be frothy, because then it is not solid nourishment, and moreover, may cause nausea. Regarding its quality, milk should be white, not yellowish, green, red, or dark. It should smell good, not acrid, sour, tart, or salty, but sweet. Regarding quantity, it should not be too abundant, because if this were the case, the baby would fill up too quickly, which leads to indigestion and many other ailments, as we will discuss. And this is why, *frontosa*, you who have so much milk, note than you should always feed the child with moderation. We have already discussed the age of the milk: it should neither be old nor too new. And remember, *frontosa*, that your milk is made from your blood and the blood that comes from your food, and good generates good, whereas bad generates bad. Therefore, I can tell you that the use of leeks, garlic, onions, and similar things, which you eat gluttonously, causes many ailments for the baby. And these ailments will make you suffer bitterly from many rough days and nights, because these foods may cause your baby to develop pustules, milk crust, diarrhea, vomit, and often fever. So stay away from these things as much as you can.

Having spoken of milk, the first food that babies should take as nourishment for their first year—if possible, without giving them other foods, at least until they have sprouted teeth—but before moving on to other foods, we will speak of how the wet nurse or mother should feed the baby. The authorities do not recommend that mothers breastfeed their children on the first day—because their milk is altered by their labor, the pain and efforts of childbirth—so it is better for the baby to be breastfed by someone else: and if it is possible to wait two days, this is even better.[253] Next, before the baby is given any milk, it is better to give him a bit of honey, because he will then like it all the more, and the honey will cleanse his gums and tongue and sweeten his lips, and afterwards, it will sweeten the tip of the breast, the nipple from which the child receives great pleasure and comfort. And even though it is not common practice, the authorities maintain that it is better always to give babies a little honey before breastfeeding them.

---

253. This idea that the mother ought not breastfeed right after birth seems to have been common in the Middle Ages. See, for example, Avicenna, *Canon*, Lib. I, fen 3, doctr. 1, c. 2 (p. 164): *Oportet autem ne sit eius mater, quae ipsum prius lactat: donec matris complexio temperetur* (It is necessary that his mother is not the first to breastfeed him, until her complexion is balanced again). It is found also in the Middle English *Knowing of Woman's Kind in Childing*, where it is stated the child should not nurse from his mother until it had nursed from nine other women. See Alexandra Barratt, ed., *The Knowing of Woman's Kind in Childing: A Middle English Version of Material Derived from the Trotula and Other Sources* (Turnhout: Brepols, 2001), pp. 72–73. This, of course, stands in contrast to modern views that this "first milk," the colostrum, is in fact extremely important for the child, especially because it bears antibodies that will, for a time, protect the child from various diseases.

As for the mother's nipple, some write that this gives much comfort to the infant when placed at his mouth, and it comforts him by removing all his pain: as Avicenna notes, "so that, as already proven by experience, when the mother's nipple is placed in the mouth of the infant, it comforts him greatly by removing what is causing him pain."[254] And this can be seen from experience, that when a baby cries and feels pain, and his mother or wet nurse puts her nipple in his mouth, he is immediately comforted; which is why nipples are also known as pacifiers.

And [Avicenna] notes that for several days in the morning the mother should squeeze some milk from her breast, before giving her breast to the child, because the initial drops are aqueous and wheyish, not good like the rest of it. He also recommends that, in the same way, the wet nurse should always take some milk from her breasts before beginning, so that the baby does not take great quantities of the first milk, being hungry, because the milk from her initial flow can harm the baby, especially in the first days. And this she should do, in my opinion, when she has much milk; but if she does not have enough, it would not be advisable to do so. As Avicenna notes, "further, it is necessary in the whole course of breastfeeding, and especially at the start, that some of the milk be extracted so that it flows, and so that it may be aided by this extraction, lest it happen that sucking that is too strenuous injures the child's organs and he is debilitated."[255] Once she has placed her nipple in the child's mouth, the wet nurse must consider if the child takes the milk very greedily; if he does, he will also take much air with his milk, which will cause him to regurgitate and will cause him pains, so that the wet nurse should often hold back her nipple by putting her finger in front of it.

Second, the mother should not give the child great quantities of milk all at once, but instead divide the feedings into several, spacing one lactation from the other. And if you ask how much time should come between feedings, I will first quote Avicenna, who says "sucking the breasts twice or three times a day ought to suffice,"[256] thus recommending that the child should be given the breast twice or three times a day. And this is especially true on the first day, because as Avicenna then says: "and according to many, in the first days it ought to be nursed three times per day, just as on the first day."[257] And after the first days, the feedings must be multiplied, keeping reasonable space between them; as Avicenna says, "a lot

254. In Latin in the text: *ita, ut iam experimento certificatum sit, quod extremum mamille matris in os infantis ponere, valde confert ad removendum quicquid ei nocet.* See Avicenna, *Canon*, Lib. I, fen 3, doctr. 1, c. 2 (p. 164).

255. In Latin in the text: *in tota preterea lactatione oportet, et proprie in lactatione prima, ut lactis aliquid mulgeatur, et ut fluat, et ut ipsum pressione iuvetur, ne contingat, ut ex multa suctione gule ledantur instrumenta meri, et faciant debilitari.* See Avicenna, *Canon*, Lib. I, fen 3, doctr. 1, c. 2 (p. 166).

256. In Latin in the text: *bis aut ter in die sugere mamillas debet ei sufficere.* See Avicenna, *Canon*, Lib. I, fen 3, doctr. 1, c. 2 (p. 164).

257. In Latin in the text: *et secundum plurimum in primis diebus quoque lactandus est ut in prima die ter lactetur.* See Avicenna, *Canon*, Lib. I, fen 3, doctr. 1, c. 2 (p. 166).

of milk ought not be given to suck all at once: rather, it is better that a little be given to him to suck at frequent intervals."[258] I know it is common practice that our women give milk not three but eight to ten times per day, because they have no other way to satisfy their children. But I would suggest that they hold back as much as possible, and keep a notable space between one feeding and the next, so that the babies do not incur indigestion, which causes many other problems.

The nursing mother or wet nurse should continue this nourishment [i.e. milk], if possible, according to the schedule we have proposed. If the wet nurse does not have sufficient milk, then the child should be given certain foods, which we will now discuss, cutting these foods into small morsels or preparing them in a certain way. But first, I would like to elaborate on the baby's first nourishment; later we will also discuss other foods and how we can assist the wet nurse when she does not have enough milk. And returning to the milk, we will add that wet nurses should seek to know more about how they may improve their milk: first, through their own regimen, and second, by monitoring the milk they retain— whether it is spoiled, or how thick or viscous it is.

It should be said from the start, then, that wet nurses should be blamed when they eat foods that are detrimental to the production of milk, or that spoil it. This blame may be assigned to those who are able to choose good foods rather than bad foods; but because often, unfortunately, wet nurses are impoverished women, they eat and drink whatever they can, and by so doing they harm the milk that is meant to nourish the child, causing fevers and other maladies that could lead to the child's death. These women should not be trusted when they say that they are able to digest properly foods such as leeks, onions, etc., and are used to eating them: because, as Avicenna says, these foods are converted into bad milk, and they later may lead to various ailments. He says, "but those who digest bad foods should not be deceived by this, because after some days bad humors will be generated in the baby, making him sick."[259]

Therefore, *frontosa* to whom her child is dear, take note of these remarks when you breastfeed, when you are pregnant, and when you give your child to a wet nurse. It is important that the wet nurse not be greatly impoverished; and remember, too, as we have said, that she must be well-mannered and have some means of support, because she must be nourished with good foods that generate good blood for the health and long life of the baby. She should be especially careful to forgo celery, which causes falling sickness, as well as rue and rocket, which upset the milk, provoke menses, and upset the blood. Certainly every mother

---

258. In Latin in the text: *neque multum lac una vice ad sugendum dandum: imo melius est ut parum ei detur ad sugendum sepius interpositis spatiis.* See Avicenna, *Canon*, Lib. I, fen 3, doctr. 1, c. 2 (p. 166).

259. In Latin in the text: *ille vero in quo mala digeruntur nutrientia, ob hoc non decipiatur quare post dies in ipso mali generabuntur humores, egritudines facientes et provocantes.* See Avicenna, *Canon*, Lib. I, fen 3, doctr. 2, c. 7 (p. 175).

should breastfeed her child when possible and not fear the burden, just as she doesn't fear the burden when she goes out dancing, for in that she takes great pleasure. Instead, she should take great pleasure in helping her child, given that breastfeeding is so useful and beneficial to him, as has been said.

In the second treatise we discussed at length what foods are nutritious and make good blood, and which foods are good especially for the pregnant woman and generate good blood. Now we note further that the wet nurse should not eat acrid foods, like onions, garlic, leeks, scallions, mustard, and similar things; nor foods that are too hot, like pigeon, duck, strong wine, or pepper; nor foods that easily decay, like fruits, clams, oysters, freshwater fish, and milk, especially after meals; nor foods that may corrupt or inflame the blood, especially rocket more than other greens. And even though mint soothes the stomach, nevertheless, because it incites coitus, which greatly upsets the milk, the wet nurse should stay away from mint, especially if she is a widow.[260]

As Avicenna says, intercourse upsets milk significantly; he says, "in no way should anyone have intercourse with her: it corrupts the menstrual blood and the smell of the milk, and diminishes its quantity: so much the worse should she be made pregnant, which would thus cause harm to both [the child she is nursing and the newly-conceived fetus]."[261] O *frontoso* and *frontosa*, who love your carnal pleasure more than your child, take heed of the warning of so great and reputable a man: he claims that the wet nurse should not lie with a man at all, since such activity corrupts the blood, gives a bad smell to her milk, and reduces its quantity. Note, *frontosa*, that if you become pregnant, your pregnancy harms the child that you are nursing as well as the one in your body. I don't know what else to say, seeing how people despise and ignore these rules and follow common customs recklessly; but yet it is right and useful to bring this up, especially for those who are prudent and desire the welfare of their children. In sum, widows make the best wet nurses when they have the aforementioned qualities specified, and when they are well-mannered and chaste, and not in love with any man, because they will then give all their heart to the well-being of the baby.

260. As already mentioned, the church advised against sexual intercourse during lactation. Medical advice warned against coitus while breastfeeding as well: not only because it was thought to spoil the milk, but also as it could lead to a new pregnancy that would completely cut off the milk supply (to the detriment of the child at the breast), and harmed the newly conceived fetus. Since this was true for all women, the reason why Savonarola took care to especially warn widows against the use of mint must be sought in the medical conviction of their supposed greater eagerness for coitus. Since the time of Hippocrates and Galen, widows—as well as young virgins—were considered prone to uterine ailments caused by the retention and corruption of the menses and seed. Coitus was considered a kind of cure in this case, and the desire for coitus was explained by doctors precisely with the natural need of these women to get rid of accumulated superfluities.

261. In Latin in the text: *Nec ullo modo aliquis cum ea coeat: hic corumpit sanguinem menstruum et lactis odorem, et ipsius minuit quantitatem: imo fortasis impregnatur, et sic fit nocumentum filiis duobus.* See Avicenna, *Canon*, Lib. I, fen 3, doctr. 1, c. 2 (p. 166).

The good wet nurse should behave like a good head of household, who gives all his heart to his family, who tries his best to nourish his family with good food so that they avoid illness, who takes into account all the needs of the family. For this reason, she must often consider the condition of her milk, if it is insufficient or spotty or too viscous or too watery or if it has any other undesirable qualities. She should provide for the child as the head of household serves wine to his guests, decanting it from one vessel to another when it is too warm.

For example, if the wet nurse recognizes that her milk is too viscous and thick, then she should turn to things that will dilute it and things that are sharp, like oximel or vinegar sweetened with honey. She should take hyssop and oregano in her foods, stay away from pastries, as well as fatty and aged meats and from everything glutinous; she should drink light white wine that is not turbid, and eat red chickpeas, always adding saffron to these. And similarly, if her milk is hot, she should partake of cool foods: lettuce, endive, squash, and similar things. And if it is cold, she should eat warm foods. If her milk is too thin, she should eat heavy foods, and avoid heavy exercise, which tends to thin out the humors, but exercise moderately; and she should drink young wine in this case, which will be beneficial, and also sweet wine; and she will benefit more from sleep than from staying awake.

And if the wet nurse smells a foul odor in her milk, she should consume fragrant wines and foods that generate good blood and stay away from foods that provoke menses, as well as foods that diminish the blood, of which we have spoken in the second book. And if the wet nurse should become ill with diarrhea or any other communicable disease, she should give the child to a healthy wet nurse until she recovers her health. And similarly, if it is necessary for the wet nurse to take a laxative, for that day the child should be breastfed by another, or he should be given food without milk.

But *frontosa* may say, "Oh my maestro, you provide sound and beautiful teachings on raising and caring for newborn babies. But who is able to observe these rules? Who will be able to observe so many of them? It is so easy to propound the rules, but observing them seems so difficult to me. So how is it that babies live when their caretakers fail to follow so many regulations?" My reply is that yes, indeed, it is truly difficult to observe all these rules, and many babies live although these regulations are not all followed; but on the other hand, I tell you that many die or are sickly and unwell from not having been treated according to these regimens. Therefore I have laid out these rules before you as a mirror, so that in it you may see the errors that you and other wet nurses commit in raising and nourishing babies, and so that babies are better cared for.

And if you ask how long a child should be breastfed, I say that the natural time period, as Avicenna says, is two years, especially in males—this is because their life expectancy is higher than in females—and females should be breastfed until they are eighteen to twenty months old. But people often disregard these timelines, and either because of expense or for another reason, they abbreviate them. There are also some physicians who abbreviate these timelines and others who extend them significantly, but what has been said remains the common practice. And in weaning, Avicenna advises putting myrrh on the nipple, while common practice is to apply aloe or theriac.

And before moving on to the cure for the diminution of milk and ailments suffered by children, we will proceed to the other five non-naturals, such as movement and rest, sleeping and waking, repletion and evacuation, and the accidents of the soul, saying first that the child of one or two months, until he starts walking, can be exercised in three ways.

First, by rocking the cradle. After being given the breast he should be placed in his cradle, as is the common practice, and it should be softly rocked, so that the milk he has received does not become excessively agitated in his stomach, and so that he does not receive harm from this rocking. This is why nurses that rock the cradle with force or those who rock the cradle on an uneven floor are to be reprimanded, because in doing this they shake the child excessively. Similarly, when nurses wrongly allow other children to rock the cradles, those who rock without discretion, they often overturn the cradle and the children fall to the ground, and from this the child may damage some of his parts, and this accident may leave the child lame or deformed.

Second, babies should be left to cry a bit before they are given their milk, because such crying is good for them and is to be considered good exercise.

Third, in the arms of the wet nurse, the baby should be shown objects that give him pleasure, like a bird, a rose, or something similar. The nurse should put this object before him, and make him turn from side to side, so that he turns his eyes and his head, neck and shoulders. And similarly she should grab the baby's little hands, gently moving his arms, and make him laugh by tickling him, doing other things, like lifting him on his feet and jiggling him one or two times, so that his whole body moves, and only after this should she give him his milk. And this could be exercise for those who cannot yet walk; and having said this, we will later discuss exercise for children who are able to walk.

Of sleep, we say that babies should sleep more than they are awake, because sleep comforts the powers of the body more than wakefulness, as Averroes notes: "sleep binds the virtues together, and comforts them."[262]

On retention, it has already been said that babies should not be given excessive quantities of milk. But it is also true that some are greater feeders than others; so this quantity is not easily measured and prescribed, but instead it is best left to the discretion of the wet nurse.

---

262. In Latin in the text: *sompnus est ligamentum virtutum, confortatioque earum.* See Averroes, *Colliget*, II.21 (fols. 16vb–17ra).

On his evacuation, when the baby is constipated, we will say for the moment that you may treat this condition with barley sugar or honey, or beet sugar, or some mouse dung, which is a stronger remedy. If necessary you may use a clyster of broth with honey and butter, or of pure milk with sugar, or of broth and sugar.

And on the accidents of the soul, I say that one should never frighten the child. We will later explain the reason. Instead one should sing softly to him, for song delights him, and the pleasure it gives is very beneficial to the child and comforting to his spirits.

This is the regimen that should be followed for children until their teeth come in. Before this they should not be given anything to eat except milk, if possible. But if for whatever reason you cannot do this, you may give him some well-cooked pap, as moist as possible, made with oil or almond milk or broth with just a little saffron. And because necessity does not follow rules, I do not add further rules for this age.

As soon as the babies' teeth start to come in, when they are eight or nine months old more or less—I say this because some children delay, while others anticipate dentition—at this point they should be given other foods that will offer them more nourishment than milk; for at this stage, it would be wrong to keep them on just milk. As Avicenna notes, "after the incisor teeth begin to appear, the child must be led to nourish himself in a progressive way on food, which makes him stronger. However, he must not chew on hard things, so at first let the nurse chew his bread for him."[263]

Thereupon, it is important that the baby be given small morsels of food, well chewed, as is common practice, and that he be given this at regular intervals, not often, like milk. But take note, *frontosa* who has an old mother who has rotten teeth and whose breath often stinks, do not allow her to pre-chew the food for your child. And also when you are ill, do not pre-chew it for him; but have someone else do this for him, some young healthy maiden. Next, I recommend that when you want to pre-chew food for your baby, wash your mouth with wine or water, then chew a morsel and spit it out and rinse your mouth again, and then you may proceed to give him the morsel; this is because your mouth, especially in the morning before having eaten, is filled with bad vapors that have arisen from the stomach or of catarrh descended from the head. Next, give the baby pap you have made with sweetened water. This is good to cleanse him and help him to grow. Other good foods are bread moistened with watered wine, and pap made with milk, or even thoroughly cooked rice with milk.

---

263. In Latin in the text: *Postquam duales aparere inceperint dentes, ipse ad nutriens movendus est ordinate, quo fit fortis. Res tamen dura ad masticandum non erit danda, imo detur ei primo panis quem masticavit nutrix.* See Avicenna, *Canon*, Lib. I, fen 3, doctr. 1, c. 2 (p. 166).

But here I wish to remind you of a rule for children, which you should remember. In nourishing children, you must make certain that their foods are moist. This is because, in order to grow, they need moisture, which promotes growth, while dryness, its opposite, stunts growth. Also, the child's constitution at this age is humid, which is why he needs moist things, although in moderation. And this is why the wise old sage Hippocrates says, "A moist diet is beneficial in all fevers, especially in the case of children and of those used to such a diet."[264] And Avicenna notes that "the infant's regimen is moist, for it suits his complexion, and he needs it for nutrition and growth."[265]

Proceeding with these recommendations, it helps children to grow if you continue with frequent baths, as the authorities strongly recommend. I advise that when they are three to four years old until the age of six, they should be bathed from three to four times per month, even if this is not the common practice. Furthermore, it is not good for children to live on bread alone, as is the common practice, or on morsels made from bread with just nuts, which do not stimulate his growth, but instead a morsel made of bread and almonds is much better for him. Second, a morsel soaked in wine, diluted in a good amount of water is also very good, and feeding him this type of morsel is also common practice especially among the impoverished.

Wealthy women err in giving the baby bread soaked in fine wine, saying that it strengthens his head and that it protects him against worms. O foolish ladies, remember what Avicenna, the great authority, says: "to give wine to children is like adding fire to fire in flammable wood."[266] Children should not be given wine at all, or as little as possible. Using wine causes fevers and then you, foolish ladies, attribute the cause of the fevers to other reasons.

However, broths and brothlike foods made from quality meats and meat morsels are good for him, as is diluted wine. And as has been said, the child should not be overfed, because eating too much may lead him to vomit and fatten his belly, which is why he should be kept from certain foods that should be given to him only sparingly.

Regarding the child's exercise, I advise that it should be moderate. As I have previously stated and remind you once more here, the bath stands in for exercise, and encourages the child's growth; this is why Avicenna often reminds us that children should be given a bath regularly. Therefore, from three to four months

---

264. In Latin in the text: *humide diete omnibus febricitantibus conferunt, et maxime pueris, et aliis sic assuetis refici.* See Hippocrates, *Aphorisms*, I.16 (pp. 106–7).

265. In Latin in the text: *infantis regimen est humectatio, propterea quod eius complexio ad hoc est conveniens, et quod ea in sui indiget nutrimento et augmento.* See Avicenna, *Canon*, Lib. I, fen 3, doctr. 1, c. 2 (p. 166).

266. In Latin in the text: *dare vinum pueris est sicut addere ignem igni in lignis debilibus.* See Avicenna, *Canon*, Lib. I, fen 3, doctr. 2, c. 8 (p. 180).

until they can walk, bathing children at least once a week is very healthy. This also, as we have said, is not common practice, but it is reasonable and recommended.

Moreover, when children reach the age when they have teeth, and they begin almost to chew, it is still necessary to assist them, to mitigate the pain in their gums and to help their teeth to sprout, by rubbing in fats like that from hare's brain, butter, or chicken fat, two times a day, in the morning and evening. Later, when the child begins to speak, you should often rub his tongue with salt and honey; rubbing his neck and throat with oil is also beneficial. It is also good to give him barley broth to drink and to rub this broth on his gums. And when his gums become sore, which you will know when he begins to put his finger in his mouth, and also when he begins to bite, at this point, you should take a bit of root of blue lily, not too dry, and make him chew on this: this will be very beneficial, mitigating the pain of his gums, healing their ulcerations, while protecting his gums from further ulceration. Continuing to rub the child's mouth with salt and honey greatly helps to prevent pain in his gums. And when all his teeth are in, the child should chew licorice root, not too dry. And when he begins to speak, you should rub the child's teeth with salt and a little honey.

Not to repeat myself, I will briefly speak of the child's regimen until the age of seven, which should be as follows. First, regarding air, he should be protected against drafts. Of food, as he grows and his chewing is stronger, he may be given more solid foods as long as they are of good quality, such as quality meats and bread that has not been soaked. Of wine, the child should drink only small amounts, diluted more or less depending on its strength and the age of the child, since older children may drink less-watered wines. White is better than dark wine. Another wine that is good for them is the *gorreto* or *gauro* wine.[267] And children should be supervised in their eating, kept away from fruits and similar foods that physicians consider harmful, and fed a variety of foods so that they grow accustomed to the diversity of foods that they will encounter in their lives; and care should be taken that they eat moderately. In the summer and winter, children should eat when they wake up, then have lunch, a snack, and supper, as is common practice.

Also children should be put to bed at a good hour, so that they can wake up at a good hour, since certainly, *frontosa*, an early riser is a good worker; however, if the child wants to sleep more, he should be left to sleep and not forced to get up from bed. On exercise, we have discussed those exercises for children who cannot yet walk; but here, so as not to be repetitious, I will continue with advice on exercise for small children from the ages of three to four. At the end of this book, we will discuss with regard to the well-being of their souls the exercise regimen for children aged five to seven.

---

267. *Gorreto*, also called *gauro*, refers to a light wine. See Treatise Two, note 128.

When, therefore, the child begins to walk, he should be leaned against a bench, as is common practice, and the wet nurse should always stand behind him; and she should not lead him by the arms, because through such leading a sudden movement could dislocate his arms. And if such a bench or table is round, so that the nurse may keep an eye on him from all sides, the child will be safer, because the nurse can follow him from all sides. And when the child feels confident about moving his little legs and walking, the wet nurse should then distance herself from him, and call him, coaxing him, until he feels confident in walking without leaning; but someone should always be behind him, so that he does not take a bad fall. Later, when the child is more sure of himself, he may walk behind a cart. Once the child is comfortable walking with this cart, put it against a wall that is far away, and then throw either a ball or an apple or something else far away from him, and coax him to walk over to fetch it. And then, surely, little by little, he will begin to walk. From twenty months or two years onward, he should be allowed to play with other children, climbing on logs, as is common practice, running, etc., or playing catch with a ball that makes him run from one place to the other. And this should go on till he reaches the age of three, as is common practice. From the age of three to five, a child should learn restraint and be made to stay more still; and in this quieter time, you may begin to introduce him to moral lessons, as we will discuss in the last chapter.

But here I will not overlook the advice of Avicenna, who advises that children should be bathed often till they reach the age of seven; he says, "when the child is roused from sleep, let him be bathed, and then let him be left to play for an hour; afterwards let him be given a little something to eat, then let him be left to play freely; and afterwards bathed again, and then fed."[268] Although this is not common practice among us, I mention this, so that it be done twice a week or at least once, as this would be beneficial. Young children should not be overfed, as mentioned before. And if they are constipated, they should be assisted, as said before, either with remedies or clysters. At the end of this book, where we will deal with behavior for children until the age of fourteen,[269] we will discuss the accidents of the soul, such as anger, sadness, happiness, fear, and similar things.

And now that the requirements for the wet nurse and the importance of a child's nourishment have been discussed, since often good nourishment is lacking, which causes great harm to children, and desiring to provide aid to those who need it, I will add here a third chapter, that will be on the causes of the reduced production of milk, and its treatment.

---

268. In Latin in the text: *cum autem puer a sompno excitatur, balneandus est, deinde dimittendus ludere hora una, postea ad comedendum aliquid ei dandum, deinde dimettendus ludere prolixius, postea balneandus, deinde cibetur.* See Avicenna, *Canon,* Lib. I, fen 3, doctr. 2, c. 4 (p. 169).

269. On the inconsistency of referring to a paragraph on the behavior of children up to the age of fourteen, which Savonarola does not actually deal with, see in this volume the Introduction, note 135.

Chapter Three
On the reduced production of milk and its treatment

Frontosa, since this often happens to the wet nurse and can be of harm to children, and since also I want to be helpful to women and appreciated by them, my intention being to assist them as much as possible, I have decided to expand on this topic significantly in this chapter. I hope that such verbosity will not be considered at all tedious to my readers, first, because it will not be too prolonged, and second, because this section will be useful and even entertaining. To begin, since milk increases due to an increase in blood, then milk also decreases when the amount of blood decreases. However, the blood, from which milk is made, may decrease for many reasons. First of all, it may decrease from lack of nourishment, as when the wet nurse does not have enough to eat and when she drinks only water. And take note, *frontosa*, you who do not mind giving your child to a wet nurse so as to rid yourself of the burden of breastfeeding, and you, *frontoso*, who disregard the fact that the wet nurse is impoverished as long as you get her for a good price, O wicked parents, you should expect to be punished severely for this, first by God, and secondly by the many problems that will result from the bad nourishment that these wet nurses provide your child.

Even if she has enough to eat, problems arise when the wet nurse eats things that diminish blood, such as millet bread, bread made from bran, sorghum, favas, or lentils; or when she has too much vinegar, watery greens, greens such as purslane, and similar things. These foods are too moist and could diminish milk, especially in phlegmatic nurses, although those who are choleric and with hot dispositions may take these things more safely. Cold and dry foods such as lentils, millet, fava, panicum, salted cheeses, and similar things also cause problems. Moreover, blood becomes scarcer with age, as is generally said, and this scarcity reduces milk; this is why the wet nurse should not be too old. Therefore, he who wants his children to survive, and to be healthy and robust, he should have them fed by a wet nurse who eats good food and fine wine; I don't mean great and fancy wine, just good, wholesome table wine.

If it happens, moreover, that because of a bodily defect, the wet nurse should suffer from an imbalance either of cold or heat, she should regulate herself by taking the opposite things. For example, if she is imbalanced by heat, she should take barley water and eat barley pancakes; she should add seeds to her pap with sugar, mallow leaves, spinach, chard, and lettuce. And if she is imbalanced by cold, she should eat hot foods like rice, fennel, wild thyme, wheat pancakes with sugar, spelt, and sweet almonds, and also broth made with choice meats, eggs, etc. And similarly if she is imbalanced by dryness, she should take moist things.

And this kind of imbalance explains why we often see wet nurses dry out. If her breasts have too dry a complexion, her breasts will harden and become smaller; and if her blood is too watery, her milk, too, will be watery; and if her complexion is very dry, her milk will be too dense. And if choler is mixed with her blood, the milk becomes less nutritious than it should be, and will be yellowish, and bitter in taste; if her blood is mixed with phlegm, the milk will be very watery and will taste vinegary and be white in color; and if it is mixed with melancholy, the milk will be dark, thick, murky, and very scant compared to the dense or watery milk previously mentioned. And note, *frontosa*, as Christ says, *a sad spirit dries the bones*,[270] so know that melancholy reduces milk.

And if she suffers from partial or complete obstruction of the passages that lead to the breasts, then her breasts will deflate, and produce very watery, weak milk, and her urine will also be watery and weak. In this case she should take broth made of red chickpeas, fennel, melon and watermelon seeds, and similar appetizing foods, cold or hot, as necessary. Moreover, this condition could arise from the breasts catching cold from being uncovered for too long; this is why, *frontosa*, you should be modest and keep them covered; if necessary, warm them with chamomile oil and with a warm cloth or also a cloth infused with a decoction of chamomile flowers and dill.

The wet nurse may also run out of milk if she suffers from a discharge of blood from the nose or from hemorrhoids, or if she loses blood from another place;[271] or if she has ulcerations or fevers that cause dehydration; or if she has performed too much physical labor, tiring herself by tilling the soil all day in the fields like a peasant, or spending too much time weaving at the loom.

And so, *frontosa*, you have nine causes that explain why the wet nurse may lack milk. The first is a deficiency in her nourishment. The second is the consumption of things that decrease or dry out the blood, or cause an imbalance of heat, of cold, or of humidity, which alters the complexion of the blood. The third is when the body of the wet nurse is generally imbalanced. The fourth is when her blood is mixed with different humors, such as choler, phlegm, and melancholy, making the milk less nourishing. The fifth is the obstruction of the passage of blood to the breasts. The sixth is the bad complexion of the breasts. The seventh is if the wet nurse suffers blood loss. The eighth is if she has ulcerations and fever. The ninth is if she is too tired, which spoils the blood that must be converted into milk.

To these we could also add a tenth, *frontosa*, for an incantation or spell might cause the milk not only to lessen, but even to completely disappear. In the

---

270. Proverbs 17:22: *spiritus tristis exicat ossa*. The Vulgate reads: *Animus gaudens aetatem floridam facit; spiritus tristis exsiccat ossa*. These words are not spoken by Christ.

271. On vicarious menstruation, and particularly on nosebleeds, as perceived by ancient and medieval physicians, see Gabriella Zuccolin and Helen King, "Rethinking Nosebleeds. Gendering Spontaneous Bleedings in Medieval and Early Modern Medicine," in *Blood Matters: Studies in European Literature and Thought, 1400–1700*, ed. Eleonor Decamp and Bonnie Lander Johnson (Philadelphia: University of Pennsylvania Press, 2018), 79–92.

Slavonic regions within the Venetian domain, women possessed by the devil use incantations or spells to steal each others' milk. And for this act they accuse each other before a judge or magistrate, and the judge for this behavior imposes a fine on them, without any other revenge or punishment; and in this way milk is restored to the woman from whom it has been taken. And this anecdote is most certainly true. I have told it not because it has anything to do with medicine, but because it tells of an amazing and diabolical act, as well as for the pleasure of the reader.

And since we have so many causes with so many remedies, we will proceed to discuss the treatment for this condition, recalling many helpful cures. And since we are writing for women I will create an epilogue that gives some simple remedies to correct a woman's lack of milk. We say, therefore, that if it is due to paucity of food, then the quantity of her food should be increased, and it should be good food, generative of good blood; but if it is because of the bad complexion of the wet nurse or of the milk or of the breast, this must be corrected with opposites; and if caused by the mixture of humors with the milk, these humors must be removed; and if she lacks milk because of loss of blood, it should be stanched; and if because of ulcerations, they should be cured; and so on.

Now we come to the remedies that help produce milk. The first is very effective: take two eighths [of an ounce] of ground sesame seeds with a glass of sweetened wine, drink it warm, in the morning, three hours before getting up, then sleep a bit more. Another valuable remedy is wheat pancakes made with water where fennel seeds had previously been boiled, with chicken fat or butter and hot sugar, or a light broth of capon or chicken, etc., with eggs and sugar. You can also take chickpeas previously soaked for four hours in an infusion of sheep's or cow's milk, and later dried.

Another helpful remedy is four ounces of rice washed four times and dried barley, well-ground, and peeled wheat, three ounces of each, plus one ounce of peeled almonds, and one and one-half ounces of white poppy seeds; of this mixture one half should be taken and it should be well-cooked in milk, and the rest boiled until a third of it evaporates; and it should be given to the wet nurse warm and with sugar every day three hours before she rises, and she should then sleep, and take it again three hours after getting up; and this should be repeated for four to five days: and this is an effective remedy.

Also, take honeycomb, the home of bees, two and one-half ounces, one ounce of fennel leaves, one-half ounce of purslane, one and one-half ounces of crushed wheat, crushed chickpeas and dried barley, one ounce of each, and six dried figs; bring all of these ingredients to a boil in fourteen pints of water until three-fourths of it has evaporated, so that little more than three pints remain; and this drink should be given to the wet nurse in the morning with some sugar as prescribed, four ounces at a time, and this treatment should be continued for four or five days.

Now if her milk should return quickly, the wet nurse can stop taking this remedy right away; but if her milk doesn't come back, she should continue taking these remedies, alternating between one and the other, and she should interpose one or two days between each cure depending on her progress. The following are also recommended to increase milk production: wild thyme, rosemary, radish, rutabaga, candhar leaves, anise, fennel, dried chickpeas, cardamom, savoy, lettuce, mallow, barley, pennyroyal, and poppy seeds. But perhaps *frontoso* will object that Avicenna says, "and among those things diminishing the milk is poppy seed."[272] But I believe that he means poppy seed when it is used for an external plaster, because its coldness and dryness diminish it. At this point I think we have said enough about this particular condition.

Now I shall go on to the cures for the ailments of children, to be discussed in the fourth chapter, by the grace of God.

Chapter Four
On the treatment of small children[273]

Since I am writing more for women than for men, I shall put forth several cures for certain ailments which typically occur in infants while they are breastfeeding and when they are in the arms of their wet nurse. However, if they become sick after this period, then their fathers should take primary responsibility, seeking the help of skilled physicians. But this does not exclude providing women with remedies that they can use to succor older children.

If I wished to describe all the possible ailments that could afflict a child, I would need to translate all of medicine into the vernacular, and this would not only be impractical for women, but also for those who are illiterate. Moreover, it would be a huge burden for me; and besides, it might result in more deaths than

272. In Latin in the text: *et ex minorantibus lac est semen papaveris*. For poppy seeds as milk reducing substances, see Avicenna, *Canon*, Lib. III, fen 12, c. 3 (p. 687): *et omnes medicinae minorantes sperma, sunt minorantes lac. Illae autem, quae ex eis sunt frigidae, sunt sicut semen papaveris, et lentes* (and all medicines that decrease sperm also decrease milk. Among these, those that are cold are poppy seed and lentils). Confirming Savonarola's point is instead Avicenna's conflicting recommendation of poppy seed to increase milk production at Lib. III, fen 12, c. 2 (p. 686): *et scias quod omne quod exuberare facit sperma, exuberare facit in pluribus corporibus lac, sicut semen lactucae et semen papaveris* (and know that everything that increases the sperm also increases the milk in most bodies, like lettuce and poppy seed).

273. Savonarola titles this section on pediatrics *De curis puerorum*, following Rhazes, his main source: *On the Treatment of Small Children* (*De curis puerorum*): *The Latin and Hebrew Translations*, ed. and trans. Gerrit Bos and Michael McVaugh (Leiden and Boston: Brill, 2015). This work was also known as *Practica puerorum*, *De morbis puerorum*, and *De egritudinibus puerorum*.

recoveries, because novices would recklessly attempt to practice medicine solely by following recipes, as the charlatans do who do not fear God, not understanding the rules that teach how these recipes should be applied.

Therefore I will write about a few of the illnesses that usually afflict children, omitting those illnesses that are less common, together with their cures, dealing with the medications for children that are most effective. But since the first thing that a physician should do is investigate the cause of the ailment, I will begin by saying that often children experience illnesses that may be linked to the wet nurse, or that are caused by the humors that are deficient in the infants themselves.

Therefore, if an ailment is caused by a problem with the wet nurse, who may have corrupted blood, and since this may lead to the infant being filled with bloody boils or pustules, it would then be best to first bleed the wet nurse, and later adjust her regimen to a quantity less than what she is used to, so that she will generate good blood. Afterwards she may be purged of phlegm or other humors that corrupt the blood. And if some fear that bloodletting will diminish the production of milk, then a cupping glass may be used on the wet nurse. Similarly, if she is filled with other humors, as we will later discuss, then it would be necessary to evacuate her, increasing the humor that is deficient. And similarly, if the baby were to suffer because of any other problem of the wet nurse—constipation or diarrhea or chest pains or a cough, or anything else—the wet nurse should first be cured, and then the baby should be taken care of. Furthermore, if possible, the baby should be breastfed in the meantime by a healthy wet nurse. Therefore, to conclude, if the child's infirmity is being caused by a problem of the wet nurse, the problem of the wet nurse should first be addressed.

But if the infant's ailment is caused by a defect of the blood or of the humors of the infant's own body, for he might have been formed from defective blood—defective, that is, because of the presence of salty phlegm or choler or black bilious melancholy—then a diet of opposites should be prescribed to the wet nurse. For example, since blood combined with salty phlegm may cause milk crust in infants, then the wet nurse should take things that are cold and humid to rectify the defective blood. And similarly, if the ailments arise from other causes, it is necessary to modify the regimen so as to oppose them.

Take note, *frontosa*, that the use of onions, garlic, scallions, leeks, rocket, mustard greens, salted cheeses, peppers, strong wine, and similar things spoil the blood, making it hot, pungent, and salty: therefore, if you become pregnant while these foods are in your regimen, you will tarnish your own blood and the good seed of your husband. Furthermore, the infant will be born with a disposition to develop milk crust, boils, and similar ailments. This is because the infant's body will naturally separate out the good, not vitiated, part of the blood sent for its nourishment, and the rest will be sent to places on the surface of the body, and be converted into milk crust, boils, and similar ailments, which will make your suppers and evenings as miserable as your luncheons were gluttonous. Therefore, ladies who are carrying children should refrain from eating garlic, onions, etc., and these types of vegetables should be left unpicked in the vegetable garden, and instead these ladies should eat a nice capon: heed my good advice.

Now, *frontosa*, I don't want to skip over this topic in silence, because it should be noted. As we have said, infection of the blood causes sickness in children: therefore, *frontosa* and *frontoso*, keep in mind that when the Marquis is galloping through,[274] you should refrain from "hunting" [coitus], because the "hunted bird" [the resulting fetus] could be born diseased or leprous: infected children are born "from infected blood, such as comes from *saphati* and leprosy, which frequently happens from intercourse at the time of menstruation."[275] Whereas Avicenna says, "and sometimes it [leprosy] occurs on account of heredity and because of the complexion of the embryo, a complexion which is either his own, [or which is acquired in the womb because of the womb's disposition], as is the case when conception takes place during menstruation."[276] This is why the Old Testament instructs *do not approach the menstruating woman.*[277] O scabious *frontosa*, tie this string around your finger: if your scab itches, do your best to find alternative ways to scratch it, even if you must plunge your arms into cold water. I am sure you understand.

And having already said enough on this topic, I will begin to present in order the afflictions and infirmities that occur commonly in newborn children, taking them one at a time, each under a separate heading, for the sake of brevity. But first recall that even though these are ailments that women themselves are able to treat, I want to warn the ladies that in applying these remedies they should

---

274. On the "Marquis" as an euphemism for menstrual period, see Treatise One, note 36.

275. In Latin in the text: *ex sanguine infecto sicut fit saphati ita et lepra, que frequenter fit ex coitu tempore menstruationis.* To make but one example, the medieval medical dictionary titled *Concordances* by the French physician Pierre de Saint-Flour (fl. 1350) clearly states the connection between sexual intercourse during the menstrual cycle and the birth of sick, particularly leprous children. This belief that must have been widespread in the Middle Ages, on the basis of religious prohibitions to approach the impure menstrated woman, will be reaffirmed even more strongly in the Renaissance. *Saphati* or *sahaphati* is a term introduced into Latin in the twelfth century by Gerard of Cremona in his translations of the works of Avicenna and Rhazes. It refers to a skin disease characterized by small pustules. On the idea that both leprosy and *saphati* might be sexually transmitted, see Danielle Jacquart and Claude Thomasset, *Sexualité et savoir médical au Moyen Âge* (Paris: Presses universitaires de France, 1985), 244.

276. In Latin in the text: *et quandoque accidit propter hereditatem et propter complexionem embrionis, ex qua creatus est in se propter complexionem que est ei, **aut acquisitam in matrice propter dispositionem que est ei**, sicut si accidit ubi fit conceptio in dispositione menstruorum.* See Avicenna, *Canon*, Lib. IV, fen 3, tract. 3, c. 1 (p. 134). Savonarola omits the important phrase bolded here, and supplied in the text in brackets.

277. Ezekiel 18:6: *ne accesseris ad menstruatam.* The Vulgate reads: *In montibus non comederit, et oculos suos non levaverit ad idola domus Israel: et uxorem proximi sui non violaverit, et ad mulierem menstruatam non accesserit.*

not be overly confident, but act prudently and cautiously, and when they have access to a physician, seek counsel on these matters: by so doing, if there are any complications with the health of the infant, they will not be sorry.

Now I would also like to remind you that, as mothers are often the cause of the ailments of infants who develop milk crust, pustules, eczema, and other infirmities—by neglecting themselves, and sating their appetites for things that generate bad humors, as has been said, eating garlic, onions, and worst of all, eating ashes, as my baker used to do, eating harmful foods because her poverty did not allow her to pay for good foods—these mothers pay dearly in consequence, having to suffer through bad nights with their sick children. O *frontosa* who pays no attention to these things, you must remember that when you are the cause of great harm to your child and even his death, as is often the case, you will be held responsible on Judgment Day. Therefore, *frontosa*, be careful, and do what you can to not cause your child such harm, and such harm to yourself, insofar as you are responsible for both your own soul and body, and your child's.

We will begin now by discussing the first category of children's illnesses, ailments of the head, that organ which, according to Plato, is first and chief organ, which is also the most prominent and most susceptible to affliction.

On the milk crust that appears on the heads of children.[278] Certain pustules, called milk crust by the common people, often appear on the heads of children, from which they suffer greatly and quickly make their wet nurses suffer, too. We will proceed in the following manner on the treatment of this ailment, first discussing the causes, and after, the cures.

We say then that this milk crust that appears on the heads of infants, and sometimes on their whole body, is caused by bad humors that are sharp, corrosive, salty, and humid, or dry, black, and melancholic humors, which are mixed with the blood that is supposed to nourish the child. This is because the substance of the organs receives benefits from nourishment and, retaining these benefits, it sends the bad and superfluous things, because of their lightness, to the head; and they ascend in this way since they are hot and sharp, thus contributing greatly to this condition of the head while the infant is in the mother's belly, where his head is declined between his knees, as we have said.

The cure, then, for this infirmity consists in these rules, or canons. The first is the modification of the diet; the second is the dissolution of the humor, which involves separating the bad humor from the good humors, so that this bad complexion is corrected; the third is the evacuation of the humor; the fourth is the application of local substances, that is, remedies that should be applied topically, such as leeches, cupping glasses, rubbing medications, ointments, and similar things.

---

278. The Italian words used by Savonarola are *lactume* and *croste*.

And explaining the first cure, which is the modification of the diet, I say that first the nourishment taken by the infant, which is the milk, must be corrected by making the wet nurse consume things contrary to the causes of the problem. For example, at first she should take cold and humid things, such as lettuce and pomegranate wine that has been watered down a lot; and with meals she should add things like purslane, squash, squash or melon seeds, and barley flour, so that her regimen tends to the cold and humid. And similarly, if the little child eats, he should also be given similar fresh foods; and if you give him eggs, which is common practice, first boil them, then allow the boiled eggs to soak in cold water for several hours; give him pap or softened bread or purslane, or lettuce, which will modify his diet. And this kind of cure should be preferred by physicians, because the tender bodies of infants do not always react well when subjected to medicines; which is why Rhazes says, who seems otherwise more disposed than others to using medicines, "for the bodies of children are defective bodies: but bodies which are defective do not need strong medicine, but only what can be provided through diet."[279] While Avicenna says, "when the child has a fever, rectify his mother's milk."[280]

And moving on to the second cause, the dissolution of the humor, the wet nurse should take the watery part of milk, that is the whey serum, in the morning in place of syrup, or she should take the water of fumitory plant, or fumitory syrup with its water. And then she should make the infant drink this water and also thoroughly boiled barley water, and even better, with this she should make his pap. Next, she should regularly add boiled borage to his food and also for the wet nurse, lettuce, purslane, and similar things: and she should make sure that he eats these things. As the third cure, have the wet nurse take fumitory pills twice a week, taking them early in the morning, first giving milk to the child; and then, she should wait five hours before giving him milk again, having someone else give him milk in the meantime, or keeping him fed with some other food. And if by these actions of the wet nurse, the body of the infant could have a bowel movement, but not an excessive one, this would be very beneficial.

And if this does not happen after the second day, I prescribe that he be given the following pill: take one-half drachm of socotrine aloes, one drachm of

---

279. In Latin in the text: *nam corpora puerorum sunt corpora defecta: modo corpora que defecta sunt non indigent forti medicamine, sed solum eo quod est per dietam.* This exact passage has not been located, but a similar statement is found in Rhazes, *On the Treatment of Small Children*, ch. 18 (p. 27): *Et cura eius est cum eis que sunt cibus et medicina, isti enim non debent curari cum forti vel vehementi medicina* (And his treatment is done through substances that are both food and medicine. They are not to be treated with a strong and powerful medicine).

280. In Latin in the text: *cum puer febricitat, retificetur lac matris eius.* Avicenna, *Canon*, Lib. I, fen 3, doctr. 1, c. 3 (p. 167). See also at Lib. I, fen 3, doctr. 1, c. 3 (p. 168): *Et accidunt ei febres, et tunc melius est ut nutrix regatur* (And they are prone to fevers, in which case it is better to take care of the nurse's diet).

citrine myrobalans, and one-half drachm of thyme dodder; fifteen pills should be made, then dried, covered in sugar, and toasted over a fire; afterwards, put one in his mouth and right after this, give him the nipple. And if this doesn't work, apply a cerate [unctious external preparation] of mouse dung or of honey or of chard, or a clyster made from a decoction of beets, fumitory, and thyme dodder, butter, and a little salt.

On the next day, put leeches behind the baby's ears and let them draw quite a bit of blood: and if he is over six months old, you may apply a cupping glass, and scarify, as prescribed by Avicenna and Rhazes.[281] And on the next day, in the morning, apply a rubbing medication to is head with a rough cloth so that he will bleed. Later in the evening of that same day, wash his head with water made from the decoction of mallow and barley. Pour this over the baby's head and keep rubbing it with your hands or with a warm cloth, and then next, after his head is dry, anoint his head with egg oil or wheat germ oil or with burnt oak gall and oil of wallflowers. This local remedy, often recommended by Avicenna, is believed to be the ultimate remedy. And oil of tartar is also very effective, as are mustard seeds crushed with vinegar: but note that this is a strong remedy and should be used only with older children. And also the root of blue lilies mixed with rose oil and a little vinegar is recommended. And even while following this step, it is important to continue with this prescribed regimen and with good nutrition and evacuation.

It is also true that Master Guglielmo da Saliceto[282] claims to have cured this ailment on several occasions, having followed these prescriptions. With warm chamomile oil he anointed the head of an infant, who was first washed with a rinse made from a decoction of chamomile, roses, and fenugreek seeds: and this is certainly a very domestic remedy and may be prepared with confidence. And I also would like to add about such milk crust and crusts, that since crusts are not as wet as milk crust, all the aforementioned remedies should verge more on the humid, as should all the remedies to be applied to choleric wet nurses, but not the phlegmatic ones.

But since I had decided to include at the end of each section the treatments for children about which Rhazes wrote a few brief pages, I will note here his recommended cure for an ailment he called *saphati*.[283] He says that, first, the diet of the wet nurse must be corrected; next, the hair of the child should be removed with a depilatory, not with a razor; finally, the following ointment should be applied: take white lead and litharge, two drachms of each; three drachms of lye made of the ashes of a vine; one drachm of rose oil; one ounce of wax; melt the

281. It does not appear that Avicenna and Rhazes prescribe these kinds of treatments for milk crust.

282. Guglielmo da Saliceto (1210–1276/1280) was an Italian physician and surgeon, famous for his handbook *Chirurgia* (1275) and his *Summa conservationis et curationis* on hygiene and therapy.

283. *Saphati* is the first ailment listed by Rhazes in his brief treatise on children's diseases, *De curis puerorum*. See Rhazes, *On the Treatment of Small Children*, ch. 1, 20.

wax and mix it with rose oil, then add two roasted egg yolks to this mixture; and then rub this ointment on the head of the child.

A type of *saphati* called "honeycomb" is also encountered, with which some flaky eczema appears on the ulcerations, causing a great itch, and descending from these ulcerations is a thick yellowish liquid, like honey. For this condition, I include here the following ointment prescribed by Rhazes:[284] take litharge and white lead, two drachms of each; sulfur and quicksilver [mercury], one drachm of each; rose oil, two parts; vinegar, one part; mix these things together, and then add wax to make the ointment. Every day the head should be washed with savory water, horehound, and marjoram, of a temperature slightly warmer than tepid, after which the ointment should be applied to the head, and this should be done twice a day, in the morning and evening.

Personally, I do not recommend the use of quicksilver. I include it, however, with the blessing of Rhazes and I emphasize all of his cautions, because it is numbered among the poisons; and although it is true that quicksilver mixed with sputum is not as dangerous, it is always better to choose the safer option in cases of doubt.[285] And since I am writing for women, I will tell them the story of what I saw as a child of ten or so: those excavating the foundations of a sacristy near the churchyard of Saint Lucia in Padua found the head of a young woman, still intact with all its hair. When a little boy threw a pebble that hit this head, it immediately discharged great quantities of quicksilver, leading the authorities working there to conclude that when she was alive, she had used quicksilver as a cosmetic, and that poisoned in this way, the poor thing died an early death.

On the spasm of the jaws, the infant suffering from which is said by women to be sgramolato.[286] This condition often occurs when newborn infants, because of humor or cold, cannot connect with the nipple of the breast, and therefore cannot lactate, and because of this many die. The infant cannot clench his jaw to draw milk, and is said to have a dislocated jaw. In this case I recommend a leather or

---

284. Savonarola uses the term *favositas mellis,* as does Rhazes. See Rhazes, *On the Treatment of Small Children,* ch. 2, 20: *Passio que dicitur favositas mellis est species sahaphati* (the condition called *favositas mellis* is a kind of *saphati*).

285. The first recorded account of animal experimentation on the toxicity of mercury comes from Rhazes (ninth century). Avicenna (eleventh century) had the foresight to recommend the use of mercury only as an external remedy: quicksilver ointments were indeed used by the Arabs in treating skin diseases. Nonetheless, there was a persistent belief that the poisonous nature of mercury was moderated by skillful administration, for example when the substance was mixed with oil or, as in this case, sputum. See Rhazes, *Liber continens* (Venice: Johannes Hamman, 1529), *sub vocem* De argento vivo, Lib. XXII, vol. 2 (fol. 364).

286. The adjective *sgramolato* derives from the Italian noun *gramola,* a kneading tool used to knead natural textile fibers. The TLIO attests the existence of a figurative sense of the word, which also means jaw. The privative letter "s" at the beginning of the adjective can only indicate a malfunction in the correspondence between the upper jaw and the lower jaw, or mandible. See TLIO, *sub vocem* gramola.

fabric plaster that could also be made of satin only, one *pechione* in length, to be placed over the spot where the brain or cranium is most tender. Then galbanum, spread over a leather strip wider than the one made of satin, should be applied to the nape or backside of the head. Next, moisten strips of fabric in chamomile oil and place them, warm but not too hot, externally over the jaws, tying them with hemp cloth and a small band; and refresh this two or three times a day. And when he is healed, you may remove this medication. Also, a lighter remedy is to take a little cotton with the satin, put it on his head as mentioned, and later anoint his nape and jaws, and cover them with hemp cloth.

On teething. Often infants have a difficult time teething. One should squeeze the gums with their fingers, and softly rub the gums and do the same to the palate, and keep them moist with hare's brain, which is appropriate for this, or with butter or with good olive oil; and this should be done twice a day. It is also appropriate to moisten them with bitch's milk, or, also very effective, to anoint and rub the gums with chicken fat.

On the sores or pustules that appear in the mouths of infants. Often small sores like pustules appear on the tongues and palates of small children, generated by salty, putrefied phlegm, named *alcola* by the authorities:[287] these are often caused by the milk of the wet nurse. But since in some cases these sores are so serious that they ulcerate the tongue and the palate, their treatment should be left to physicians; so I will only speak of those that are not ulcerated. And of these, some are red and bloody, others yellowish, others black, and many are white salty phlegmatic. And an abundance of drool or spittle flows continually from the mouth.

In order to cure this ailment, first it is necessary that the wet nurse be willing to eat foods that oppose it: for example, since this condition is caused by hot, salty matter, she should eat cold and humid foods, such as those mentioned earlier. Here I will offer some remedies that are usually effective, leaving other treatments to the physicians for cases in which they intervene.

Therefore, following the advice of our authorities, we will say that if the *alcola* is white and generated from salty phlegm, then it is beneficial for the child to take strained rose honey, mixed together with a little sweetened alum, rubbed on his tongue and palate twice a day. For this condition, it is also very beneficial for you to pre-chew lentils, and once chewed, put them in the infant's mouth; or place there a little starch soaked with rose water. Mild and strong pomegranate seeds, and the juice of quinces also help to alleviate this condition.

On the excessive wakefulness of infants. It is often the case that small children do not sleep as much as they should, staying awake more than is good for them. Since no other cause is apparent, we must accuse the corruption of the milk they are taking, which perhaps, because of its intensity, is too stimulating. Therefore,

---

287. In Avicenna's *Canon*, *alcola* is always synonym for *aphtas*, i.e. aphthous ulcers, open sores in the mucous membrane of the mouth.

the first thing to do is to correct the milk of the wet nurse, and later move on to other remedies. And although it may be taken for granted, for it has often been said, the wet nurse's diet must always be considered first. I will move on to discuss the remedies for this condition, naturally incorporating the theories of my teachers and the authorities who have written on these topics.

When the child does not sleep as he should, and he cries, you should anoint his temples and his nose with this oil: take one spoonful of white poppy seeds, one and one-half spoonfuls of juice of lettuce, half a spoonful of hyoscyamus seeds, two and one-half ounces of oil of violets; and mix these together and bring them to a boil, and afterwards, strain this mixture well. Also populeon ointment may be beneficial. If you need to strengthen this recipe, ask a physician. Also, the milk of white poppy seeds may be beneficial mixed with the mother's milk and with violet water, giving him one spoonful at a time, three times a day. And if the infant eats, mix some of these seeds, or powder made from poppy seeds, into his pap. Also, if possible give him some poppy syrup before he goes to sleep, more or less, depending on his age: for example for a child of three to six months, one eighth [of an ounce of poppy syrup] mixed with three [eighths] of water lily water; for a child of six months to a year, two [eighths of poppy syrup]; for a child of one to two years, three [eighths of poppy syrup] with three [eighths of water lily water]; for a child of two to three years, half an ounce [of poppy syrup] with one ounce of water lily water. It is also common practice to give him in this instance a *requies*,[288] although I hesitate to praise this fully. If necessary, give him only a tiny amount.

On night terrors that small children experience in their sleep, called by some mater puerorum.[289] Some small children experience night terrors in their sleep and they cry out in great fear. This happens because they have overeaten and because of the corruption of their food. Therefore, it is better to give them less food, and not put them to bed immediately after they have eaten, and to make them take before their meal a bit of warm honey-infused water, if you can afford it. If they are a little older, give them a pill of washed aloe or simple *hiera*,[290] covered in sugar with egg as mentioned: for example, for a six-month-old, a pill as big as

---

288. *Requies* (Latin noun for rest, stillness, quiteness) might indicate a mild sedative, but nothing more specific about this remedy is found in Savonarola's sources.

289. The term "mother of children" (fear) in the Latin and Hebrew translations of *De curis puerorum* by Rhazes is a loan-translation from the Arabic. According to some scholars, it always means "epilepsy" in Arabic medical literature, with the exception of the work by Rhazes, where it is used in the sense of *pavor nocturnus*. For a detailed and insightful discussion of this condition, including references to its treatment in Hippocrates and Galen, see Rhazes, *On the Treatment of Small Children*, commentary to ch. 8 (pp. 76–77).

290. *Hiera* (ἱερά) is a name that can be given to various purgative compounds in ancient and medieval medical practice. Mesuae, for example, describes many different types of *hiera*, which "is *sacred*, because of its divine and miraculous effects," including one he had invented himself, under the heading *De medicamentis purgantibus compositis*. See Mesuae, *De re medica*, Lib. III.5 (pp. 258–68).

one grain of millet; if he is older, a little bigger; for those who are two years old or close to this age, a pill as big as one grain of sorghum. Theriac is also highly recommended given with milk, but not often.

On the eyes. Often the eyes of infants may swell, and they can swell to the point that the child cannot open his eyes. This is caused by the descent of humors from the head to the eyes. The child may also be red in the face and overheated. In this case, mix together the juice of horned poppies and of roses, one ounce of each, one eighth [of an ounce] of pulverized myrrh, and half an eighth [of an ounce] of crushed saffron. Soak strips of cloth in this mixture and place them on his forehead and over his eyes, refreshing the strips often, until he opens his eyes. However if there is no redness or heat, then take one part saffron, and two parts myrrh, aloe, and rose powder, and mix them together with good wine and apply this remedy in the same way as has been described.

On fluid in the ears and on earaches. Often fluid from the brain will drain out of the ears of small children. When this happens, take some wool and make a small plug out of it. Dip this in honey, mixed with a little wine and a little saffron and warm it slightly, then put it in his ear. You should do this twice a day, morning and evening; but make sure to clean his ears before inserting this plug.

Earaches are also caused by fluids and gases. Take a little oregano and a little myrrh and bring them to a boil in bitter almond oil, and while it is still warm, apply two drops of this to his ears, and plug the hole with a cotton ball; do this twice a day, and make sure to clean his ear out before doing this. This is a most potent remedy. Before doing this, start with just oil with a little saffron; this is a lighter remedy. And also clean the ear out often with soft cotton. Also, Rhazes praises wine that has first been infused with nitre.[291]

And if the infant has ulcerations around his ears, treat them by applying honey water and cleaning these ulcerations with honey water; and also to heal them, after cleaning them, add to the honey preparation the powder of myrtle or oak gall.

On sneezing. Small children may sneeze often, and this may be from a lesion in their brains. If this is the case, a physician should be consulted because the cure is more complicated as fever can set in and their eyes may become hollow; but if they are sneezing from excessive gases or humors, then simply make the child blow his nose a bit.

On coughing. Small children may become very agitated from coughing. It is beneficial for them to take some tragacanth, quince seeds, and licorice juice in equal parts, and mix these ingredients together with barley sugar and incorporate this mixture with his mother's milk three or four times a day. Also rub the following ointment on the child: butter two parts, sweet almond oil one part, violet oil one-half part. This ointment should be made with white wax and it should

---

291. See Rhazes, *On the Treatment of Small Children,* ch. 9 (p. 23).

be applied to his chest, after which you should cover this with clean uncombed or unwashed wool. You can also give him sweet almond milk mixed with water in which fennel was first boiled, twice a day; and if he should have a fever, add some sweet pomegranate juice. And likewise: take the seeds of white poppy and tragacanth, one-half eighth [of an ounce] of each, seeds of washed and crushed squash, one eighth [of an ounce], and mix these together with the water in which was cooked a little *sebesten*.[292]

Another treatment that works is raisins, first warmed in a stone pot and then mixed with barley sugar: give this remedy to him in the evening and morning in the quantity of a small nut. Cotton seed given with cooked egg is also helpful. Also, if you want, give him as he goes to sleep a *hiera* pill with sweetened agaric as prescribed, between two to six grains in weight, increasing or decreasing the dose depending on his age, at the discretion of the caretaker, who should always consult with the physician. I recommend the use of turpentine with barley sugar for small children until the age of seven, one eighth [of an ounce] for the little ones and three eighths [of an ounce] for the bigger ones. And because coughing is often a sign of the more serious diseases smallpox or measles, called by Italians *fersa*, from "fervor," the next section will be on smallpox and measles.

On smallpox and measles. Small children tend to contract smallpox and measles, with pustules of different sizes, appearance, and seriousness even though all of them come from residual menstrual blood in the veins of the child's body. Measles are less grave an ailment; this is why Avicenna says that the smallpox is more dry and more serious.[293]

Therefore, *frontosa*, when you hear the baby groaning with back pain, and he often scratches his nose, and he wakes from slumber screaming in fear, and he moans because he feels a pricking sensation all over his body, and his face begins to get red, and his eyes to tear, and he yawns frequently, and he begins coughing and has congestion in his chest, and his voice goes hoarse and his head hurts and his throat is inflamed, and his mouth becomes dry, and he has a constant high fever, then you should suspect smallpox. But if together with these signs, you see his eyes tear up more greatly and he has a higher fever, then you should suspect measles, which will appear early and all across the face. But if it is smallpox, it will not appear as early: today one bump may appear, the next day two, and so on.[294]

---

292. The Arabic *sebesten* names the fruit of an East Indian tree, often used medicinally for pectoral ailments.

293. See Avicenna, *Canon*, Lib. IV, fen 1, tract. 4, c. 8 (p. 74): *Et morbillus est minor variolis*. The belief that smallpox arose from residual maternal menstrual blood that remained in the child after birth was a staple of Islamic views on the disease since at least the tenth century. See, for example, Rhazes, *A Treatise on the Smallpox and Measles*, ed. and trans. William Alexander Greenhill (London: Sydenham Society, 1848).

294. This description of the onset of smallpox is the nearly exact translation of the one made by Rhazes in his aforementioned treatise.

Now if at first you suspect the child has smallpox and later you are certain that he does, you should become knowledgeable about this illness and pay careful attention to three things: first, the child's diet; second, protecting the body parts that usually suffer greater harm from smallpox and are more greatly endangered; and third, administering medicines, which we will discuss afterwards.

There are four body parts that may be affected by smallpox: the eyes, the throat, the lungs, and the intestines. Our experience shows us that eyes are often lost because of smallpox, but this is less of a risk with measles. As for damage to the throat, which becomes congested with superfluous material, young children often die from suffocation: this is why Avicenna says, "and many of those who die from smallpox die suffocating from quinsy."[295] As for the lungs, they may ulcerate, and this can lead to consumption. As for the intestines, which may also ulcerate, causing diarrhea that may lead to the death of the child: where Avicenna says, "and sometimes they die because of the loss of strength from dysentery and diarrhea."[296]

So first, pay attention to the child's regimen, which consists in the six things called by physicians non-natural: that is air, food and drink, movement and rest, sleep and wake, repletion and evacuation, and accidents of the soul. We will cover all of these briefly, beginning with the air. You should take great care, *frontosa*, that the child not be exposed to the cold or drafts, but instead keep him warm, more or less depending on the weather. For example in the winter, more; in the autumn less; and in summer even less: and keep him in a well-ventilated place, and not in the dark. He should be wrapped in red, not black, cloth. He should rest and sleep more than he is awake. Keep him on a good diet, at least for the first four to seven days with as little food as possible, but do this with discretion. Don't upset him; but instead treat him with sweetness and kindness.

On food, when you suspect the onset of smallpox or measles, and even before you are sure, you should give him cooling foods, like barley porridge or porridge made of starch, twice-boiled lentils (even better if they are boiled three times), panicum, squash, purslane, lettuce, endive, common seeds, pap made from lentil broth or made with water in which lettuce or purslane has been boiled. Also, although you cook with these ingredients as you usually do, make sure that all foods are acidified with vinegar or cooled with pomegranate wine and seeds, or verjuice. You may also prepare hulled spelt cooked with the milk of sweet almonds or with the milk of common seeds, or farro with cooked lettuce. All foods should either be acidified or pomegranate wine should be added. And this should be done at the first onset of the illness.

---

295. In Latin in the text: *et plurimi eorum, qui moriuntur per variolas, moriuntur prefocati ex squinantia*. See Avicenna, *Canon*, Lib. IV, fen 1, tract. 4, c. 6 (p. 73). Quinsy (*squinantia*) was variosly understood in the Middle Ages both as a kind of abscess or tumor in the throat.

296. In Latin in the text: *et quandoque moriuntur propter casum virtutis cum raxura et fluxu ventris*. See Avicenna, *Canon*, Lib. IV, fen 1, tract. 4, c. 6 (p. 73).

But if the baby doesn't want to take this food, which is often the case, he will not refuse eggs cooked as I will describe—especially when the infant is weak and does not want to take food, as is often the case: crack an egg into the water in which lettuce, purslane, or similar cold foods have been boiled, and give him eggs cooked this way with the white and the yolk, with pomegranate wine or verjuice with a little bit of vinegar on top, and not too cold. These recipes are prescribed by authorities that women should model themselves after, and they should make sure to stick to the food regimen that is most beneficial to the infants. In this case, no matter what, do not give him oil or any fats, or anything inflammatory. Do not feed him meat, if possible, unless it is chicken cooked with the cool ingredients mentioned earlier, which should only be eaten when prepared with verjuice, pomegranate wine, or wine. And this should be done until at least the fourth day. Then you may ease the strictness of the food regimen somewhat, but always proceed with prudence. Give him boiled barley water tempered with pomegranate wine to drink, and if you like, add a little bit of sugar or rose or violet julep, which will not harm him.

When he begins to develop smallpox or measles, then you must protect the small child from cold air and drafts. Continue giving him the aforementioned foods, little by little decreasing their frigidity, that is, with less vinegar, less verjuice, pomegranates, and similar things, perhaps being a little less strict with the meat and eggs, which don't have to be cooled so much. With such foods you should cook parsley root, fennel, and similar things. Also, you may give him a few grains of red chickpeas with sugar. But nevertheless, as he begins to recover from the ailment and the fever, the frigidity of the food must be lowered.

Pap made with broth with a little bit of saffron and common seeds is beneficial. And then give him water boiled with dried figs to drink, for example in one *ingistara*[297] add three or four figs, depending on their size and shape; and he should drink this water with meals, before meals, and afterwards, since drinking this is advantageous for this condition. This is why Avicenna says, "and water of figs is very good, for figs encourage strong expulsion from the body."[298] And if in this water you boil hulled lentils with fennel seeds with a little tragacanth, it will become like a syrup, and should be given to him at the hour of the syrups,[299] and if possible, he should drink it hot. You cannot err in giving him this drink until

---

297. An *ingistara* is a unit of measure for liquid capacity (around 1 liter), chiefly employed in medieval Verona, Venice and Vicenza, derived from the word *agrestara*, *inguistara* or *anguistara* (carafe), attested in Italian since the thirteenth century. See TLIO, *sub vocem* anguistara.

298. In Latin in the text: *et aqua ficuum est bona valde: ficus enim sunt vehementis expulsionis ad exteriora.* See Avicenna, *Canon*, Lib. IV, fen 1, tract. 4, c. 10 (p. 74).

299. It has not been possible to determine when this "hour of syrups" might be, as Savonarola prescribes syrups both in the morning and in the evening. See, for example, the section on the milk crust ("in the morning in place of syrup," 194), and the section on the excessive wakefulness of infants ("give him some poppy syrup before he goes to sleep," 198).

the pustules of smallpox or measles have completely maturated; and when they are completely out, you may give him a little bit of white wine, either tempered with boiled barley water or without, and return to his normal diet little by little. And I believe this will suffice with regards to the first of the three things of which you must be aware.

Regarding the second, know that the ulceration left by smallpox on the body parts mentioned may be followed by the corruption of the functioning of these parts, making the child lose his sight, smell, and hearing, or possibly making him consumptive and damaging the intestines, as mentioned before; therefore remember that you are responsible for protecting these from the start. For example, first for the eyes, sprinkle rose water on them frequently; and if you happen to have sumac water, adding a few drops of this to each eye is even better. For his throat, give the child pomegranate seeds, or have him often drink pomegranate wine, or give him mulberry juice or quince or medlar juice. For his lungs, give him lentil water and some poppy seed milk or some *diapapaver*,[300] having him sip on it little by little. For the nose and ears, keep them moist with a cloth infused with vinegar, or make the child smell the vinegar: this is very beneficial. Or anoint his nose and ears with the oil of myrtle or rose oil mixed with sandalwood. For his stomach, since small children tend to resist taking medicines by mouth, I recommend a clyster made with plantain juice with chilled water; I mean, cook the plantain in chilled water, and make the clyster with this and with the fat of a gelding. I also recommend the decoction of tragacanth with roses and wax.

And now arriving at the third item, medications to be employed, I say that when you first see the signs of smallpox, bloodletting will be very useful, especially when children are fleshy. Even though this is not common practice, still it is proposed and commended by all the medical authorities. And if you do not bleed him, instead you may place cupping glasses over his buttocks: since this, as Avicenna says, may act as a substitute for phlebotomy. It is true that Avenzoar, a physician himself, had his five-year-old son bled and he immediately recovered from his fever. But once the smallpox pustules appear, one should definitely not apply cupping glasses.

On the efficacy of medication by mouth, I have my doubts. This is because with smallpox, as well as with measles, diarrhea often develops; and then physicians discourage strong laxatives. But because of necessity, they permit manna, cassia, tamarind, and similar things. Instead, *frontosa mia*, I recommend clysters when necessary, made with the broth of meat made from water in which mallow has been cooked, and violet stems with butter.

Also, I warn you that often smallpox bumps take longer than they should to break. Because pus remains, leaving a pock in the flesh, and later, scars and pocks remain, and these can greatly ruin the beauty of the infant, especially of baby girls,

300. This term was used to indicate an electuary containing poppy seeds.

for which you must be particularly careful because this can hurt her beauty and impede her chances of marriage. So I am warning you, turn to the physician. And if the physician can't see you, take a needle, or a stylet that is sharp like the tip of a needle, and pop the pox. Once they are popped, the pus will drain and then you should apply to them fava or red chickpea flour with litharge and aloe. And if you ask when they should be popped, I say that from when they first appear to the seventh day: after seven days have passed, they can be lanced if they do not pop. And if these pox should become ulcerated, consult a physician: but if you are not able to, take white ointment, that is some white lead with litharge, and anoint the spot.

Smallpox is very dangerous, and conditions can become very serious and at times fatal: in such a case, therefore, you should consult a physician. For example, smallpox that appear greenish in color, or purplish, or close to black are dangerous; similarly, white ones when they are all clumped together and appear in many parts of the body; also those pox that take long in developing; from all of these young children often die. Wherefore, *frontosa*, when you hear the child recover his voice and his good breathing, and his chest is clear and decongested, this is a good sign and you can hope for his recovery, as Avicenna says, "for these two, when they remain good, is a sign of health."[301] And when you see the child weaken, especially if he develops diarrhea with tearing of the intestines, or if he pisses blood, and he often gets anxious, take this as a sign that he may die, and make sure to turn to the physician.

And that is all I wanted to say about smallpox and measles, and of these illnesses we shall write more extensively, God willing, in our *Canonica de febribus*.[302]

On the stomach and hiccups. If the child's stomach is upset, give him some powdered clove and some *galia muscata*, rose powder, and quince juice. Soak some wool cloth in this mixture, warm it, and lay it on him in the evening and the morning. Infants often develop hiccups. Give them strained rose honey with a little mint syrup, or cook honey in water with a little mint, and while warm, make him drink this, or he may lick it until he swallows it.

301. In Latin in the text: *nam ipsa duo* [anhelitus et vox] *cum remanent bona, est res salva.* See Avicenna, *Canon*, Lib. IV, fen 1, tract. 4, c. 6 (p. 73).

302. The future tense of this verb (*scriveremo*, "we shall write") poses some problems with the internal chronology of Savonarola's works, because the *Practica canonica de febribus* (written in 1439; *editio princeps* Bologna: Dionigi Bertocchi, 1487) was apparently composed some twenty years before the *De regimine pregnantium,* when the physician was still teaching in Padua; see Tiziana Pesenti Marangon, *Professori e promotori di medicina nello studio di Padova dal 1405 al 1509: Repertorio bio-bibliografico* (Padua and Trieste: Lint, 1984), and Segarizzi, *Della vita e delle opere di Michele Savonarola.* One possibility is that Savonarola translated this sentence into the vernacular from one of his own earlier Latin works, without adjusting the verb to the past tense. Possibilities would be his *Directorium ad actum practicum,* written ca. 1420, or his *De pulsibus, urinis et egestionibus,* written before 1439 (cited in *Works by Michele Savonarola,* #1 and #3), although a search for a corresponding Latin sentence in these works has been unsuccessful. The source was not Savonarola's *Practica maior* (1440–1446), as that work, unlike the *Mother's Manual,* has no section on childcare, pediatrics, and pedagogy.

On vomiting. Infants often vomit for many reasons, especially because of too much milk. And the wet nurse is well aware of this, saying "he is one *gran tetone*":[303] so when this is the case, she should give him a smaller quantity of milk and she should leave him to cry a bit before lactation. In addition, there are also problems arising from the corruption of milk, which should be well-examined for its color and taste, if it is sour or bitter or yellowish or similar; and this problem should be addressed right away by correcting the diet of the wet nurse; and for this you should consult a physician. Now if the child's vomit comes from weakness of the stomach, as is often the case, especially in very weak infants, then anoint his stomach with the following ointment: take mastic, aloe, acacia, oak gall, *olibanum*,[304] toasted bread, one drachm of each; prepare this with rose oil, and place it over his stomach. But because this condition may come from many other causes, I advise the wet nurse to consult an old physician, not a young one. Avicenna also highly recommends three grains of pulverized cloves, given with milk in the morning and evening.[305]

On the disposition of the stomach, with regard to pain, diarrhea and constipation. Stomachache, when it comes from gas, is often caused by milk, because milk is gas inducing, especially when it is watery, perhaps because of the poor diet of the wet nurse. In this case we advise that first the wet nurse must correct her diet with things that restore heat, but not too much; and keep the baby warm, anointing his belly with dill oil in which cumin was boiled, and laying warm strips of cloth on top of him. Also, you should have the wet nurse take cumin or aniseed in her food, and she should forgo cold and gas-inducing foods, a practice that Avicenna praises highly. She should take cumin and oregano, three grains of each pulverized, and have her drink this warm in wine with a little sugar.[306]

Diarrhea occurs in young children, especially when they are teething, because children are debilitated by the great pain that comes with teething, and are not able to digest as they should, and the result of this is diarrhea. When it is a mild case, it does not need to be treated; but if it is strong, then it needs to be treated with an embrocation made with a sponge infused with chilled water in which the seeds of roses or cumin were boiled, and also place over his stomach a plaster made of roses, cumin, and spelt flour. And if he still is not better, give him the sixth part of an eighth [of an ounce] of rennet with cold water, and make sure the wet nurse avoids foods that are lubricative.

---

303. "one great breast-sucker."

304. *Olibanum* is the the medieval Latin term for frankincense.

305. See Avicenna, *Canon*, Lib. I, fen 3, doctr. 1, c. 3 (p. 169): *Et est cum infanti accidit vomitus fortis, cui forsan dabitur medietas davic unius gariophylli* (And since the child may suffer from severe vomiting episodes, he should be given for example half a *davic* of cloves). One davic corresponds to six grains. The half of it (*medietas*) is three grains, as specified by Savonarola.

306. See Avicenna, *Canon*, Lib. I, fen 3, doctr. 1, c. 3 (p. 169).

Moreover, diarrhea often comes from choler, and the feces appear yellow-ish. In this case, make the wet nurse eat cold or unheated foods tending to the cold and humid, like spinach, etc. And if the problem stems from phlegm, the child will writhe in pain, and the feces will tend to the white or viscous.

If the problem stems from choler, give him rose syrup with a little mint. Also: Take *lapathum*[307] seeds and arils of dried raisins, four drachms of each; acorns and white poppy seeds, two drachms of each; and a dash of saffron; and grind them into a powder. And you may give this to the child mixed with the juice of quinces or rose syrup, giving him one to two drachms of it according to his age; and this is an advantageous remedy. If the diarrhea comtinues, place the following reliable plaster over his stomach, making sure to cover the part below his navel: take white lead and acacia, one drachm of each; the seventh part of one drachm of opium poppy; shape a lint with rose honey, and place this plaster over his stomach. It is always better to begin with a lighter medication; perhaps sumac mixed with barley or millet flour softened with water in which sumac was boiled will suffice as an effective plaster.

If the diarrhea comes from cold or phlegm, place the following plaster on his stomach: take saffron, myrrh, and wax, and mix these ingredients with wine, and if you want, add some incense, which is good. But if the child is over the age of one and one half, he will have to be treated differently, according to physicians, because the diarrhea is from a different cause. This type of ailment often leaves physicians perplexed. Excessive cold may also cause tenesmus; for this condition, you should make a clyster with old butter and a little nasturtium and cumin, boiled in water.

On constipation or tightening of the stomach. As said earlier, it can be re-lieved with the treatment of barley sugar or with mouse dung, or with the powder of mouse dung and barley sugar which is even stronger. It is also beneficial if the wet nurse takes one or two pills of washed aloe. Clysters are also beneficial for the relief of constipation, especially clysters made with honey, chard, or the root of lily (which is stronger). Avicenna praises turpentine, given in one or two chickpea-sized quantities, depending on the age of the child.

On worms. As the intention here is to write about the regimen of children until the age of seven, I will not only write of the extenal medicines, which are use-ful for those, like infants younger than one year old, who cannot take medications by mouth, but also for those who do take their medications by mouth. No doubt that in doing so I will be considered long-winded, but since many die from this affliction, what I write may not be too prolix, but rather too brief. But anyone who wishes to be further informed should read the treatise I have written on worms, or what I have written in my *Practica*.[308]

---

307. *Lapathum* is the Latin name for dock or sorrel.

308. See Michele Savonarola, *De vermibus* (Venice: Ottaviano Scoto per Boneto Locatello, 1498; *editio princeps*); cited in *Works by Michele Savonarola*, #4. This Latin work on worms, dedicated to Zanardo

And to please you, my ladies, I will first note the things that produce worms, concerning which women need to take great caution in giving to their children, especially things that are phlegmatic and viscous, such as cooked wheat, fresh cheese, especially milk, favas, beans, pastries, greens, apples, pears, grapes and similar fruits; the meat of swine, goose, duck, quail, fish, fatty foods and foods difficult to digest; as well as excessive drinking, overeating, excessive exercise, and all those things that may impede digestion, such as cold air and cold wind; and all those things that impair digestion, especially in autumn. During this season, worms may multiply in the stomachs of infants, and also in March, because of the winds: therefore, in the springtime and in the autumn, be sure to give children things that prevent worms, and keep them from things that produce worms.

And to satisfy the desires of those of my ladies who are very eager to learn of such things, in this chapter I will proceed, briefly, discussing this regimen, saying first that they should make sure to feed their children good food, and keep them from those that produce worms as mentioned earlier. They must avoid overeating, cold, drafts, etc., and heavy wines, especially indigestible ones. Instead I prescribe light and subtle wines, etc.

Having discussed this regimen for eating, I will now provide a regimen of medications, given in three sections: first, I will name those medicines to be taken by mouth; second, those to be taken from below; and last, those to be applied externally. By mouth we mean drinks, pills, solid confections, electuaries; taken underneath are suppositories and clysters; applied externally, fomentations, ointments, poultices, and plasters. And we will discuss each of these without too much elaboration, leaving a more detailed discussion to attending physicians.

We will now proceed to the first section, medicines taken by mouth, dividing that into preventive and curative. Preventive medications are used to prevent the generation of worms. And given what was discussed earlier, one should, at the times of greatest risk such as at the beginning of autumn—that is at the end of August—and at the end of February, keep children purged and clean, taking care that they are not exposed to winds or drafts, and that they eat and drink properly: and you should feed them foods that are comforting to the stomach and give them things that purge humors that are apt to generate worms, such as phlegmatic humors.

At these times, then, it is beneficial to give the child a simple syrup of wormwood water, making him take this for ten to twelve days, in the morning two hours before getting up: either the wormwood water by itself, or that of southernwood, or, better, with syrup. And if you do not have money, *frontosa*, take a little honey and some vinegar and make the water recommended equally sweet and acrid, and give this to the child warm. And you can give him more or less depending on his age; for example: for those who are two, two ounces; for four-year-olds, up to

---

Cambiatore da Reggio, was composed before 1440. Also see Savonarola, *Practica maior*, tract. VI, c. 16, rubr. 23 (fols. 212vb–215ra).

three to four ounces. Later give him the following pills: take aloe, one and one-half drachms; myrrh, one drachm; saffron, one-half drachm; dittany, one scruple; cabbage seeds, one-half drachm; mix these ingredients together with aromatic wine; for those who are two years old, twelve pills should be made per eighth [of an ounce]; for those older, ten pills should be made out of one eighth [of an ounce], and you may give them one or two or three as you think best depending on the strength of the child, or the constipation of his stomach. This remedy may also be taken once every eight days, when the child has an upset stomach. Also recommended is scutch grass water, or oil given with malmsey; and impoverished women may use water from the decoction of scutch grass and rye with a little dittany. It is also common practice to give *somentina* pear with honey, likewise tortelli of santonica (or wormseed) cooked in oil served with a little good wine. Theriac is good especially in the cold weather.

A powerful electuary: Take santonica (or wormseed), one-half ounce; pellitory of Spain, toasted bread soaked in vinegar, one ounce of each; burnt deer horn, two drachms; cabbage seeds, one-half ounce; nigella, nasturtium, and red coral, one-half drachm of each; wormwood, one drachm; mix these together with honey. Of this electuary, give him more or less, but no more than one eighth [of an ounce] for the older children, and for the younger ones six grains, and for those in the middle, half way between these two doses depending on their ages.

Preparation for worms: Take centaurea flowers, caraway seeds, one drachm of each; colocynth, one-half drachm; purslane seeds, one drachm; indic myrobalans, one-half drachm; root of pomegranate and myrtle, one and one-half drachms of each; for every six eighths [of an ounce], add a pound of sugar. These should be used in their proper time. Of this preparation give him one drachm, that is an eighth [of an ounce], to two drachms, depending on his age.

When the child is sick and he has a fever, take some wormwood or southernwood with roses and pomegranate rind with a little bit of horehound and some mint; boil these ingredients in vinegar for a good bit, until they are reduced by a fourth; later take a sponge and soak it in this vinegar and while it is still warm, place it on the child's stomach, and when it cools off, warm it up and then anoint the child with the ointment prescribed here.

Take note that when you wish to administer a clyster or suppository, place this sponge on the child's stomach at least once, and then, after an eighth of an hour has passed, administer the clyster of meat broth with honey or milk and sugar, which is certainly an optimal remedy. And note: never give him a clyster with oil, because oil is the enemy of worms and makes them ascend [in the intestine]; and as it has been stated, in place of oil, it is more beneficial to use butter. I also recommend a wholesome plaster of rose water, bugloss, wormwood, and borage, with a little saffron, applied over his heart with strips of linen cloth.

Ointment: Take mint juice, one ounce; centaurea flowers, caraway seeds, and lupins, one drachm of each; felwort and wormwood, one and one-half drachms of each; orange juice, one-half ounce; toasted bread soaked in vinegar, one drachm; prepare with citrine wax; anoint the stomach, his temples, his nostrils, and repeat this often.

I have provided this brief instruction to keep my promise not to be long-winded, although certainly such a subject is worthy of much longer explanation. But anyone who wishes to be instructed further by me should consult the treatise on worms that I have compiled according to the authorities, or they may read about this in my *Practica*, where I have written extensively on such matters.[309]

On hernias. At times, children may develop hernias. Take equal parts of each of the following: the rind of pomegranates, myrtle, roses, dried acorn shells, burnt horn powder, Yemen alum, balusters, oak gall; bring to a boil so that all the water evaporates; and while this decoction is still lukewarm, have the child soak in it. This is a strong treatment. And repeat this two or three times throughout the day, as often as it seems necessary.[310]

On fissures and weakening and rupture of the abdominal muscles. Often ruptures are caused in children by great and long fits of weeping. Such young children should certainly not be cut open: for I have myself seen in my day two-year-olds die from such surgery, and even older children are in great danger. So this is why it is recommended that they be cured with medicine.

For the moment, I suggest only one poultice, which is effective in such cases: take three drachms of alum; two drachms of oak gall; grind these ingredients together, and add wine to your preparation until it thickens; and put this poultice over the injured spot. When the intestine returns to its place, take a sponge dipped in vinegar and lukewarm water, apply with pressure, and tie it with a bandage; and change this dressing daily. And when the intestine is reduced, apply on the belly some paste made out of chorion, and keep this on as long as it lasts: and when this is gone, replace it with another. And also you should make a ligature with some cotton.

These remedies are also good for the relaxation [of the abdominal walls]: that is, when there are not actual fissures, but there seems to be a rupture, because the intestines protrude on account of the relaxation of the peritoneum.

---

309. See note 308 at 206.

310. This section on hernias is oddly abbreviated. Hernias were normally the province of the surgeon, not the physician, being treated with surgery or cautery. But Savonarola is clear that surgery ought not be performed on young children. For the development of surgical procedures, see Michael McVaugh, "Cataracts and Hernias: Aspects of Surgical Practice in the Fourteenth Century," *Medical History* 45 (2001): 319–40, and McVaugh, *The Rational Surgery of the Middle Ages* (Florence: SISMEL, Edizioni del Galluzzo, 2006).

On the fissures or ulcerations of the thighs and buttocks. These areas ulcerate because of the great acidity of the urine. This is why it is important first to correct the milk, and then anoint the area with white lead, rose oil washed three times in plantain water, and white wax. It is also helpful if you perfume this substance with the water in which violet stems were boiled, mallow, and grains of barley. But take note, *frontosa*, that sometimes in these places pustules and ulcerations result not from the acidity of the urine, but because of the corruption of the milk, and sometimes they are so malignant, especially when they are black, that they can kill infants. For these, I shall leave the cure to the expert physician.

On falling sickness or epilepsy. Although this very serious infirmity deserves a lengthy and learned discussion devoted exclusively to the topic, the least I can do here, so as not to pass by without acknowledging it among the other infirmities that children suffer, is to discuss it briefly, proposing just a few but certain remedies that can help children of every age.

First we advise that when this infirmity is congenital,[311] then the milk the child is given should be altered to the opposite of the cause, which is excessive frigidity and humidity. In this case, it is said to be a natural form of epilepsy, and it may be expected to resolve, with the prescription of good regimens, as the child gets older. And if growing up he does not recover from this ailment, it should be expected he will die with it.

But if he develops this infirmity after his birth, he will be able to recover. And in curing this ailment, it is important to pay attention to the regimen of the wet nurse. She should be purged, keeping her away from all things that increase phlegm; and she should nurse the child with the smallest amount of milk possible, then be diligent and cautious that the food does not corrupt in his stomach. She should also make sure that the child holds mint in his hand, and smells it often; and she should keep some root of peony, or emeralds, tied close to his collar; coral tied to the neck of the child is also useful, and this is common practice. Also useful is the pulverized bone of the head of a man given to him in his food or with wine or sugar.[312] At times give him theriac. Also useful is Mesue's confection of diamusk.[313]

---

311. On epilepsy and other diseases considered hereditary in the Middle Ages, see Maaike van der Lugt, "Les maladies héréditaires dans la pensée scolastique, XIIe–XVIe siècle," and Carlos López-Beltrán, "Les *haereditarii morbi* au début de l'époque moderne," both in *L'hérédité entre Moyen Âge et époque moderne: Perspectives historiques*, ed. Maaike van der Lugt and Charles de Miramon (Florence: SISMEL, Edizioni del Galluzzo, 2008), respectively 273–320 and 321–51.

312. On this specific substance for the treatment of epilepsy, see for example Valentina Giuffra and Gino Fornaciari, "Pulverized Human Skull in Pharmacological Preparations: Possible Evidence from the "martyrs of Otranto" (Southern Italy, 1480)," *Journal of Ethnopharmacology* 160 (2015): 133–39.

313. See Mesuae, *De re medica*, Lib. III.5 (p. 232): *Electuarium dulce ex moscho*.

Let this suffice at the moment, reminding you, with regard to this and other infirmities, that what I have written is brief in respect to what needs to be written on these topics, including an explanation of their causes and the rules to be followed in their treatment. Because I have written this for women, I have included familiar and light remedies, those that may be necessary and be of assistance at the first onset of the infirmity. But once these ailments become more serious, I recommend that the expert physician be called. Certainly if I had set out to write all that should be said, I would have composed a much longer volume. Anyone who wishes to study these ailments further should read Avicenna and the other authorities who have written more extensively on these illnesses. I will stop here also because I have dealt with these ailments at length in my longer *Practica*. Therefore, we give thanks to God for this brief discussion of these topics.

Chapter Five
On how to care for the well-being of the soul and body of the child

The words contained in this chapter are nothing more than moral instructions, so that the child may grow in dignity and morality and bodily health: because certainly, as Avicenna says, "the safekeeping of the health of both soul and the body consists in the moderation of habits."[314] Therefore, fathers and mothers should exert great diligence and effort in rearing their children, and begin early: so that the children may accustom themselves to these habits, and because the more they take in when they are young, the stronger they will be when they are adults; this is why they say: "what youth is used to, age remembers."[315]

And if ever it were necessary to begin early, now is the time, because our generation has declined so much compared to the past, so that children who are three years old at the present are as astute as five- and six-year-olds used to be, and those who are five behave like seven- or eight-year-old children. We certainly see that life spans are getting shorter now than they were long ago: now few men and women reach the age of seventy, whereas in the past they lived to be more than one hundred. And if you ask, *frontoso*, the cause, even though it is not the main concern of this chapter, I will discuss this briefly, hoping that my readers will enjoy learning about this topic, because certainly this is something worth knowing, and as you will recognize, it is not far from our purpose.

But before doing this, I would like to explain the saying of Avicenna, because it greatly serves our purpose, which also relies on his authority. The matchless Avicenna advises that fathers should always strive to better the morals of their children. Accordingly, he suggests that children be raised with great prudence and

---

314. In Latin in the text: *in temperamento igitur morum custodia sanitatis anime et corporis simul constitunt.* See Avicenna, *Canon,* Lib. I, fen 3, doctr. 1, c. 4 (p. 169).

315. In Latin in the text: *quod nova testa capit, inveterata sapit.*

kindliness, and encouraged to pursue their healthy appetites, and not forced to do the opposite, so that they will not feel upset or threatened. When they are too often scolded with threats, they develop bad habits, and they become wrathful and fearful, and so distress their complexion, which is changed by the heat caused by anger, or the melancholic humor caused by fear and sadness. This is why Avicenna said that the health of the body and soul consists in maintaining a moral mean.

I will now return, *frontoso*, to a question often asked by the medical authorities, especially the Paduan Peter of Abano: whether it is true that our life expectancy is now shorter than in the past, remembering here the lives of our ancient forefathers: Adam who lived to be 930 years old, Noah who reached the age of 700, Methuselah 900, and many others who lived hundreds of years. And rather than continue to cite ages, to be brief, I will respond by agreeing with my fellow citizen Peter of Abano, briefly saying that there are two causes for the brevity of our lives. One cause derives from the conjunctions of the stars, which induce various effects on earthly things; however, since this would require too long an explanation, I shall not enter upon it. The other cause is itself earthly, and is governed by the free will of men: and this we will divide in two.

First, we will note that men and women in our times are very prone to gluttony, much more than the ancients. We read that our forefathers were satisfied by eating simply acorns and chestnuts, as Galen writes in the second book of his treatise *On the Properties of Foodstuffs*.[316] Since they nourished themselves mainly with coarse and harsh foods, their bodily humors as well as their spirits were made compact and strong; hence their bodies became much stronger than ours today. This is why in the past Hippocrates and other physicians prescribed powerful medicines—like hellebore, euphorbia, mezereon, and scammony—in great quantities, which in the present we cannot use because of the weakness of our bodies, brought on by our over-refined and extravagant lives.

Because we eat foods that are delicate, soft, and liquid, which are easily dissolved, making our humors softer and more easily dissolved in consequence, the composition of our bodies becomes loose and rarified, and the same is true for the spirits. And as even the slightest wind blows us to the ground, we are not able to sustain great toil, or strong medicines. This is why air has more power over us than in the past, and the stars also have more effect on us than they once had; therefore we can no longer tolerate these things as bodies of the past used to, and this is why we die earlier. Therefore, *frontoso* delicate gentleman, and you *frontosa* delicate lady, leading the life you lead, you will die much earlier than workers and peasants. This is why you should accustom your children little by little, and with discretion, to eating course foods, if you love them and you wish them to have a

---

316. Galen, *On the Properties of Foodstuffs*, Book II, ch. 38 (p. 98); =Kühn, 6:621. Galen writes that the Arcadians nourished themselves in this way "for a very long time, although all present-day Greeks use cereals."

long life. I say "little by little" because they are delicate when they are babies; hence in this process it is necessary to use great wisdom.

O *frontosa*, think that if this first explanation seems pertinent, how much more you will appreciate the second explanation of the cause of our present decline—for it concerns the sexual intercourse of men and women. *Frontosa*, you should know that in the olden days, by which I mean until less than two hundred years ago, young men did not marry before the age of twenty-five, as was said at the beginning of this book, and women were at least eighteen years old. Since they married when they were both mature, and their principal bodily parts were strong and well formed, nature did not debilitate them in the act of intercourse; thus the semen of both parents was complete and strong, and generated a stronger fetus. Today, however, people copulate before the appropriate time; and the nourishment that should contribute to the strength of their limbs dissipates in superfluity. As a result, they are feeble and produce weak seed, which generates a fetus that is weak and vulnerable, and dies earlier.

Nowadays, we are so lascivious and so ready and desirous for coitus that men behave like beasts, engaging often in this act, with food in their stomachs, and in every other way [disregarding sound advice], thus debilitating their seed. O drunkard, in this way you will generate yet another drunkard; and for this reason you must be sober in the act of coitus. Nowadays, men are not satisfied with their wives; they also want young maids. Keep in mind what Aristotle says, that to lie with a woman other than a wife goes against nature, because the offspring that are born are not looked after and they are ill-bred, and because of them, nature is vilified. O filthy ruffian, tie a string around your finger and remember this.

It seems, therefore, that the solution to the question that has been posed about human degeneration is now evident: since, given the decline of the natural human condition, infants who are currently five years old are like those who were seven long ago, these children should be sent to school earlier, and they should be educated earlier than in the past.

We will now move on to our main concern, the morals that children should learn from their parents. There are two regimens the child should follow: first, that which instills the moral principles necessary for civil existence; and second, that which nourishes his spiritual life.

At the time when the little child starts to talk and to understand more, that is usually from one to two years, you should speak to him with kindness and with tact, calling him "my dear child," and using his name. And at this moment you should have on hand things that he enjoys, so you can say "I will give you this, if you say what I say," and in this manner name one object after another. And in doing this, most women are well-skilled.

It is also important not to instill great fear in children, making them timid, and causing them to become melancholic; as Hippocrates says, "if fear and pusillanimity last a long time, they are made melancholic."[317] Similarly, do not anger them, nor let them stay idle; instead, let them go out and play.

But when they begin to pronounce words, from two to three years of age, this is when you should guide their tongues and actions to moral words and ways. Teach children to obey their father and mother and others in their station; and especially make sure that, with their little knees planted on the floor, they reverently proffer these names, "Yhesu, Maria," teaching them the Ave Maria and the Lord's Prayer, and making them recite these prayers daily, and teaching them how to make the sign of the cross, and similar things, which Christian matrons know well how to teach.

Now when they reach the age of five, children should start with a tutor, if you can afford one. The tutor should be able to educate children in good manners and letters, neither holding them back nor continuously compelling them, but instead, after they have been schooled enough, letting them play and exercise. The tutor should take good care of the youngsters, sending them home at least one hour or more before the older children, aged fourteen or more, and they should manage the children's education with few blows and much praise. The tutor should not behave erratically, but instead he should be old-fashioned and wise. Children should feel great reverence for the tutor because of his age and wisdom, and they should feel this way more from the great respect they have for him than from fear of blows. Surely such tutors, when they are well-trained and well-mannered, deserve great respect. And now turning to the spiritual life, I advise fathers and mothers to take their children to church, so that they will become familiar with the ceremonies performed in praise of God, and so that they become fully accustomed to these and keep God in the highest reverence. Children should regularly be taken to worship on the appropriate days, to attend sermons and vespers and other occasions, and parents should often demonstrate the importance of all matters pertaining to religion, so that when the children grow up they will remember this instruction and observe it effortlessly. Also it is important to bring them before a discreet confessor who will guide them toward the good and warn them of the bad. Parents should take special care that their children speak honorably, and protect them from the company of children who are spoiled and wayward.

After the child masters the Ave Maria and Paternoster, teach him the Creed above all else, because it is the foundation of our faith, by which we are saved, and encourage the child to continuously repeat it. O *frontosa*, there is no greater power than that which comes from the true love that man acquires towards God. For he who truly loves God is absolved of all sins, holding all sin in abomination, because sin is contrary to God, the sum of all virtues. This is why philosophers

---

317. In Latin in the text: *si timor et pusillanimitas multum tempus habitant, melancolicum perficiunt.* See Hippocrates, *Aphorisms*, VI.23 (p. 184).

write that virtue is man's eternal and enduring possession. And what endures more eternally than God?

Of course, I also condemn those good-for-nothing slacker fathers—they should be stoned!—who do not esteem holy matrimony and lie with wretched women and so give birth to wretched children. O my dear children, how much grace you receive from God when you are born of a legitimate marriage and of proper parents who take good care of you! Those who are born illegitimately are like counterfeit coins: that is, completely without worth.

Because certainly, *frontosa*, taking good care of your children will ensure that later they will be well-disciplined, and without good discipline they cannot be virtuous. This is because virtue is not in us by nature. We must acquire it through discipline and good habits, that prepare us to receive it in our souls, just as soil ploughing will cause the seed to produce much better fruit, as long as the seed is good and not spoiled. This is why you must be very careful not to say improper words or tell improper stories in front of the child, so that you do not plant a bad seed in his soul, but instead speak of worthy and fruitful topics. As the poet so aptly says: "while the child is young, instill him with worthy morals."[318]

And here I emphasize again, it is important to make sure that the tutor or pedagogue is of good upbringing and that he values the child more greatly than the money he makes. You understand what I mean, *frontoso*. For if you are not diligent from the start in your search for the appropriate tutor, it then follows that once they are grown, children who have been badly reared will run after prostitutes and gamble, causing you great pain and suffering, and you will spend much more money for them than if you had found a good and moral tutor from the start.

Children must, therefore, be pushed to acquire good habits, so that they can acquire good virtues, something that everybody can acquire and make his own, as I have demonstrated in that little book *De non dictandis filiis*.[319] And as we have stated, children should be taught these virtues with kind words and with praise, together with fear and blows, thus balancing rewards with discipline; so if you first shame them, later you should find room for praise as well, alternating the two, as long as you keep the praise in check. Also, it is important when they are very young, not to overwork them, as many parents do, wanting their children to

318. In Latin in the text: *dum tener est gnatus, generosos instrue mores.* This saying is attributed to the ancient elegiac poet Phocylides.

319. This is Savonarola's only mention of this lost work (written before 1460). In the edition of *De regimine praegnantium*, Belloni—following the Vatican manuscript—writes *dietandis*, but he notes that the Venice manuscript has *dictandis* instead. The third manuscript (Reggio Emilia, Biblioteca Panizzi, Codice Turri C 12), unknown to Belloni, also has *dictandis*. The second reading, the one discarded by Belloni, is preferred, resulting in the title *On What Should Not Be Prescribed to Children*, rather than *On Diets that Ought Not Be Given to Children*. See also in this volume the Introduction, note 121, and *DRP*, 198.

exceed others; or halfway through their lives, they might perhaps fall. Children need, as we have said, space to play.

And certainly, it is also imperative that you stay involved in your child's rearing and you should examine daily your child's exercises and work, in a much more diligent way than if you have employees on salary. How can you possibly prioritize checking the work your employees have completed and not take an interest in what your own child has done and learned? O beastly and blind *frontoso*, tie this string around your finger and remember the common saying, a business thrives under the eye of its owner.

Above all, father, and you, tutor, ensure that the child exercises his memory, which is the mother of the muses—that is, of the sciences—which rest in her arms.

Children should be forbidden to engage in empty talk and they should be condemned if they do so. They should also be steered away from anger, but taught to be docile and benevolent, and keep their hands to themselves and not injure others, walking the streets throwing stones. And it is especially important to make sure they do not tell lies.

O father, O mother, you with demonic and wicked morals, what sort of models will you be for your children and what terrible vices will they inherit from you? Learn to and force yourselves to be modest, to discipline and honor your children, exposing them to good examples and removing them from all reprehensible vices. Make sure to exercise moderation when beating, reprehending, and rebuking your children, and support them with good words and do not rush to spankings.

So definitely, he who observes the aforementioned rules will have good children and will be a good parent.

Therefore, my Ferrarese ladies, to whom I have also addressed this little book, you should read and study my words. Do not fear the effort, and put it to good use for yourselves and for your infants. Perhaps you will ask, *frontosa*, "who could possibly follow so many rules?" I respond that these rules are put forward to help you with raising your children; and will serve as a mirror, in which parents, looking in it at their reflections, will better recognize their errors, and turn away from them.

It is true that what has been said is addressed to those who can afford to do these things, but I have also kept in mind the needy, so that they too may learn how to raise their children, and their children may grow in virtue. I want to remind them how greatly virtue exalts the human being, and how many in the past and present who were born in a low station or of lowly ancestors have become rich by their virtue alone, and, overtaking the highborn, have joined the ranks of doctors, cavaliers and great captains, cardinals, popes, and great ladies. And of these the poet says so well that "ardent virtue raised [them] up to the stars,"[320] for it

---

320. Virgil, *Aeneid* 6.130: *aut ardens evexit ad sidera virtus.*

is by virtue that humanity rises to the stars. Therefore, you impoverished readers who do not have anything material to leave your children, take care to make them virtuous and near to God.

We praise the Lord for whom this book was written and also we praise Mary, who was pregnant with him and gave birth to him, as well as to all the holy children whose blood was sacrificed for the love of Jesus.

Amen.

Bibliography

Primary Sources

Works by Michele Savonarola

Works by Savonarola are numbered for easier reference in the footnotes to the introduction and translated text. [L] and [V] signify texts in Latin or the vernacular (*volgare*). Citations of items under the heading "Studies" are in author (last name)/date format, with full citations following in the section on *Secondary Sources*.

Medical works composed in Padua
1. *Directorium ad actum practicum* (ca. 1420). Deontological treatise on the practice of medicine. [L]
    Manuscript: Munich, Bayerische Staatsbibliothek, Lat. 12021.
    Studies: Pesenti 1977; Pesenti 1984; Segarizzi 1900.
2. *Practica canonica de febribus* (before 1439). Dedicated to the physician Rainiero Siculo. On fevers. [L]
    Editions: Bologna: Dionisio Bertocchi, 1487. Other editions in 1496, 1498, 1503, 1517, 1531, 1543, 1552, 1560, 1561, 1563, 1577.
    Studies: Pesenti 1984; Segarizzi 1900.
3. *De pulsibus, urinis et egestionibus* (before 1439). On pulse, urine, and evacuations. [L]
    Editions: Venice: Christoforo de Pensis di Mandello, 1497. Other editions in 1498, 1503, 1517, 1531, 1543, 1552, 1560, 1561, 1563, 1577.
    Studies: Pesenti 1984.
4. *De vermibus* (before 1440). Dedicated to Zanardo Cambiatore from Reggio. On worms. [L]
    Editions: Venice: Ottaviano Scoto per Boneto Locatello, 1498. Other editions in 1503, 1517, 1531, 1543, 1552, 1560, 1561, 1563, 1577.
    Studies: Penso 1973, 96–98; Pesenti 1977; Pesenti 1984; Segarizzi 1900.
5. *Dialogus de contentione alei cum cepa* (before 1440). Lost work. Dialogical dispute between Garlic and Onion. [L]
    Quoted in: Segarizzi 1900.
6. *Practica maior, or Practica de aegritudinibus a capite usque ad pedes* (1440, before 1446). Dedicated to the physician Sigismondo Policastro. Started in Padua, completed in Ferrara before 1446. On diseases from head to toe. [L]
    Editions: Colle Val d'Elsa: Bono di Béthune, 1479. Other editions in 1486, 1497, 1502, 1518, 1519, 1547, 1559, 1560, 1561.

Studies: Albano 1997; Agrimi, Crisciani 1994; Demaitre 1976; Demaitre 2013; Jacquart 2011; Pesenti 1977; Pesenti 1984; Segarizzi 1900.

Medical works composed in Ferrara

7. *Libellus de aqua ardenti* (1440). On grape spirit. [L and V]
   Latin version dedicated to the jurist Antonio Roselli:
   Manuscripts: Modena, Biblioteca Estense, cod. lat. 174 [= α.O.6.15]; Munich, Bayerische Staatsbibliothek, Lat. 207.
   Vernacular version, dedicated to Leonello of Este, Marquis of Ferrara and Duke of Modena and Reggio from 1441 to 1450:
   Editions: (1) Michele Savonarola. *I trattati in volgare della peste e dell'acqua ardente.* Edited by Luigi Belloni. Milan: Stucchi, 1953. (2) Michele Savonarola. *Trattato dell'acqua ardente.* Edited by Piero Cigada. Milan: Philobyblon, 1988.
   Studies: Jacquart 1993; Pesenti 1984; Segarizzi 1900.

8. *Speculum physionomiae* (1442). Dedicated to Leonello of Este. On physiognomy. [L]
   Manuscripts: Leipzig, Universitätsbibliothek, 3472; Paris, Bibliothèque Nationale, lat. 7357; Venice, Biblioteca Marciana, Lat. VI, 156 (2672).
   Edition: Michele Savonarola. *Speculum physionomiae.* Edited by Gabriella Zuccolin. Florence: SISMEL, Edizioni del Galluzzo. Forthcoming for the series *Corpus philosophorum medii aevi* of the Unione Accademica Nazionale.
   Studies: Agrimi 2002; Denieul-Cormier 1953; Denieul-Cormier 1956; Federici Vescovini 1991; Federici Vescovini 1996; Federici Vescovini 2001; Pesenti 1977; Pesenti 1984; Segarizzi 1900; Thomann 1997; Thorndike 1934; Ziegler 2001; Ziegler 2004; Ziegler 2005a; Ziegler 2005b; Ziegler 2007; Ziegler 2008; Ziegler 2011; Ziegler 2014; Zuccolin 2012; Zuccolin 2018.

9. *De preservatione a peste et eius cura* (1444–1449). Dedicated to the citizens of Ferrara. On the plague. [V]
   Edition: Michele Savonarola. *I trattati in volgare della peste e dell'acqua ardente.* Edited by Luigi Belloni. Milan: Stucchi, 1953.
   Studies: Pesenti 1977; Pesenti 1984; Segarizzi 1900.

10. *De balneis* (1448–1449). Dedicated to Borso of Este, Marquis of Ferrara from 1450 and Duke of Ferrara and Modena from 1452 to 1471. On thermal baths. [L]
    Editions: Sergio Pasalodos Requejo. *De balneis et termis Ytalię de Michele Savonarola: Edición crítica, traducción y estudio.* PhD diss., Universidad de Valladolid, Valladolid, 2020; Ferrara: Andrea Gallo [André Belfort], 1485. Other editions in 1493, 1496, 1497, 1498, 1503, 1508, 1517, 1531, 1543, 1552, 1553, 1560, 1561, 1563, 1577.
    Studies: Chambers 1992; Gualdo 2004; Montagnani 2004; Nicoud 2002;

Nicoud 2007a; Nicoud 2011; Park 1999; Pesenti 1984; Segarizzi 1900; Thorndike 1934.

11. *De gotta* (ca. 1450). Posthumous dedication to Niccolò III of Este, Marquis of Ferrara from 1393 to 1441. On gout. [V]
Edition: Michele Savonarola. *De gotta, la preservatione e cura de essa per lo preclaro medico m. Michel Savonarola ordinata et intitulata allo illustre Marchese di Ferrara S. Niccolò da Este.* Pavia: Jacopo da Borgofranco, 1505.
Studies: Cracolici 2011; Crisciani 2003; Gualdo 2004; Pesenti 1984; Van der Lugt 2008.

12. *Libreto de tute le cosse che se magnano comunamente* (after 1452). Dedicated to Borso of Este. On dietetics. [V]
Editions: (1) Michele Savonarola. *Libreto de tute le cosse che se manzano: Un libro di dietetica di Michele Savonarola, medico padovano del secolo XV: Edizione critica basata sul Codice Casanatense 406.* Edited by Jane Nystedt. Stockholm: Gotab, 1982. (2) Michele Savonarola. *Libreto de tutte le cosse che se magnano: Un'opera di dietetica del secolo XV.* Edited by Jane Nystedt. Stockholm: Almqvist & Wiksell, 1988.
Studies: Agrimi 1984; Jacquart 1987; Alberini 1991; Bell 1999; Cracolici 2011; Nystedt 1997; Past 2011; Pesenti 1984; Segarizzi 1900.

13. *De regimine praegnantium et noviter natorum usque ad septennium* (before 1460). Dedicated to the women of Ferrara. On gynecology, obstetrics, and pediatrics. [V]
Manuscripts: Vatican Apostolic Library, Ms Reginense Latino 1142; Venice, Biblioteca Marciana, Ital. III 30; Reggio Emilia, Biblioteca Panizzi, Codice Turri C 12.
Edition: Michele Savonarola. *Il trattato ginecologico-pediatrico in volgare "Ad mulieres ferrarienses de regimine pregnantium" di Michele Savonarola.* Edited by Luigi Belloni. Milan: Stucchi, 1952.
Studies: Green 2008; Gualdo 1996; Gualdo 1999; Gualdo 2001; Marafioti 2010; Martorelli Vico 2011; O'Neill 1974; O'Neill 1975; Zuccolin 2008a; Zuccolin 2011.

14. *Consilia.* [L]
Manuscript: Florence, Biblioteca Riccardiana, 2153 (L III 12).
Studies: Belloni 1953; Pesenti 1984; Segarizzi 1900.

15. *Ricettario* [spurious]. Recipe collection.
Manuscript: Ferrara, Biblioteca Ariostea, ms Cl. II, 147.
Studies: Corrain 1985; Corrain 1987; Menini 1954–1955; Pesenti 1984; Torresi 1992.

16. *Dialogo del vilano e de la rapa* (before 1452). Lost work. Dialogue between the peasant and the turnip. [V]
Quoted in: Pesenti 1984; Segarizzi 1900.

17. *De lepra*. Dedicated to Gianpietro Gonzaga. On leprosy. [L]
     Manuscript: Florence, Biblioteca Riccardiana, 868 (LII 1), 165ra–189rb.
     Studies: Pesenti 1984; Segarizzi 1900; Thorndike 1934.

Historical works

18. *Libellus de magnificis ornamentis regiae civitatis Paduae* (1446–1447). Dedicated to the friar Antonio de Sancto Arcangelo. Encomium of Padua. [L]
     Edition: Michele Savonarola. *Libellus de magnificis ornamentis regie civitatis Padue*. Edited by Arnaldo Segarizzi. In *Rerum italicarum scriptores,* vol. 24.15 (Città di Castello: Lapi, 1902).
     Studies: Crisciani 2005a; Crisciani 2005b; Donato 1999; Donato 2000; Pesenti 1977; Pesenti 1984; Segarizzi 1900.
19. *De la decorante Ferrara* (before 1452). Lost work. Encomium of Ferrara. [V]
     Studies: Pesenti 1984; Segarizzi 1900.

Courtly works

20. *Del felice progresso di Borso d'Este / De felici progressu illustrissimi Borsii Estensis ad marchionatum Ferrariae, Mutinae et Regii ducatum comitatumque Rodigii* (ca. 1452). Dedicated to Borso of Este. Political and encomiastic work for Borso. [L and V]
     Latin version:
        Manuscript: Modena, Biblioteca Nazionale Estense, lat. α. W. 2, 15.
     Vernacular version:
        Edition: Michele Savonarola. *Del felice progresso di Borso d'Este.* Edited by Maria Aurelia Mastronardi. Bari: Palomar, 1996.
     Studies: Cracolici 2011; Mastronardi 1998; Mastronardi 2000; Samaritani 1976; Segarizzi 1900; Zuccolin 2007.
21. *De vera republica et digna saeculari militia* (ca. 1460). Dedicated to Niccolò di Leonello of Este. Political work. [L]
     Manuscript: Modena, Biblioteca Nazionale Estense, cod. lat. 114 [= α.W.6.6].
     Studies: Mastronardi 1996; Samaritani 1976; Segarizzi 1900.
22. *De nuptiis Battibecco et Serrabocca* (1466). Dedicated to the physician Niccolò Varo. Satirical work on courtly virtues and vices. [V]
     Edition: Michele Savonarola. *Peccati di lingua alla corte estense: Il "De nuptiis" di Michele Savonarola.* Edited by Paola Biamini. *Schifanoia* 11 (1992): 101–79.
     Studies: Cracolici 2011; Samaritani 1976; Segarizzi 1900.
23. *De sapiente et insipiente* (1466). Dialogue on morals and princely virtues. [L]
     Manuscript: Città del Vaticano, Biblioteca Apostolica Vaticana, ms. Vat. Ott. Lat. 1667.
     Studies: Samaritani 1976; Samaritani 1985; Zuccolin 2010.

24. *Funerary epitaph for Niccolò III of Este.* [L]
    Edition: Ferrante Borsetti. *Historia almi Ferrariae gymnasii,* vol. 1:43. Ferrara: Bernardino Pomatelli, 1735. Facsimile reprint Bologna: Forni, 1970. Studies: Bertoni and Vicini 1906, 40; Capra 1973, 198–99; Pesenti 1984; Segarizzi 1900.

Religious works

25. *Exhortatio ad Nicolaum fratrem* (before 1454). Dedicated to Michele's brother Niccolò Savonarola. Exhortation to virtue. [L]
    Manuscript: Toledo, Archivo y Biblioteca Capitular, 100.42, fols. 122v–130v.
    Edition: Sesto Prete. "Umanesimo a Ferrara nel secolo XV." *Atti dell'Accademia delle scienze di Ferrara* 43–44 (1965–1967): 65–78.
    Studies: Prete 1964; Prete 1967; Samaritani 1976.

26. *De laudibus Johannis Baptiste* (before 1458). Hymn in praise of John the Baptist. [L]
    Manuscript: Ferrara, Biblioteca Comunale Ariostea, ms. Cl. II, 147 α.
    Studies: Samaritani 1976; Segarizzi 1900.

27. *De non dictandis filiis* (before 1460). Lost work. On pedagogy.
    Studies: Samaritani 1976; Pesenti 1977; Pesenti 1984.

28. *Confessionale* I (for laymen; ca. 1461). Handbook for confession. [V]
    Manuscript: Modena, Biblioteca Estense, cod. ital. 107 [= α.T.6.1].
    Edition: Zuccolin 2018, 237–71.
    Studies: Samaritani 1976; Segarizzi 1900; Zuccolin 2008b.

29. *Confessionale* II (for clerics; ca. 1461). Dedicated to the Carthusian monks in Ferrara. Handbook for confession. [V]
    Manuscript: Modena, Biblioteca Estense, cod. ital. 117 [= α.S.7.7].
    Edition: Zuccolin 2018, 272–309.
    Studies: Samaritani 1976; Segarizzi 1900; Zuccolin 2008b.

30. *De cura languoris animi ex morbo venientis.* Dedicated to Ludovico Casella, secretary of Borso of Este. On the exercise of patience in times of sickness. [L]
    Edition: Michele Savonarola. *De cura languoris animi ex morbo venientis.* Edited by Cesare Menini. Ferrara: Istituto di storia della medicina dell'Università di Ferrara, 1955.
    Studies: Segarizzi 1900.

31. *Ad Laurentium adolescentem monacum de fortitudine et poenitentia* (before 1466). Dedicated to the novice Lorenzo. On the virtues of strength and penitence. [L]
    Manuscript: Ferrara, Biblioteca Comunale Ariostea, ms. Cl. II, 83 α.
    Studies: Samaritani 1976.

Other Primary Sources

Manuscripts

Hamburg, Staats- und Universitätsbibliothek, cod. med. 801, an. 1494, 9–130 (*Von Kranckheiten, Siechtagen und Zuval der Swangern und geberenden frowen und ihrer neugebornen Kinderen*).

Munich, Bayerische Staatsbibliothek, Clm 207 (*Antonii Cermisoni consilia* [. . .] *cum prologo Hartmanni Schedelii et effigie Cermisoni ab Hermanno Schedelio Paduae collecta et conscripta*). This ms, dated 1440–1444, also contains other *consilia* by the Italian physicians (active in Padua) Cristoforo Barzizza and Bartolomeo da Montagnana, as well as one treatise on wine by Arnaud de Villanova and the Latin version of the treatise on grape spirit by Michele Savonarola.

Munich, Bayerische Staatsbibliothek, Clm 25 (*Bartholomaei de Montagnana consilia*).

Printed works

Albert the Great [Albertus Magnus]. *De animalibus libri XXVI, nach der Cölner Urschrift*. Edited by Hermann Stadler. 2 vols. Münster: Aschendorff, 1916–1920.

Albert the Great [pseud., Albertus Magnus]. *El "De secretis mulierum" atribuido a Alberto Magno: Estudio, edición crítica y traducción*. Edited by José Pablo Barragán Nieto. Porto: Fédération internationale des instituts d'études médiévales, 2012.

Alberti, Leon Battista. *I libri della famiglia*. Edited by Francesco Furlan. New ed. Turin: Einaudi, 1994.

Aldobrandino da Siena. *Le régime du corps de Maître Aldebrandin de Sienne: Texte français du 13e siecle*. Edited by Louis Landouzy and Roger Pépin. Paris: Honoré Champion, 1911. Reprint Geneva: Slatkine, 1978.

Aristotle. *On the Generation of Animals*. Edited by Hendrik J. Drossaart Lulofs. Oxford: Clarendon Press, 1965.

———. *History of Animals, I–VI*. Translated by Arthur L. Peck. London: W. B. Heinemann; Cambridge, MA: Harvard University Press, 1965–1970; *VII–X*. Edited and translated by David M. Balme. Cambridge, MA: Harvard University Press, 1991.

———. *Metaphysics*. Edited by William D. Ross. Oxford: Clarendon Press, 1924.

———. *Nicomachean Ethics*. Edited by William D. Ross. Oxford: Clarendon Press, 1908.

———. *Physics*. Edited by William D. Ross. Oxford: Clarendon Press, 1955.

———. *Politics*. Translated by Benjamin Jowett, with introduction, analysis, and index by Henry W. C. Davis. Oxford: Clarendon Press, 1905.

————. *Prior and Posterior Analytics*. Edited by William D. Ross. Oxford: Clarendon Press, 1949.

Aristotle [pseud.]. *Problems*. Edited and translated by Robert A. Mayhew. Cambridge, MA: Harvard University Press, 2011.

Arnaldus de Villanova. *Regimen sanitatis ad regem Aragonum*. Edited by Luis García Ballester and Michael R. McVaugh, with others. Vol. 10.1 of *Opera medica omnia*. Barcelona: Publicacions i edicions de la Universitat de Barcelona, 1996.

Augustine of Hippo. *De civitate dei*. Edited by Bernhard Dombart and Alfons Kalb. Corpus Christianorum, Series Latina, 47–48. 2 vols. Turnhout: Brepols, 1955.

Averroes. *Colliget libri VII*. Supplement I (vol. 10) of Aristotle, *Omnia quae extant opera*. Venice: Giunta, 1562. Facsimile reprint, with title *Aristotelis Opera cum Averrois commentariis: Venetiis apud Junctas 1562–1574*, Frankfurt am Main: Minerva, 1962.

Avicenna. *De animalibus*. In *Avicenne perhypatetici philosophi ac medicorum facile primi opera in lucem redacta, ac nuper quantum ars niti potuit per canonicos emendata*. Venice: Ottaviano Scoto per Boneto Locatello, 1508. Facsimile reprint Frankfurt am Main: Minerva, 1961.

————. *Canon medicinae*. Edited by Giovanni Costeo and Giovanni Paolo Mongio. 2 vols. Venice: Giunta, 1608.

————. *Liber de anima, seu Sextus de naturalibus: Édition critique de la traduction latine médiévale*. Edited by Simone Van Riet. Introduction by Gérard Verbeke on the psychological doctrine of Avicenna. Vol. 2 (IV–V) of 2. Louvain: Éditions Orientalistes; Leiden: Brill, 1968.

Bacon, Roger. *Secretum secretorum cum glossis et notulis*. Edited by Robert Steele. Anglo-Norman version edited by A. S. Fulton. Oxford: Clarendon Press, 1920.

Barberino, Francesco da. *Un galateo femminile italiano del Trecento: Il "Reggimento e costumi di donna."* Edited by Giovanni Battista Festa. Bari: Laterza, 1910.

Bernardino da Siena. *Prediche volgari sul Campo di Siena 1427*. Edited by Carlo Delcorno. 2 vols. Milan: Rusconi, 1989.

Bourgeois, Louise. *Observations diverses sur la stérilité, perte de fruict, fœcondité, accouchements et maladies des femmes et enfants nouveaux naiz*. Paris: Saugrain, 1609. Multiple subsequent editions.

————. *Midwife to the Queen of France: Diverse Observations*. Edited by Alison Klairmont Lingo. Translated by Stephanie O'Hara. Toronto: Iter Press; Tempe, AZ: ACMRS, 2017.

Cermisone, Antonio. *Consilia medicinalia*. Frankfurt: ex Collegium Musarum Paltheniano, 1604.

Constantinus Africanus. *Pantechni decem libri theorices*. In *Opera omnia Ysaac*. Lyon: Bartholomeus Trot in officina Johannis de Platea, 1515.

Cordus, Valerius. *Dispensatorium pharmacorum omnium*. Nuremberg: Paulus Kaufmann, 1612.

Felici, Costanzo. *Scritti naturalistici*. Edited by Guido Arbizzoni. Urbino: Quattroventi, 1986.

Galen. *De alimentorum facultatibus*. In *Opera omnia*, 6 (1823): 453–748.

———. *Ars medica*. In *Opera omnia*, 1 (1821):305–412.

———. *Commentarii in Hippocratis Aphorismos*. In *Opera omnia*, 17,2 (1829): 345–450.

———. *On the Constitution of the Art of Medicine; The Art of Medicine; A Method of Medicine to Glaucon*. Edited and translated by Ian Johnston. Cambridge, MA: Harvard University Press, 2016.

———. *De crisibus*. In *Opera omnia*, 9 (1825): 550–768.

———. *On Diseases and Symptoms*. Edited and translated by Ian Johnston. Cambridge: Cambridge University Press, 2006.

———. *On the Natural Faculties*. Translated by Arthur J. Brock. Cambridge, MA: Harvard University Press, 1916.

———. *Opera omnia*. Edited by Karl Gottlob Kühn. 20 vols. in 22. Leipzig: Cnobloch, 1821–1833. Facsimile reprint Cambridge: Cambridge University Press, 2011.

———. *On the Properties of Foodstuffs*. Edited and translated by Owen Powell. Cambridge: Cambridge University Press, 2003.

———. *De sanitate tuenda*. In *Opera omnia*, 6 (1823): 1–452.

———. *De semine*. In *Opera omnia*, 4 (1822): 512–651.

———. *De symptomatum causis*. In *Opera omnia*, 7 (1824): 85–272.

———. *De usu partium corporis humani*. In *Opera omnia*, 3 (1822): 1–933, and 4 (1822): 1–366.

Guarini, Battista. *La didattica del greco e del latino: De ordine docendi ac studendi e altri scritti*. Edited by Luigi Piacente. Bari: Edipuglia, 2002.

Guarino Veronese [Guarino da Verona]. *Epistolario di Guarino Veronese*. Edited by Remigio Sabbadini. 3 vols. Venice: A spese della Società [di storia veneta], 1915–1919. Facsimile reprint Turin: Bottega d'Erasmo, 1959.

Hippocrates. *Aphorisms*. In *Hippocrates*, 4:97–222. Translated by William H. S. Jones. Cambridge, MA: Harvard University Press, 1931.

———. *Diseases of Women*, 1 and 2. In *Hippocrates*, 11. Edited and translated by Paul Potter. Cambridge MA: Harvard University Press, 2018.

———. *Regimen in Health*. In *Hippocrates*, 4:43–60. Translated by William H. S. Jones. Cambridge, MA: Harvard University Press, 1931.

Lawn, Brian, ed. *The Prose Salernitan Questions, Edited from a Bodleian Manuscript, Auct. F.3.10: An Anonymous Collection Dealing with Science and Medicine, Written by an Englishman c. 1200, with an Appendix of Ten Related Collections*. London: Oxford University Press for the British Academy, 1979.

Marinelli, Giovanni. *Le medicine pertinenti alle infirmità delle donne*. Venice: Francesco de Franceschi Senese, 1563.

Mercurio, Scipione [Girolamo]. *Della comare o riccoglitrice*. Venice: Giovan Battista Ciotti, 1595.

Mesuae Damasceni, Johannes [pseud.]. *De re medica libri tres*. Iacobo Sylvio medico interprete [Jacques Dubois]. Lyon: Jean de Tournes and Guillaume Gazeau, 1548.

Mondino dei Liucci [Liuzzi, Luzzi]. *Expositio super capitulum de generatione embrionis canonis Avicennae cum quibusdam quaestionibus*. Edited by Romana Martorelli Vico. Rome: Istituto storico italiano per il Medioevo, 1993.

Ovid. *Metamorphoses*. Vol. 2, Books 9–15. Translated by Frank J. Miller. Cambridge, MA: Harvard University Press, 1916. Third edition (1977) revised by G. P. Goold.

Piedemonte, Francesco. *Supplementum in secundum librum Compendii secretorum medicinae Io. Mesues [. . .]*. In *Ioannis Mesuae Damasceni medici clarissimi opera De medicamentorum purgantium delectu, castigatione et usu, Libri duo. [. . .]*, part 2. Venice: Giunta, 1623.

Ployant, Teresa. *Breve compendio dell'arte ostetricia di Madama Teresa Ployant*. Naples: Vincenzo Orsino, 1787.

Polenton, Sicco. *La Catinia, le orazioni e le epistole di Sicco Polenton*. Edited by Arnaldo Segarizzi. Bergamo: Istituto italiano d'arti grafiche, 1899.

Rhazes. *Liber ad Almansorem*. In *Opera parva Abubetri filii Zachariae filii Arasi [Rasis] que in hoc parvo volumine continentur*. Lyon: Impressa per Gilbertum de Villiers, impensis Johannis de Ferrariis, alias de Jolitis, ac Vincentii de Prothonariis, 1511.

———. *Continens Rasis*. 2 vols. Venice: Ottaviano Scoto, 1529.

———. *A Treatise on the Smallpox and Measles*. Edited and translated by William Alexander Greenhill. London: Sydenham Society, 1848.

———. *On the Treatment of Small Children (De curis puerorum): The Latin and Hebrew Translations*. Edited and translated by Gerrit Bos and Michael McVaugh. Leiden and Boston: Brill, 2015.

Rösslin, Eucharius. *Libro nel qual si tratta del parto delhuomo, e de tutte q[ue]lle cose, che cerca esso parto accadeno, e delle infermita che po[sso]no accadere a i fanciulli, con tutti i suoi rimedii posti particolarme[n]te*. Venice: Giovanni Andrea Valvassori, 1538.

———. *Der swangern Frauwen und hebammen Rosegarten*. Strasburg: Martin Flach, 1513. Facsimile reprint edited by Huldrych Martin F. Koelbing, Zurich: Verlag Bibliophile Drucke von J. Stocker, 1976.

———. *When Midwifery Became the Male Physician's Province: The Sixteenth-Century Handbook "The Rose Garden for Pregnant Women and Midwives."* Edited and translated by Wendy Arons. Jefferson, NC: McFarland, 1994.

Serapion [Johannes Serapion the Younger]. *Liber aggregatus in medicinis simplicibus.* Milan: Antonius Zarotus, 1473.

The Trotula: A Medieval Compendium of Women's Medicine. Edited and translated by Monica H. Green. Philadelphia: University of Pennsylvania Press, 2001.

Vergerio, Pietro Paolo. *The Character and Studies Befitting a Free-Born Youth.* Edited and translated by Craig Kallendorf. In *Humanist Educational Treatises,* edited by Craig Kallendorf, 2–91. Cambridge, MA: Harvard University Press, 2002.

Secondary Sources

Albano, Monica. "La metodologia della diagnostica e della terapeutica nella 'Practica maior' di M. Savonarola." *Rudiae: Ricerche sul mondo classico* 9 (1997): 319–47.

Alberini, Massimo. *Breve storia di Michele Savonarola: Seguita da un compendio del suo "Libretto de tutte le cosse che se manzano."* Padua: Editoriale Programma, 1991.

Albini, Giuliana. "I bambini nella società lombarda del Quattrocento: Una realtà ignorata o protetta?" *Nuova rivista storica* 68 (1984): 611–38.

Agrimi, Jole. *Ingeniosa scientia nature: Studi sulla fisiognomica medievale.* Florence: SISMEL, Edizioni del Galluzzo, 2002.

———. Review of Michele Savonarola, *Libreto de tute le cosse che se magnano: Un' opera di dietetica del secolo XV,* edited by Jane Nystedt (Stockholm: Gotab, 1982). *Aevum* 58 (1984): 358–65.

Agrimi, Jole, and Chiara Crisciani. "La medicina scolastica: Studi e ricerche, 1981–1991." In *Filosofia e teologia nel Trecento: Studi in ricordo di Eugenio Randi,* edited by Luca Bianchi, 381–412. Louvain-la-Neuve: Fédération internationale des instituts d'études médiévales, 1994.

Altieri Biagi, Maria Luisa. "Forme della comunicazione scientifica." In Alberto Asor Rosa, *La letteratura italiana,* vol. 3: *Le forme del testo,* 2: *La prosa,* 891–947. Turin: Einaudi, 1984.

———. *Guglielmo volgare: Studio sul lessico della medicina medievale.* Bologna: Forni, 1970.

Andretta, Elisa, and Marilyn Nicoud, eds. *Être médecin à la cour: Italie, France, Espagne, XIIIe–XVIIIe siècle.* Florence: SISMEL, Edizioni del Galluzzo, 2013.

Ariès, Philippe. *L'enfant et la vie familiale sous l'ancien régime.* Paris: Plon, 1960. New edition: Paris: Éditions du Seuil, 1973. Translated by Robert Baldick as *Centuries of Childhood: A Social History of Family Life* (New York: Alfred A. Knopf, 1962).

Arnaud, Sabine. *On Hysteria: The Invention of a Medical Category between 1670 and 1820.* Chicago: University of Chicago Press, 2015.

Ausécache, Mireille. "Une naissance monstrueuse au Moyen Age: Le 'frère de Salerne.'" *Gesnerus* 64 (2007): 5–23.

Bakos, Adrianna E. "A Knowledge Speculative and Practical: The Dilemma of Midwives' Education in Early Modern Europe." In *Women's Education in Early Modern Europe: A History, 1500 to 1800,* edited by Barbara J. Whitehead, 225–50. New York: Garland, 1999.

Barkai, Ron. *A History of Jewish Gynaecological Texts in the Middle Ages.* Leiden: Brill, 1998.

Barratt, Alexandra, ed. *The Knowing of Woman's Kind in Childing: A Middle English Version of Material Derived from the Trotula and Other Sources.* Turnhout: Brepols, 2001.

Battaglia, Salvatore, ed. *Grande dizionario della lingua italiana.* 21 vols. Turin: UTET, 1961–2009.

Bell, Rudolph M. *How To Do It: Guides to Good Living for Renaissance Italians.* Chicago: University of Chicago Press, 1999.

Beneduce, Chiara. *Natural Philosophy and Medicine in John Buridan: With an Edition of Buridan's "Quaestiones de secretis mulierum."* PhD diss., Radboud Universiteit, Nijmegen. Zutphen: Koninklijke Wöhrmann, 2017.

Berriot-Salvadore, Evelyne. *Un corps, un destin: La femme dans la médecine de la Renaissance.* Paris: Champion, 1993.

Bertoni, Giulio, and Emilio Paolo Vicini. *Poeti modenesi dei secoli XIV–XV.* Modena: Edizioni Rossi, 1906.

Bianchi, Luca. *Studi sull'aristotelismo del Rinascimento.* Padua: Il Poligrafo, 2003.

Bolton, Lesley. *An Edition, Translation and Commentary of Mustio's Gynaecia.* PhD diss., University of Calgary. Prism: University of Calgary's Digital Repository, 2015. <https://prism.ucalgary.ca/handle/11023/2252>

Boudet, Jean-Patrice, Franck Collard, and Nicolas Weill-Parrot, eds. *Médécine, astrologie et magie entre Moyen Âge et Renaissance: Autour de Pietro d'Abano.* Florence: SISMEL, Edizioni del Galluzzo, 2013.

Boudet, Jean-Patrice, Martine Ostorero, and Agostino Paravicini Bagliani, eds. *De Frédéric II à Rodolphe II: Astrologie, divination et magie dans les cours, XIIIe–XVIIe siècle.* Florence: SISMEL, Edizioni del Galluzzo, 2017.

Broomhall, Susan. *Women's Medical Work in Early Modern France.* Manchester: Manchester University Press, 2004.

Bryce, Judith. "Les livres des Florentines: Reconsidering Women's Literacy in Quattrocento Florence." In *At the Margins: Minority Groups in Premodern Italy,* edited by Stephen J. Milner, 133–61. Minneapolis: University of Minneapolis Press, 2005.

Burnett, Charles S. F. "The Planets and the Development of the Embryo." In *The Human Embryo: Aristotle and the Arabic and European Traditions,* edited by Gordon R. Dunstan, 95–112. Exeter: University of Exeter Press, 1990.

Cadden, Joan. *Meanings of Sex Difference in the Middle Ages: Medicine, Science and Culture*. Cambridge: Cambridge University Press, 1993.

Campbell, Julie D., and Anne R. Larsen, eds. *Early Modern Women and Transnational Communities of Letters*. Farnham, Surrey, UK: Ashgate, 2009.

Capra, Luciano. "Gli epitaffi per Niccolò III d'Este." *Italia medievale e umanistica* 16 (1973): 197–226.

Chambers, David S. "Spas in the Italian Renaissance." In *Reconsidering the Renaissance: Papers from the Twenty-First Annual Conference*, edited by Mario A. Di Cesare, 3–27. Binghamton, NY: Center for Medieval and Early Renaissance Studies, 1992.

Corrain, Cleto. "Alcune ricette d'interesse cosmetico in un ricettario attribuito a Michele Savonarola (1384–1468)." *Quaderni di scienze antropologiche* 11 (1985): 57–105.

———. "Alcune ricette interessanti: la cosmesi in un ricettario attribuito a Michele Savonarola (1384–1468)." *Atti e memorie della Accademia italiana di storia della farmacia* 4 (1987): 19–40.

Corriente, Federico. *Dictionary of Arabic and Allied Loanwords: Spanish, Portuguese, Catalan, Galician and Kindred Dialects*. Leiden and Boston: Brill, 2008.

Cotgrave, Randle. *Dictionarie of the French and English Tongues*. 1611; reprinted Columbia: University of South Carolina Press, 1950.

Cracolici, Stefano. "Michele Savonarola e le bizzarrie di corte." In Crisciani and Zuccolin, *Michele Savonarola*, 23–58. (2011).

Crisciani, Chiara. "*Historia* ed *exempla*: Storia e storie in alcuni testi di Michele Savonarola." In *Il principe e la storia: Atti del Convegno, Scandiano, 18–20 settembre 2003*, edited by Tina Matarrese and Cristina Montagnani, 53–68. Novara: Interlinea, 2005a.

———. "Histories, Stories, *Exempla*, and Anecdotes: Michele Savonarola from Latin to Vernacular." In *Historia: Empiricism and Erudition in Early Modern Europe*, edited by Gianna Pomata and Nancy G. Siraisi, 297–324. Cambridge, MA: MIT Press, 2005b.

———. "Michele Savonarola medico: Tra università e corte, tra latino e volgare." In *Filosofia in volgare nel Medioevo: Atti del Convegno della Società italiana per lo studio del pensiero medievale (S.I.S.P.M.), Lecce, 27–29 settembre 2002*, edited by Nadia Bray and Loris Sturlese, 433–49. Louvain-la-Neuve: Fédération internationale des instituts d'études médiévales, 2003.

———, and Gabriella Zuccolin, eds. *Michele Savonarola: Medicina e cultura di corte*. Florence: SISMEL, Edizioni del Galluzzo, 2011.

Dardano, Maurizio. "I linguaggi scientifici." In *Storia della lingua italiana*, vol. 2: *Scritto e parlato*, edited by Luca Serianni and Pietro Trifone, 497–551. Turin: Einaudi, 1994.

Daston, Lorraine J., and Katharine Park, eds. *Wonders and the Order of Nature, 1150–1750*. New York: Zone Books, 1998.

Dearnley, Elizabeth. "'Women of oure tunge cunne bettir reede and vnderstonde this langage': Women and Vernacular Translation in Later Medieval England." In *Multilingualism in Medieval Britain, c. 1066–1520: Sources and Analysis*, edited by Judith A. Jefferson and Ad Putter, 259–72. Turnhout: Brepols, 2013.

Demaitre, Luke. "The Idea of Childhood and Child Care in Medical Writings of the Middle Ages." *Journal of Psychohistory* 4 (1977): 461–90.

———. "Medical Writing in Transition: Between Ars and Vulgus." *Early Science and Medicine* 3.2 (1998): 88–102.

———. *Medieval Medicine: The Art of Healing, from Head to Toe*. Santa Barbara, CA: Praeger, 2013.

———. "Scholasticism in Compendia of Practical Medicine, 1250–1450." *Manuscripta* 20 (1976): 81–95.

De Mauro, Tullio, ed. *Grande dizionario italiano dell'uso* [GRADIT]. 8 vols. Turin: UTET, 1999–2007.

Denieul-Cormier, Anne. *Le "Speculum phisionomie" de Michel Savonarole et ses sources*. Paris: École des Chartes, 1953.

———. "La très ancienne 'Physiognomie' de Michel Savonarole." *La biologie médicale* 45 (1956): 1–107.

De Vos, Paula. "The 'Prince of Medicine': Yūḥannā ibn Māsawayh and the Foundations of the Western Pharmaceutical Tradition." *Isis* 104, no. 4 (December 2013): 667–712.

Donato, Maria M. "'Historie parens Patavum': Per una tradizione d'arte civica, dal Medioevo all'età moderna." In *Percorsi tra parole e immagini, 1400–1600*, edited by Angela Guidotti and Massimiliano Rossi, 51–74. Lucca: Pacini Fazzi, 2000.

———. "'Pictorie studium': Appunti sugli usi e lo statuto della pittura nella Padova dei Carraresi (e una proposta per le 'città liberate' di Altichiero e di Giusto al Santo)." *Il Santo: Rivista francescana di storia, dottrina e arte* 39 (1999): 467–504.

Du Cange, Charles Du Fresne. *Glossarium mediae et infimae latinitatis*. New edition by Léopold Favre. 10 vols. Niort: L. Favre, 1883–1887.

Federici Vescovini, Graziella. "L'individuale nella medicina tra Medioevo e Umanesimo: La fisiognomica di Michele Savonarola." In *Umanesimo e medicina: Il problema dell'individuale*, edited by Roberto Cardini and Mariangela Regoliosi, 63–87. Rome: Bulzoni, 1996.

———. "La medicina astrologica dello 'Speculum physiognomiae' di Michele Savonarola." *Keiron* 8 (2001), 110–15.

———. "Pietro d'Abano e la medicina astrologica dello 'Speculum physiognomiae' di Michele Savonarola." In *Musagetes: Festschrift für Wolfram Prinz zu seinem 60. Geburtstag am 5. Februar 1989*, edited by Ronald G. Kecks, 167–77. Berlin: Mann, 1991.

Ferguson, Margaret W. *Dido's Daughters: Literacy, Gender, and Empire in Early Modern England and France*. Chicago: University of Chicago Press, 2003.

Filippini, Nadia. "Levatrici e ostetricanti a Venezia tra Sette e Ottocento." *Quaderni storici* 20.58 (1985): 149–80.

Fioravanti, Gianfranco. "Un trattato medico di eugenetica: Il 'Libellus de ingenio bonae nativitatis.'" *Mediaevalia* 21 (2002): 89–111.

Fissell, Mary E. "Introduction: Women, Health, and Healing in Early Modern Europe." *Bulletin of the History of Medicine* 82 (2008): 1–17.

———. *Vernacular Bodies: The Politics of Reproduction in Early Modern England*. Oxford: Oxford University Press, 2004.

García Ballester, Luis. "On the Origin of the 'Six Non-Natural Things' in Galen." In *Galen und das hellenistische Erbe: Verhandlungen des IV. Internationalen Galen-Symposiums veranstaltet vom Institut für Geschichte der Medizin am Bereich Medizin (Charité) der Humboldt-Universität zu Berlin 18.–20. September 1989*, edited by Jutta Kollesch and Diethard Nickel, 105–15. Stuttgart: Franz Steiner, 1993.

Gentilcore, David. *Healers and Healing in Early Modern Italy*. Manchester: Manchester University Press, 1998.

Gerritsen, Willem P., and Anthony G. Van Melle, eds. *A Dictionary of Medieval Heroes: Characters in Medieval Narrative Traditions, and Their Afterlife in Literature, Theatre and the Visual Arts*. Woodbridge, Suffolk, UK; Rochester, NY: Boydell Press, 1998.

Gil-Sotres, Pedro. "Els 'regimina sanitatis.'" In Arnaldus de Villanova, *Regimen sanitatis ad regem Aragonum*, edited by Luis García Ballester, Juan A. Paniagua, and Michael R. McVaugh, 17–110. Barcelona: Publicacions i edicions de la Universitat de Barcelona, 1996.

Gislon Dopfel, Costanza, Alessandra Foscati, and Charles S. F. Burnett, eds. *Pregnancy and Childbirth in the Premodern World, European and Middle Eastern Cultures, from Late Antiquity to the Renaissance*. Turnhout: Brepols, 2019.

Giuffra, Valentina, and Gino Fornaciari. "Pulverized Human Skull in Pharmacological Preparations: Possible Evidence from the "martyrs of Otranto" (Southern Italy, 1480)." *Journal of Ethnopharmacology* 160 (2015): 133–39.

Green, Monica H. "Bodies, Gender, Health, Disease: Recent Work on Medieval Women's Medicine." *Studies in Medieval and Renaissance History* 2 (2005): 1–49.

———. "Books as a Source of Medical Education for Women in the Middle Ages." *Dynamis* 20 (2000b): 331–69.

———. "Caring for Gendered Bodies." In *Oxford Handbook of Medieval Women and Gender*, edited by Judith M. Bennett and Ruth Mazo Karras, 345–61. Oxford: Oxford University Press, 2013.

———. "From 'Diseases of Women' to 'Secrets of Women': The Transformation of Gynecological Literature in the Later Middle Ages." *Journal of Medieval and Early Modern Studies* 30 (2000c): 5–39.

———. *Making Women's Medicine Masculine: The Rise of Male Authority in Pre-Modern Gynaecology.* Oxford: Oxford University Press, 2008.

———. "The Possibilities of Literacy and the Limits of Reading: Women and the Gendering of Medical Literacy." In *Women's Healthcare in the Medieval West: Texts and Contexts*, edited by Monica H. Green, 1–76. Aldershot, UK; Burlington, VT: Ashgate, 2000a.

———. "The Sources of Eucharius Rösslin's 'Rosegarden for Pregnant Women and Midwives' (1513)." *Medical History* 53 (2009): 167–92.

Grendler, Paul F. *Schooling in Renaissance Italy: Literacy and Learning, 1300–1600.* Baltimore, MD: The Johns Hopkins University Press, 1989.

———. *The Universities of the Italian Renaissance.* Baltimore, MD: The Johns Hopkins University Press, 2002.

Grinaschi, Mario. "La diffusion du 'Secretum secretorum' ('Sirr-al'arsār') dans l'Europe Occidentale." *Archives d'histoire doctrinale et littéraire du Moyen Âge* 47 (1981): 7–69.

Gualdo, Riccardo. "Le cure e i bagni del principe nelle opere di Michele Savonarola." In *Gli umanisti e le terme: Atti del convegno internazionale di studio, Lecce, Santa Cesarea Terme, 23–25 maggio 2002*, edited by Paola Andrioli Nemola, Olga Silvana Casale, and Paolo Viti, 189–206. Lecce: Conte, 2004.

———. *Il lessico medico del "De regimine pregnantium" di Michele Savonarola.* Florence: Accademia della Crusca, 1996.

———. "Sul lessico medico di Michele Savonarola: Derivazione, sinonimia, gerarchie di parole." *Studi di lessicografia italiana* 16 (1999): 163–251.

———. "La lingua della pediatria: Il trattato di Paolo Bagellardo dal Fiume." In Gualdo, *Le parole della scienza*, 21–48. (2001).

———, ed. *Le parole della scienza: Scritture tecniche e scientifiche in volgare, secoli XIII–XV: Atti del convegno, Lecce, 16–18 aprile 1999.* Galatina: Congedo, 2001.

Hamesse, Jacqueline. *Les "Auctoritates Aristotelis": Un florilège médiéval: Étude historique et édition critique.* Louvain: Publications Universitaires; Paris: Béatrice Nauwelaerts, 1974.

Hanson, Ann E. "The Eight Month's Child and the Etiquette of Birth: Obsit Omen!" *Bulletin of the History of Medicine* 61 (1987): 589–602.

Hanson, Ann E., and Monica H. Green. "Soranus of Ephesus: Methodicorum Princeps." In *Aufstieg und Niedergang der römischen Welt: Geschichte und Kultur Roms im Spiegel der neueren Forschung*, vol. 2, part 37.2, edited by Wolfgang Haase and Hildegard Temporini, 968–1075. Berlin and New York: Walter de Gruyter, 1994.

Harris-Stoertz, Fiona. "Midwives in the Middle Ages? Birth Attendants, 600–1300." In *Medicine and the Law in the Middle Ages,* edited by Wendy J. Turner and Sara M. Butler, 58–87. Leiden and Boston: Brill, 2014.

Hellwarth, Jennifer W. "'I wyl wright of women prevy sekenes': Imagining Female Literacy and Textual Communities in Medieval and Early Modern Midwifery Manuals." *Critical Survey* 14.1 (2002): 44–63.

Hopwood, Nick, Rebecca Flemming, and Lauren Kassell, eds. *Reproduction: Antiquity to the Present Day.* Cambridge: Cambridge University Press, 2018.

Ingerslev, Emmerik. "Rösslin's 'Rosegarten': Its Relation to the Past (the Muscio Manuscripts and Soranus), Particularly with Regard to Podalic Version." *Journal of Obstetrics and Gynaecology of the British Empire* 15 (January 1909): 1–25 (part 1); and 15 (February 1909): 73–92 (part 2).

Jacquart, Danielle. "En feuilletant la 'Practica maior' de Michel Savonarole: Quelques échos d'une pratique." In Crisciani and Zuccolin, *Michele Savonarola,* 59–82. (2011).

———. "Médecine et alchimie chez Michel Savonarole (1385–1466)." In *Alchimie et philosophie à la Renaissance: Actes du colloque international de Tours, 4–7 décembre 1991,* edited by Jean-Claude Margolin and Sylvain Matton, 109–22. Paris: Vrin, 1993.

———. "Naissance d'une 'pédiatrie' en milieu de cour." *Micrologus* 16 (2008): 271–94.

Jacquart, Danielle, and Claude Thomasset. *Sexualité et savoir médical au Moyen Âge.* Paris: Presses universitaires de France, 1985. Translation by Matthew Adamson as *Sexuality and Medicine in the Middle Ages* (Oxford: Polity Press; Princeton, NJ: Princeton University Press, 1988).

Jarcho, Saul. "Galen's Six Non-Naturals: A Bibliographic Note and Translation." *Bulletin of the History of Medicine* 44 (1970): 372–77.

Jones, Peter M. "Medical Literacies and Medical Culture in Early Modern Vernacular Medicine." In Taavitsainen and Pahta, *Medical Writing in Early Modern English,* 30–43. (2011).

King, Helen. *Midwifery, Obstetrics and the Rise of Gynaecology: The Uses of a Sixteenth-Century Compendium.* Aldershot, Hampshire, UK; Burlington VT: Ashgate, 2007.

———. "Once upon a Text: Hysteria from Hippocrates." In *Hysteria Beyond Freud,* edited by Sander L. Gilman, 3–90. Berkeley: University of California Press, 1993.

———. *The One-Sex Body on Trial: The Classical and Early Modern Evidence.* Farnham, Surrey, UK; Burlington, VT: Ashgate, 2013.

King, Margaret L. "Concepts of Childhood: What We Know and Where We Might Go." *Renaissance Quarterly* 60, no. 2 (2007): 371–407.

Kristeller, Paul Oskar. "Umanesimo e Scolastica a Padova fino al Petrarca." *Medioevo* 11 (1985): 1–18.

Kruse, Britta-Juliane. "Neufundeiner handschriftlichen Vorstufe von Eucharius Rößlins Hebammenlehrbuch 'Der schwangeren Frauen und Hebammen Rosengarten' und des Frauenbüchleins Ps.-Ortolfs." *Sudhoffs Archiv* 78 (1994): 220–36.

———. *Verborgene Heilkünste: Geschichte der Frauenmedizin im Spätmittelalter.* Berlin: Walter de Gruyter, 1996.

Kudlein, Fridolf. "The Seven Cells of the Uterus: The Doctrine and its Roots." *Bulletin of the History of Medicine* 39 (1965): 415–23.

Legaré, Anne-Marie, and Bertrand Schnerb, eds. *Livres et lectures des femmes en Europe entre Moyen Âge et Renaissance.* Turnhout: Brepols, 2007.

Lie, Orlanda S. H. "What Every Midwife Needs to Know: The Trotula." In *Women's Writing from the Low Countries, 1200–1875: A Bilingual Anthology*, edited by Lia van Gemert et al., 138–43. Amsterdam: Amsterdam University Press, 2010.

López-Beltrán, Carlos. "Les *haereditarii morbi* au début de l'époque moderne." In *L'hérédité entre Moyen Âge et époque moderne: Perspectives historiques*, edited by Maaike van der Lugt and Charles de Miramon, 321–51. Florence: SISMEL, Edizioni del Galluzzo, 2008.

Marafioti, Martin. "The Prescriptive Potency of Food in Michele Savonarola's 'De Regimine Pregnantium.'" In *Table Talk: Perspective on Food in Medieval Italian Literature*, edited by Christiana Purdy Moudarres, 19–33. Newcastle upon Tyne: Cambridge Scholars Publishing, 2010.

Marland, Hilary, ed. *The Art of Midwifery: Early Modern Midwives in Europe.* New York and London: Routledge, 1993.

Martorelli Vico, Romana. "Madri, levatrici, balie e padri: Michele Savonarola, l'embriologia e la cura dei piccoli." In Crisciani and Zuccolin, *Michele Savonarola*, 127–36. (2011)

———. *Medicina e filosofia: Per una storia dell'embriologia medievale nel XIII e XIV secolo.* Milan: Guerini e associati, 2002.

Mastronardi, Maria Aurelia. "L'immagine di Ferrara nella letteratura estense." In *Acta Conventus Neo-Latini Abulensis: Proceedings of the Tenth International Congress of Neo-Latin Studies, Avila, 4–9 August 1997*, edited by Jenaro Costas Rodriguez et al., 423–30. Tempe, AZ: Arizona Center for Medieval and Renaissance Studies, 2000.

———. " . . . *Redeunt Saturnia regna*: Città ideale ed età dell'oro nella Ferrara estense." *Annali della facoltà di lettere e filosofia dell'Università degli studi della Basilicata* 8 (1998): 153–81.

McClive, Cathy. *Menstruation and Procreation in Early Modern France.* Farnham, Surrey, UK; Burlington, VT: Ashgate, 2015.

McTavish, Lianne. *Childbirth and the Display of Authority in Early Modern France.* Aldershot, Hampshire, UK; Burlington, VT: Ashgate, 2005.

McVaugh, Michael R. "Cataracts and Hernias: Aspects of Surgical Practice in the Fourteenth Century." *Medical History* 45 (2001): 319–40.

———. *The Rational Surgery of the Middle Ages*. Florence: SISMEL, Edizioni del Galluzzo, 2006.

Menini, Cesare. "Su di un ricettario attribuito a Michele Savonarola." *Acta medicae historiae patavina* 1 (1954–1955): 55–85.

Montagnani, Cristina. "Ferrara e dintorni: Le acque degli Estensi." In *Gli umanisti e le terme: Atti del convegno internazionale di studio, Lecce, Santa Cesarea Terme, 23–25 maggio 2002*, edited by Paola Andrioli Nemola, Olga Silvana Casale, and Paolo Viti, 175–88. Lecce: Conte, 2004.

Musacchio, Jacqueline. *The Art and Ritual of Childbirth in Renaissance Italy*. New Haven: Yale University Press, 1999.

Nagel, Silvia. "*Puer* e *pueritia* nella letteratura medica del XIII secolo." *Quaderni Fondazione Feltrinelli* 23 (1983): 87–107.

Nicoud, Marilyn. "*Inventio, experimentum* e perizia medica nel 'De balneis' di Michele Savonarola." In Crisciani and Zuccolin, *Michele Savonarola*, 83–112. (2011).

———. "Les médecins italiens et le bain thermal à la fin du Moyen Âge." *Médiévales* 43 (2002): 13–40.

———. *Le prince et les médecins: Pensée et pratiques médicales à Milan, 1402–1476*. Rome: École Française de Rome, 2014.

———. *Les régimes de santé au Moyen Âge: Naissance et diffusion d'une écriture médicale en Italie et en France, XIIIe–XVe siècle*. Rome: École Française de Rome, 2007b.

———. "Les vertus médicales des eaux en Italie à la fin du Moyen Âge." In *Bains curatifs et bains hygiéniques en Italie de l'Antiquité au Moyen Âge: Actes du colloque réuni à Rome, 22, 23 mars 2004*, edited by Marie Guérin-Beauvois and Jean-Marie Martin, 321–44. Rome: École Française de Rome, 2007a.

Nystedt, Jane. "La dimensione sociale nei 'Regimina sanitatis' di Michele Savonarola." In *Il Friuli e le cucine della memoria fra Quattro e Cinquecento: Per un contributo alla cultura dell'alimentazione*, edited by Cesare Corradini, 83–100. Udine: Forum Edizioni, 1997.

O'Neill, Ynez V. "Giovanni Michele Savonarola: An Atypical Renaissance Practitioner." *Clio Medica* 10 (1975): 177–93.

———. "Michele Savonarola and the *fera* or Blighted Twin Phenomenon." *Medical History* 18 (1974): 222–39.

Paravicini Bagliani, Agostino. *Medicina e scienze della natura alla corte dei Papi nel Duecento*. Spoleto: CISAM (Centro Italiano di studi sull'alto Medioevo), 1991.

Park, Katharine. "Natural Particulars: Medical Epistemology, Practice and the Literaure of Healing Springs." In *Natural Particulars: Nature and the Disciplines in Renaissance Europe*, edited by Anthony Grafton and Nancy G. Siraisi, 347–67. Cambridge, MA: MIT Press, 1999.

———. *Secrets of Women: Gender, Generation, and the Origins of Human Dissection*. New York: Zone Books, 2006.

Past, Elena. "Una ricetta per *longo* e *iocundo* vivere: Il 'Libreto de tutte le cosse che se magnano.'" In Crisciani and Zuccolin, *Michele Savonarola*, 113–25. (2011).

Pazzini, Aldo. *Crestomazia della letteratura medica in volgare dei due primi secoli della lingua*. Rome: Università degli studi di Roma, Scuola di perfezionamento in storia della medicina, 1971.

Pelling, Margaret. *Medical Conflicts in Early Modern London: Patronage, Physicians, and Irregular Practitioners, 1550–1640*. Oxford: Clarendon Press, 2003.

Penso, Giuseppe. *La conquista del mondo invisibile: Parassiti e microbi nella storia della civiltà*. Milan: Feltrinelli, 1973.

Pesenti Marangon, Tiziana. *Marsilio Santasofia tra corti e università: La carriera di un "monarcha medicinae" del Trecento*. Treviso: Antilia, 2003.

———. "Michele Savonarola a Padova: L'ambiente, le opere, la cultura medica." *Quaderni per la storia dell'Università di Padova* 9–10 (1977): 45–102.

———. *Professori e promotori di medicina nello studio di Padova dal 1405 al 1509: Repertorio bio-bibliografico*. Padua and Trieste: Lint, 1984.

Pibiri, Eva, and Fanny Abbott, eds. *Féminité et masculinité altérées: Transgression et inversion des genres au Moyen Âge*. Florence: SISMEL, Edizioni del Galluzzo, 2017.

Pomata, Gianna. *Contracting a Cure: Patients, Healers and the Law in Early Modern Bologna*. Baltimore, MD: The Johns Hopkins University Press, 1998.

Prete, Sesto. "Humanismus und Humanisten am Fürstenhofe der Este in Ferrara während des XV. Jahrhunderts." *Arcadia* 2 (1967): 125–38.

———. *Two Humanistic Anthologies*. Città del Vaticano: Biblioteca Apostolica Vaticana, 1964.

———. "Umanesimo a Ferrara nel secolo XV." *Atti dell'Accademia delle scienze di Ferrara* 43–44 (1965–1967): 65–78.

Rankin, Alisha M. *Panaceia's Daughters: Noblewomen as Healers in Early Modern Germany*. Chicago: University of Chicago Press, 2013.

Rapisarda, Stefano. "Appunti sulla circolazione del 'Secretum secretorum' in Italia." In Gualdo, *Le parole della scienza*, 87–105. (2001).

Rather, Lelland J. "The 'Six Things Non-Naturals': A Note on the Origins and Fate of a Doctrine and a Phrase." *Clio medica* 3 (1968): 3373–47.

Reisert, Robert. *Die siebenkammerige Uterus: Studien zur mittelalterlichen Wirkungsgeschichte und Entfaltung eines embryologischen Gebärmuttermodells*. Pattensen, Germany: Horst Wellm, 1986.

Richards, Jennifer. "Reading and Hearing 'The Womans Booke' in Early Modern England." *Bulletin of the History of Medicine* 89, no. 3 (2015): 434–62.

Ridolfi, Roberto. *Vita di Girolamo Savonarola.* 6th ed. Florence: Le Lettere, 1997. Previously published Florence: Sansoni, 1981. Original Rome: A. Belardetti, 1952.

Saif, Liana. "The Universe and the Womb: Generation, Conception, and the Stars in Islamic Medieval Astrological and Medical Texts." *Journal of Arabic and Islamic Studies* 16 (2016): 181–98.

Samaritani, Antonio. "Michele Savonarola riformatore cattolico nella corte estense a metà del secolo XV." *Atti e memorie della deputazione provinciale ferrarese di storia patria* 3, no. 22 (1976): 44–85.

———. "Il 'De sapiente et insipiente' di Michele Savonarola." *Memorie domenicane* 16 (1985): 305–24.

Schmitt, Charles B. *Aristotle and the Renaissance.* Cambridge, MA: Harvard University Press, 1983.

———. *La tradizione aristotelica: Fra Italia e Inghilterra.* Naples: Bibliopolis, 1985.

Segarizzi, Antonio. *Della vita e delle opere di Michele Savonarola, medico padovano del secolo XV.* Padua: Gallina, 1900.

Smith, Helen. *"Grossly Material Things": Women and Book Production in Early Modern England.* Oxford: Oxford University Press, 2012.

———. "More Swete vnto the Eare/Than Holsome for ye Mynde: Embodying Early Modern Women's Reading." *Huntington Library Quarterly* 73, no. 3 (2010): 413–32.

Smoak, Ginger L. "Midwives as Agents of Social Control: Ecclesiastical and Municipal Regulation of Midwifery in the Late Middle Ages." *Quidditas: Online Journal of the Rocky Mountain Medieval and Renaissance Association* 33 (2012): 79–96.

Snook, Edith. *Women, Reading, and the Cultural Policy of Early Modern England.* Aldershot, Hampshire, UK; Burlington, VT: Ashgate, 2005.

Soergel, Philip M., ed. *Sexuality and Culture in Medieval and Renaissance Europe.* New York: AMS Press, 2005.

Taavitsainen, Irma, and Päivi Pahta, eds. *Medical Writing in Early Modern English.* Cambridge: Cambridge University Press, 2011.

———. "Vernacularisation of Medical Writing in English: A Corpus-Based Study of Scholasticism." *Early Science and Medicine* 3, no. 2 (1998): 157–85.

Taglia, Kathryn. "Delivering a Christian Identity: Midwives in Northern French Synodal Legislation, c. 1200–1500." In *Religion and Medicine in the Middle Ages,* edited by Peter Biller and Joseph Ziegler, 77–90. Woodbridge, Suffolk, UK; Rochester, NY: York Medieval Press, 2001.

Tavoni, Mirko. "Il Quattrocento." In *Storia della lingua italiana: Il Quattrocento,* edited by Francesco Bruni, 29–34. Bologna: il Mulino, 1992.

Thijssen, Johannes M. "Twins as Monsters: Albertus Magnus's Theory of the Generation of Twins and Its Philosophical Context." *Bulletin of the History of Medicine* 61 (1987): 237–46.

Thomann, Johannes. *Studien zum "Speculum physionomie" des Michele Savonarola*. PhD diss., University of Zurich, Zurich, 1997.

Thomasset, Claude. "La natura della donna." In *Storia delle donne in Occidente: Il Medioevo*, edited by Christiane Klapisch-Zuber, 56–87. Bari: Laterza, 1994.

Thorndike, Lynn. "Michael Savonarola." In Thorndike, *A History of Magic and Experimental Science*, 4:183–214. New York: Columbia University Press, 1934.

Torresi, Antonio P., ed. *Pseudo-Savonarola: A far littere de oro: Alchimia e tecnica della miniatura in un ricettario rinascimentale*. Ferrara: Liberty House, 1992.

Van der Lugt, Maaike. "Les maladies héréditaires dans la pensée scolastique, XIIe–XVIe siècles." In *L'hérédité entre Moyen Âge et époque moderne: Perspectives historiques*, edited by Maaike Van der Lugt and Charles de Miramon, 273–320. Florence: SISMEL, Edizioni del Galluzzo, 2008.

———. "Nature as Norm in Medieval Medical Discussions of Breastfeeding and Wet-Nursing." *Journal of Medieval and Early Modern Studies* 49, no. 3 (2019): 563–88.

———. *Le ver, le démon et la Vierge: Les théories médiévales de la génération extraordinaire: Une étude sur les rapports entre théologie, philosophie naturelle et médecine*. Paris: Les Belles Lettres, 2004.

Van 't Land, Karine. "Sperm and Blood, Form and Food. Late Medieval Medical Notions of Male and Female in the Embryology of *Membra*." In *Blood, Sweat and Tears: The Changing Concepts of Physiology from Antiquity into Early Modern Europe*, edited by Manfred Horstmanshoff, Helen King, and Claus Zittel, 363–92. Leiden and Boston: Brill, 2012.

Vázquez de Benito, María Concepción, and María Teresa Herrera. *Los arabismos de los textos médicos latinos y castellanos de la Edad Media y de la Modernidad*. Madrid: Consejo superior de investigaciones cientificas, 1989.

Wack, Mary F. "The Measure of Pleasure: Peter of Spain on Men, Women and Lovesickness." *Viator* 17 (1986), 173–96.

Whitehead, Barbara J., ed. *Women's Education in Early Modern Europe: A History, 1500 to 1800*. New York: Garland, 1999.

Williams, Steven J. "The Early Circulation of the Pseudo-Aristotelian 'Secret of Secrets' in the West: The Papal and Imperial Courts." *Micrologus* 2 (1994): 127–44. Reprinted in *The "Secret of Secrets": The Scholarly Career of a Pseudo-Aristotelian Text in the Latin Middle Ages*, edited by Steven J Williams, 109–40. Ann Arbor: University of Michigan Press, 2003a.

———. "Giving Advice and Taking It: The Reception by Rulers of the Pseudo-Aristotelian 'Secretum Secretorum' as a 'Speculum Principis.'" In *Consilium: Teorie e pratiche del consigliare nella cultura medievale*, edited by Carla

Casagrande, Chiara Crisciani, and Silvana Vecchio, 139–56. Florence: SIS-MEL, Edizioni del Galluzzo, 2004.

———. "The Vernacular Tradition of the Pseudo-Aristotelian 'Secret of Secrets' in the Middle Ages: Translations, Manuscripts, Readers." In *Filosofia in volgare nel Medioevo: Atti del Convegno della Società italiana per lo studio del pensiero medievale (S.I.S.P.M.), Lecce, 27–29 settembre 2002*, edited by Nadia Bray and Loris Sturlese, 451–82. Louvain-la-Neuve: Fédération internationale des instituts d'études médiévales, 2003b.

Wilson, Adrian. *The Making of Man-Midwifery: Childbirth in England, 1660–1770*. London: UCL Press, 1995.

Worth-Stylianou, Valerie. *Pregnancy and Birth in Early Modern France: Treatises by Caring Physicians and Surgeons, 1581–1625: François Rousset, Jean Liebault, Jacques Guillemeau, Jacques Duval, and Louis de Serres*. Toronto: Iter Press and Centre for Reformation and Renaissance Studies, 2013.

———. *Les traités d'obstétrique en langue française au seuil de la modernité: Bibliographie critique des "Divers travaulx" d'Euchaire Rösslin (1536) à l' "Apologie de Louyse Bourgeois sage femme" (1627)*. Geneva: Droz, 2007.

Wright, Thomas. *Dictionary of Obsolete and Provincial English*. 2 vols. London: H. G. Bohn, 1857.

Ziegler, Joseph. "Hérédité et physiognomonie." In Van der Lugt and Miramon, *L'hérédité entre Moyen Âge et Époque moderne*, 245–71. (2008).

———. "Measuring the Human Body in Medieval and Renaissance Physiognomy." *Micrologus* 18 (2011): 349–68.

———. "Médicine et physiognomonie du XIVe au début du XVIe siècle." *Médiévales* 45 (2004): 87–105.

———. "Philosophers and Physicians on the Scientific Validity of Latin Physiognomy." *Early Science and Medicine* 12 (2007): 285–312.

———. "*Phisionomia est lex nature*: On the Nature of Character and Behaviour in Late Medieval Physiognomy." In Van der Lugt, *La nature comme source de la morale au Moyen Âge*, 359–81. (2014).

———. "Sexuality and the Sexual Organs in Latin Physiognomy, 1200–1500." In Soergel, *Sexuality and Culture in Medieval and Renaissance Europe*, 83–107. (2005a).

———. "Skin and Character in Medieval and Early Renaissance Physiognomy." *Micrologus* 13 (2005b): 511–35.

———. "Text and Context: On the Rise of Physiognomic Thought in the Later Middle Ages." In *"De Sion exibit lex et verbum domini de Hierusalem": Essays on Medieval Law, Liturgy, and Literature in Honour of Amnon Linder*, edited by Yitzhak Hen, 159–82. Turnhout: Brepols, 2001.

Zuccolin, Gabriella. *I gemelli nel Medioevo: Questioni filosofiche, mediche e teologiche*. Pavia: Ibis, 2019.

———. "Gravidanza e parto nel Quattrocento: Le morti parallele di Beatrice d'Este e Anna Sforza." *Quaderni di artes* 2 (2008a): 111–45.

———. "Medici a corte e formazione del signore." In *Costumi educativi nelle corti europee, XIV–XVIII secolo,* edited by Monica Ferrari, 77–102. Pavia: Pavia University Press, 2010.

———. *Michele Savonarola "medico humano": Fisiognomica, etica e religione alla corte estense.* Bari: Edizioni di Pagina, 2018.

———. "Nascere in latino ed in volgare: Tra la 'Practica' e il 'De regimine.'" In Crisciani and Zuccolin, *Michele Savonarola,* 137–210. (2011).

———. "Princely Virtues in 'De felici progressu' of Michele Savonarola, Court Physician of the House of Este." In *Princely Virtues in the Middle Ages, 1200–1500,* edited by István P. Bejczy and Cary J. Nederman, 237–58. Turnhout: Brepols, 2007.

———. "Il ruolo dell''exemplum' nella produzione medica e religiosa di Michele Savonarola (1385–1466)." In *Exempla medicorum: Die Ärzte und ihre Beispiele, 14.–18. Jahrhundert,* edited by Mariacarla Gadebusch Bondio and Thomas Ricklin, 109–28. Florence: SISMEL, Edizioni del Galluzzo, 2008b.

———. "The 'Speculum phisionomie' by Michele Savonarola." In *Universalità della ragione: Pluralità delle filosofie nel Medioevo [. . .]: XII Congresso internazionale di filosofia medievale, Palermo, 17–22 settembre 2007,* vol. 2, edited by Alessandro Musco, with Carla Compagno, Salvatore D'Agostino, Giuliana Musotto, 873–87. Palermo: Officina di studi medievali, 2012.

Zuccolin, Gabriella, and Helen King. "Rethinking Nosebleeds: Gendering Spontaneous Bleedings in Medieval and Early Modern Medicine." In *Blood Matters: Studies in European Literature and Thought, 1400–1700,* edited by Eleonor Decamp and Bonnie Lander Johnson, 79–92. Philadelphia: University of Pennsylvania Press, 2018.

Index

Note: Page numbers in italics indicate figures.

The Other Voice in Early Modern Europe: The Toronto Series

SENIOR EDITOR Margaret L. King

SERIES EDITORS Jaime Goodrich, Elizabeth H. Hageman

Series Titles